Genitourinary Tract Disease (Fourth Series) Test and Syllabus

Harold A. Mitty, M.D.
Section Chairman

N. Reed Dunnick, M.D.
Peggy J. Fritzsche, M.D.
Stanford M. Goldman, M.D.
Carl M. Sandler, M.D.

 American College of Radiology
Reston, Virginia   1992

Sets Published

Chest Disease
Bone Disease
Genitourinary Tract Disease
Gastrointestinal Disease
Head and Neck Disorders
Pediatric Disease
Nuclear Radiology
Radiation Pathology and
   Radiation Biology
Chest Disease II
Bone Disease II
Genitourinary Tract Disease II
Gastrointestinal Disease II
Head and Neck Disorders II
Nuclear Radiology II
Cardiovascular Disease
Emergency Radiology
Bone Disease III
Gastrointestinal Disease III
Chest Disease III
Pediatric Disease II
Nuclear Radiology III
Head and Neck Disorders III

Genitourinary Tract Disease III
Diagnostic Ultrasound
Breast Disease
Bone Disease IV
Pediatric Disease III
Chest Disease IV
Neuroradiology
Gastrointestinal Disease IV
Nuclear Radiology IV
Magnetic Resonance
Radiation Bioeffects and
   Management
Genitourinary Tract Disease IV

Sets in Preparation

Head and Neck Disorders IV
Musculoskeletal Disease
Pediatric Disease IV
Diagnostic Ultrasonography II'
Breast Disease II
Chest Disease V
Neuroradiology II
Gastrointestinal Disease V

Note: While the American College of Radiology and the editors of this publication have attempted to include the most current and accurate information possible, errors may inadvertently appear. Diagnostic and interventional decisions should be based on the individual circumstances of each case.

SET 33:
Genitourinary Tract Disease (Fourth Series) Test and Syllabus

Editor in Chief

BARRY A. SIEGEL, M.D., Professor of Radiology and Medicine and Director, Division of Nuclear Medicine, Mallinckrodt Institute of Radiology, Washington University School of Medicine, St. Louis, Missouri

Associate Editor

ANTHONY V. PROTO, M.D., Professor of Radiology and Chairman, Department of Radiology, Medical College of Virginia, Virginia Commonwealth University, Richmond, Virginia

Section Editor

HAROLD A. MITTY, M.D., Professor of Radiology and Urology and Director of the Divisions of Interventional Radiology and Uroradiology, Mount Sinai School of Medicine, City University of New York, New York

Co-Authors

N. REED DUNNICK, M.D., Professor and Chairman, Department of Radiology, University of Michigan Medical Center, Ann Arbor, Michigan

PEGGY J. FRITZSCHE, M.D., Medical Director, Riverside MRI, Riverside, and Clinical Professor of Radiology, Loma Linda University School of Medicine, Loma Linda, California

STANFORD M. GOLDMAN, M.D., Radiologist-in-Chief, Francis Scott Key Medical Center; Professor of Radiology and Urology, Johns Hopkins University School of Medicine; Adjunct Professor of Radiology, University of Maryland School of Medicine; and Clinical Professor of Radiology, Uniformed Services University of the Health Sciences, Baltimore, Maryland

CARL M. SANDLER, M.D., Professor of Radiology and Surgery (Urology), University of Texas Medical School; Chief, Radiology Service, Lyndon B. Johnson General Hospital; and Adjunct Professor of Radiology, Baylor College of Medicine, Houston, Texas

AMERICAN COLLEGE OF RADIOLOGY
PROFESSIONAL SELF-EVALUATION AND CONTINUING EDUCATION PROGRAM

Publishing Coordinators:	*G. Rebecca Haines Gardner and Thomas M. Rogers*
Administrative Assistant:	*Lisa Lantzy*
Production Editor:	*Sean M. McKenna*
Copy Editors:	*Yvonne Strong and John N. Bell*
Text Processing:	*Fusako T. Nowak*
Composition:	*Karen Finkle*
Index:	*Editorial Experts, Inc., Alexandria, Va.*
Lithography:	*Lanman Progressive, Washington, D.C.*
Typesetting:	*Publication Technology Corp., Fairfax, Va.*
Printing:	*John D. Lucas Printing, Baltimore, Md.*

Library of Congress Cataloging-in-Publication Data

Genitourinary tract disease (fourth series) test and syllabus / Harold A. Mitty, section chairman ; N. Reed Dunnick ... [et al.]

    p. cm. — (Professional self-evaluation and continuing education program ; set 33)

    On cover: Committee on Professional Self-Evaluation and Continuing Education, Commission on Education, American College of Radiology.

    Includes bibliographical references and index.

    ISBN 1-55903-033-X : $175.00. — ISBN 1-55903-000-3 (series)

    1.   Genitourinary system—Radiography—Examinations, questions, etc. I. Mitty, Harold A.   II. Dunnick, N. Reed.   III. American College of Radiology. Commission on Education. Committee on Professional Self-Evaluation and Continuing Education.   IV. Series.

    [DNLM: 1. Genital Diseases, Male—diagnosis—examination questions. 2. Urologic Diseases—diagnosis—examination questions.

W1 PR606 set 33]

    RC874.G458   1992

    616.6'07572'076—dc20

    DNLM/DLC   92-21930

    for Library of Congress   CIP

v

Additional Contributors

MAY KINALY, M.D., Radiology Assistant, Loma Linda University School of Medicine, Loma Linda, California

MARK McKINNEY, M.D., Radiology Resident, Loma Linda University Medical Center, Loma Linda, California

JANICE W. SEMENKOVICH, M.D., Instructor of Radiology, Mallinckrodt Institute of Radiology, Washington University School of Medicine, St. Louis, Missouri

Section Chairman's Preface

It has only been 6 years since the publication of the last self-evaluation volume on genitourinary disease, the ACR's *Genitourinary Tract Disease (Third Series) Syllabus*. Even so, major advances in imaging technology have led to substantial modifications in the radiologic approach to a variety of diseases. The decreased utilization of excretory urography in favor of sonography or computed tomography has been evolving for some time. The rapid growth in our understanding of the roles of MRI and duplex Doppler imaging has led to the inclusion of these modalities in some of the cases presented here. The contributions of new techniques to our understanding of disease are occurring at such an astonishing pace I often have the feeling that I should not take a vacation for fear of missing some new innovation.

Since my activities occur in a large metropolitan teaching hospital, I may have a somewhat biased view of what is important. I tried to include here standard diagnostic problems that may be looked upon in a new light in view of new clinical information, new modality evaluation, or new therapeutic options (i.e., interventional radiologic management). Areas in which many of our practices have little direct involvement, such as trauma, are also included so as to broaden general knowledge. Several actively emerging areas—such as prostate imaging, percutaneous interventions, the evaluation of impotence, and the management of stone disease—are also included in this volume.

I must admit that I approached this project with some trepidation. I remember the sessions involved in producing the last genitourinary disease syllabus, under the able guidance of Dr. Howard Pollack. It is a difficult exercise to produce sensible questions with meaningful discussions. Yet, it is also a stimulating process that brings together a group of active radiologists who critically question one another's knowledge and who examine data and beliefs regarding disease, imaging, and therapy. Often, seemingly solid ideas and opinions are based on limited available data. The process of self-evaluation inevitably makes us all think in a more rational fashion. The committee was shepherded, cajoled, and—most importantly!—enlightened by the editors of the self-evaluation series, Dr. Barry A. Siegel and Dr. Anthony V. Proto. We have all learned to think more clearly as a result of their constructive involvement in this project.

The staff at the American College of Radiology has provided guidance and support through every phase of the development and printing of this volume. Ms. Rebecca Haines Gardner, Director of ACR Publications, ably led the way for us during the early stages of this effort. Mr. Thomas

Rogers, the ACR Associate Director of Publications, kept all of the manuscripts moving between contributors and is responsible for getting all of this material into print. His literary witticisms were greatly appreciated.

Finally, I am very grateful to the members of the *Genitourinary Tract Disease IV* committee: Dr. Stanford M. Goldman, Dr. Peggy J. Fritzsche, Dr. N. Reed Dunnick, and Dr. Carl M. Sandler. These outstanding radiologists took many hours from their already busy professional lives to contribute to this volume. In the 2 years since writing of this syllabus began, many personal and professional changes occurred for the members of this committee. Nevertheless, their collective fortitude and wisdom brought this project to a successful conclusion.

Harold A. Mitty, M.D.
Section Chairman

Editor's Preface

The publication of the *Genitourinary Tract Disease (Fourth Series) Test and Syllabus*, the 33rd volume in the series of diagnostic radiology syllabi, marks the 20th anniversary of the American College of Radiology's Professional Self-Evaluation and Continuing Education (PSECE) Program. The subject matter chosen for this syllabus clearly illustrates the diversity of clinical problems addressed by genitourinary radiologists, as well as the wide array of diagnostic examinations and imaging methods now routinely employed to solve these problems. Several case discussions focusing on interventional radiologic procedures of the genitourinary system are included here in recognition of the ever-increasing role that radiologists play in the treatment, as well as diagnosis, of many diseases. It is the intent of the editors to include interventional topics in future self-evaluation packages whenever it is logical to do so. This reflects our desire to ensure that each syllabus will contain material that represents a balanced cross-section of new developments in a particular radiologic subspecialty.

The fundamental approaches used in the development of this test and syllabus are essentially unchanged from those used in preceding volumes published in recent years. The authors and editors have been guided in their efforts by one principal objective: the test cases should represent credible, clinically relevant problems of the type faced daily by diagnostic radiologists. Recognizing that a multiple-choice examination and syllabus can only aspire to reproduce real clinical situations, we nonetheless hope that the format of the book makes for a challenging and enjoyable course of self-evaluation and self-instruction.

My co-editors and I are deeply grateful to Dr. Harold A. Mitty for his consummate efforts in developing this self-evaluation package. The College was indeed fortunate to have such an able clinician, editor, and leader in the role of section chairman for this volume. We are equally indebted to Drs. Stanford M. Goldman, Peggy J. Fritzsche, N. Reed Dunnick, and Carl M. Sandler for their long hours of voluntary effort to ensure the continuing success of the PSECE Program. Working with such devoted radiologists of such high caliber was a distinct pleasure for me.

Thanks are also due to many other individuals who contributed directly or indirectly to this project. Dr. Anthony V. Proto served expertly as co-editor of this volume and kept us on track (and on schedule) in his simultaneous role as Chairman of the PSECE Committee. The support of the other members of the PSECE Committee—Drs. Jack Edeiken, Harold G. Jacobson, David H. Stephens, Elias G. Theros, and Jerome F.

Wiot—continues to be essential to maintaining the momentum of the program. The support and encouragement of Dr. Joseph Ferrucci and the College's Commission on Education is also gratefully acknowledged. As always, G. Rebecca Haines Gardner, Thomas M. Rogers, and the other members of the staff in the ACR Publications Department ultimately are the *sine qua non* of the PSECE Program and are key contributors to the quality of each volume.

The editors hope that this self-evaluation package will prove as popular as those that came before it. The enthusiastic support of radiologists has been the driving force of the PSECE Program since its inception 20 years ago. Striving to contribute to the educational needs of both practicing radiologists and those in training remains as this program's principal goal.

Barry A. Siegel, M.D.
Editor in Chief

Genitourinary Tract Disease (Fourth Series) Test

For you to derive the maximum benefit from this program, you should complete the following test, and send your answer sheet to the ACR for scoring, before you proceed to the syllabus.

If for any reason you refer to the syllabus material, or any other references, in answering the questions, please be sure to so indicate when answering Question 148, the first demographic question. Your score will then not be used in developing the norm tables.

NOTE: You must return your answer sheet for scoring, whether or not you use reference materials, in order to claim the 20 hours of Category I credit.

Category I credit is valid for this publication from October 1992 through October 1995. Category I credit review will be conducted in October 1995 and every three years thereafter.

CASE 1: Questions 1 through 4

History withheld. You are shown a radiograph (Figure 1-1) centered at the symphysis pubis of a 24-year-old man. You are also shown a urethrogram (Figure 1-2).

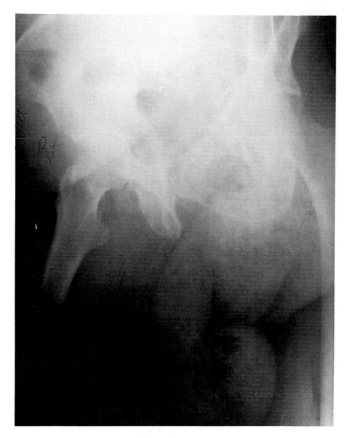

Figure 1-1

1. Which *one* of the following is the MOST likely diagnosis?

    (A) Scrotal hernia
    (B) Torsion of the testis
    (C) Epididymo-orchitis
    (D) Scrotal gangrene
    (E) Decompression sickness

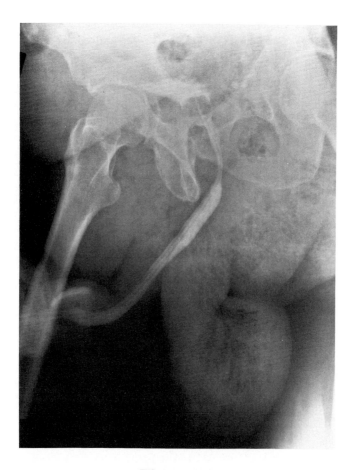

Figure 1-2

2. On gray-scale ultrasonography of the scrotum, a scrotal hernia is MOST likely to be confused with which *one* of the following?

   (A) Hydrocele
   (B) Varicocele
   (C) Spermatocele
   (D) Sperm granuloma
   (E) Adenomatoid tumor of the epididymis

CASE 1 (Cont'd)

QUESTIONS 3 AND 4: MARK YOUR ANSWER SHEET TRUE
(T) OR FALSE (F) FOR EACH OF THE RESPONSE CHOICES.

3. Concerning testicular torsion,

    (A) at 6 hours, a peritesticular rim of intensely increased
        activity is usually seen on scintigraphy
    (B) it is most often seen in men in their late twenties
    (C) color-flow Doppler ultrasonography reliably distin-
        guishes it from epididymitis
    (D) after 24 hours the likelihood of testicular salvage is
        approximately 50%
    (E) gray-scale ultrasonography reliably differentiates it
        from contusion

4. Concerning scrotal gangrene,

    (A) mortality exceeds 60%
    (B) cultures most commonly contain *Clostridium welchii*
    (C) the infection is most common in elderly diabetic pa-
        tients
    (D) the testes are rarely involved
    (E) effective treatment requires both antibiotics and exten-
        sive debridement

This 6-month-old boy presented with difficulty in voiding. You are shown an abdominal radiograph (Figure 2-1) and a cystogram (Figure 2-2).

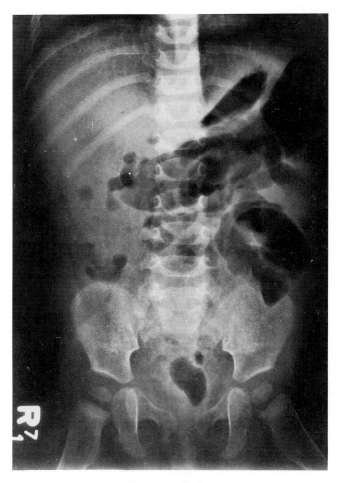

Figure 2-1

5. Which *one* of the following is the MOST likely diagnosis?

   (A) Sacrococcygeal teratoma
   (B) Lymphoma
   (C) Rhabdomyosarcoma
   (D) Neurofibromatosis
   (E) Neuroblastoma

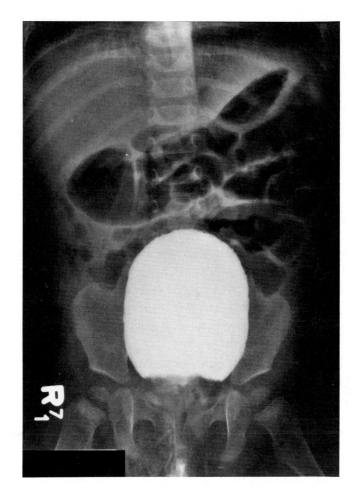

Figure 2-2

CASE 2 (Cont'd)

QUESTIONS 6 THROUGH 8: MARK YOUR ANSWER SHEET TRUE (T) OR FALSE (F) FOR EACH OF THE RESPONSE CHOICES.

6. Concerning pelvic lymphoma in children,

   (A) it is most common in children under 2 years of age
   (B) hematuria is a common presenting feature
   (C) it usually arises in the pelvic floor
   (D) multiple filling defects in the bladder are typical on cystography
   (E) non-Hodgkin's lymphomas predominate

7. Concerning rhabdomyosarcomas,

   (A) they are the most common tumors affecting the bladder in the first decade of life
   (B) in childhood, they most commonly arise in the bladder and prostate
   (C) those of the prostate characteristically cause elongation of the prostatic urethra
   (D) those of the bladder typically arise in the dome
   (E) radiation therapy is the treatment of choice for those of the bladder and prostate

8. Genitourinary tract findings in patients with neurofibromatosis include:

   (A) clitoral hypertrophy
   (B) renal artery stenosis
   (C) extrinsic masses deforming the floor of the bladder
   (D) polypoid filling defect in the membranous urethra

This 33-year-old woman was evaluated for infertility. Her pelvic sonogram was normal. You are shown a hysterosalpingogram (Figure 3-1).

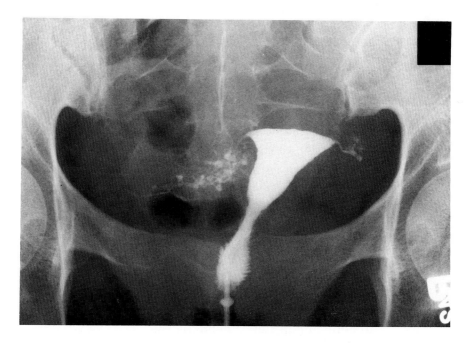

Figure 3-1

9. Which *one* of the following is the MOST likely diagnosis?

   (A) Tuberculosis
   (B) Endometriosis
   (C) Salpingitis isthmica nodosa
   (D) Maternal exposure to diethylstilbestrol
   (E) Pelvic inflammatory disease

CASE 3 (Cont'd)

QUESTIONS 10 THROUGH 13: MARK YOUR ANSWER SHEET TRUE (T) OR FALSE (F) FOR EACH OF THE RESPONSE CHOICES.

10. Concerning tuberculosis of the female genital tract,

    (A) it is usually spread via periureteric and periuterine lymphatics
    (B) it is associated with an increased incidence of tubal neoplasms
    (C) it is most commonly caused by *Mycobacterium bovis*
    (D) fistulization to the bladder is common
    (E) adnexal calcification suggests the diagnosis

11. Concerning endometriosis,

    (A) the ultrasonographic pattern is specific
    (B) there is a correlation between the extent of the disease and the severity of symptoms
    (C) MRI appears to be more sensitive than ultrasonography in detecting diffuse endometriosis
    (D) it is discovered in about 20% of patients undergoing gynecologic laparotomy
    (E) it is more common in Caucasian than in non-Caucasian patients

12. Concerning salpingitis isthmica nodosa,

    (A) it is commonly associated with tubal obstruction
    (B) the ultrasonographic findings are characteristic
    (C) it represents congenital Wolffian rests
    (D) it is associated with an increased frequency of ectopic pregnancies
    (E) it is not associated with primary infertility

13. Concerning pelvic inflammatory disease,

    (A) ectopic pregnancy is a common complication
    (B) it is commonly seen in patients with a bicornuate uterus
    (C) it usually can be differentiated from endometriosis on ultrasonography
    (D) its development can be prevented by the use of an intrauterine device
    (E) transuterine fallopian tube recanalization is an effective mode of therapy for associated infertility

CASE 4: Questions 14 through 17

This 54-year-old woman presented with hematuria. You are shown a bladder image from an excretory urogram (Figure 4-1) and a CT scan (Figure 4-2).

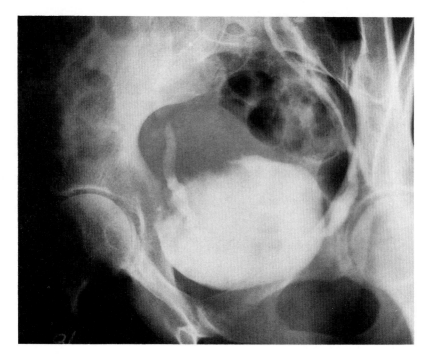

Figure 4-1

14. Which *one* of the following is the MOST likely diagnosis?

    (A) Transitional cell carcinoma of the bladder
    (B) Crohn's disease
    (C) Squamous cell carcinoma of the bladder
    (D) Schistosomiasis
    (E) Urachal carcinoma

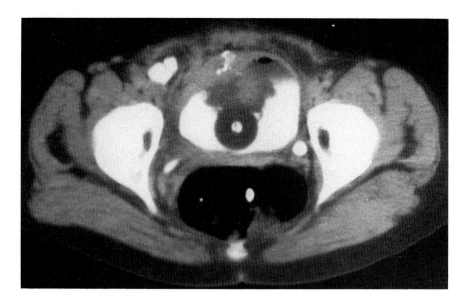

Figure 4-2

QUESTIONS 15 THROUGH 17: MARK YOUR ANSWER SHEET TRUE (T) OR FALSE (F) FOR EACH OF THE RESPONSE CHOICES.

15. Factors predisposing to the development of transitional cell carcinoma of the bladder include:

   (A) exposure to aniline dyes
   (B) cigarette smoking
   (C) exstrophy of the bladder
   (D) schistosomiasis
   (E) malakoplakia

16. Concerning Crohn's disease,

    (A) the most common type of associated calculus is struvite
    (B) it is the most common cause of a fistula between the small bowel and the bladder
    (C) the bladder is the most common site of urinary tract involvement
    (D) the right and left ureters are affected with equal frequency
    (E) it most commonly involves the mid-ureter

17. Concerning urachal carcinoma,

    (A) the bulk of the tumor is extravesical
    (B) it is more common in men than in women
    (C) it is most commonly an adenocarcinoma
    (D) calcification is common
    (E) it has a 5-year survival rate similar to that of transitional cell carcinoma of the bladder
    (F) voided urine often contains mucus

CASE 5: Questions 18 through 25

This 19-year-old man presented with chronic renal failure. You are shown two CT sections (Figure 5-1).

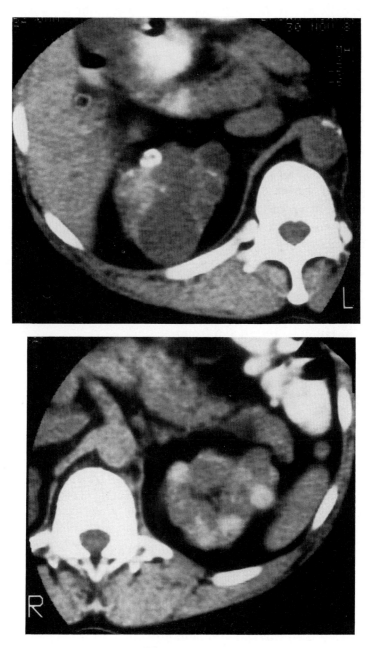

Figure 5-1

18. Which *one* of the following is the MOST likely diagnosis?

    (A) Autosomal dominant polycystic disease
    (B) Medullary cystic disease
    (C) Acquired cystic renal disease
    (D) Autosomal recessive polycystic disease
    (E) Von Hippel-Lindau syndrome

For each numbered cystic disease listed below (Questions 19 through 22), select the *one* lettered pattern of inheritance (A, B, C, or D) that would be MOST closely associated with it if first diagnosed in the third decade of life. Each lettered pattern may be used once, more than once, or not at all.

19. Multicystic dysplastic kidney
20. Medullary sponge kidney
21. Medullary cystic disease
22. von Hippel-Lindau syndrome

    (A) Autosomal dominant
    (B) Autosomal recessive
    (C) Sex linked
    (D) No known hereditary pattern

QUESTIONS 23 THROUGH 25: MARK YOUR ANSWER SHEET TRUE (T) OR FALSE (F) FOR EACH OF THE RESPONSE CHOICES.

23. Concerning medullary cystic disease,

    (A) cortical cystic changes are noted in about 10% of cases
    (B) the angiographic pattern is indistinguishable from that of adult autosomal dominant polycystic disease
    (C) a thin cortical rim is identifiable on ultrasonography
    (D) it is a salt-wasting nephropathy

24. Concerning acquired cystic kidney disease,

    (A) it is seen only after hemodialysis
    (B) there is an increased risk of renal cell carcinoma
    (C) dystrophic calcification is often present
    (D) patients should be monitored by CT or ultrasonography
    (E) it is commonly seen in transplanted kidneys

25. Concerning autosomal dominant polycystic disease,

    (A) approximately 50% of patients have associated hepatic cysts
    (B) hemorrhage into one or more cysts is common
    (C) the gene penetrance approaches 85%
    (D) it occurs as a spontaneous mutation in approximately 10% of patients
    (E) dystrophic calcification is common

This newborn presented with a distended abdomen. You are shown an abdominal radiograph (Figure 6-1) and longitudinal sonograms of both kidneys (Figure 6-2A and B).

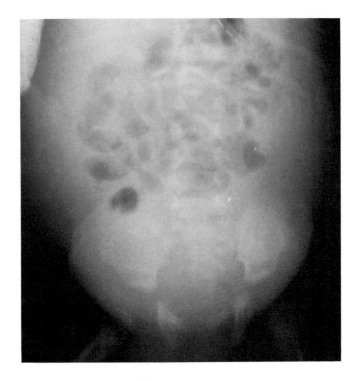

Figure 6-1

26. Which *one* of the following is the MOST likely diagnosis?

   (A) Posterior urethral valves
   (B) Multicystic dysplastic kidney
   (C) Neurogenic bladder
   (D) Megacystis-microcolon syndrome
   (E) Prune belly syndrome

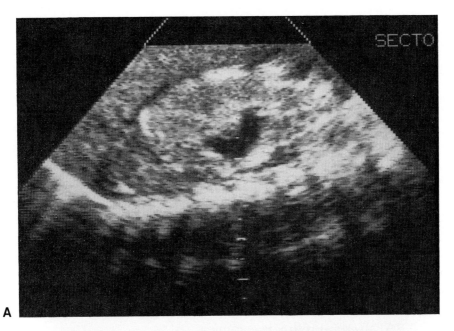

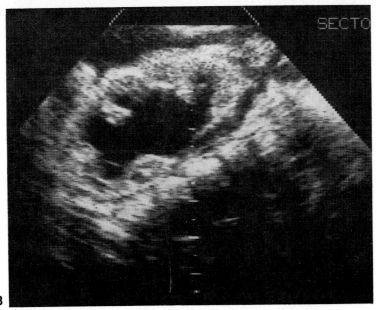

Figure 6-2

CASE 6 (Cont'd)

QUESTIONS 27 THROUGH 29: MARK YOUR ANSWER SHEET TRUE (T) OR FALSE (F) FOR EACH OF THE RESPONSE CHOICES.

27. Concerning posterior urethral valves,

    (A) they are associated with "spinning-top" urethra
    (B) the most common type extends just distal to the verumontanum as a circumferential diaphragm
    (C) hypertrophy of the external sphincter is common
    (D) retrograde urethrography is the most accurate method of diagnosis
    (E) they are usually associated with renal dysplasia

28. Concerning prune belly syndrome,

    (A) ureteral reflux is common
    (B) maternal oligohydramnios is usually present
    (C) bilateral cryptorchidism is present
    (D) renal dysplasia is not a significant feature
    (E) on voiding cystourethrography, urethral valves are usually present

29. Concerning multicystic dysplastic kidney,

    (A) it is predominantly an abnormality of the metanephros
    (B) children with higher ureteral obstructions have a better prognosis than do those with lower ureteral obstructions
    (C) contralateral ureteropelvic junction obstruction is present in about 40% of live-born infants
    (D) it is difficult to distinguish from severe ureteropelvic junction obstruction by ultrasonography alone
    (E) the risk of malignant degeneration necessitates nephrectomy

This 60-year-old man presented with oliguria. You are shown a CT scan obtained 24 hours after administration of contrast material for an excretory urogram (Figure 7-1).

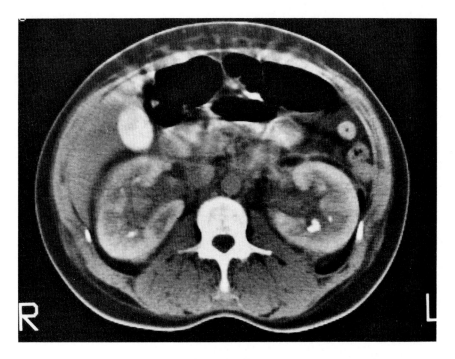

Figure 7-1

30. Which *one* of the following is the MOST likely diagnosis?

    (A) Bilateral ureteral obstruction
    (B) Lymphoma
    (C) Renal sinus hemorrhage
    (D) Uric acid nephropathy
    (E) Shock

QUESTIONS 31 THROUGH 33: MARK YOUR ANSWER SHEET TRUE (T) OR FALSE (F) FOR EACH OF THE RESPONSE CHOICES.

31. Concerning bilateral ureteral obstruction,

(A) ureteral dilatation on sonography establishes the diagnosis
(B) it is usually due to tumor
(C) antegrade placement of stents is preferable to retrograde placement
(D) early dialysis is recommended

32. Concerning renal sinus hemorrhage,

(A) it is often related to anticoagulation
(B) the suburothelial tissue is not involved
(C) surgical decompression is indicated
(D) it is often associated with perinephric hemorrhage

33. Causes of dense nephrograms include:

(A) acute tubular necrosis
(B) uric acid nephropathy
(C) renal vein thrombosis
(D) multiple myeloma
(E) amyloidosis

This 56-year-old man developed anuria and hypertension 1 day after extracorporeal shock wave lithotripsy (ESWL) for a calculus in a solitary kidney. You are shown a left retrograde pyelogram with the catheter tip just below the ureteropelvic junction (Figure 8-1).

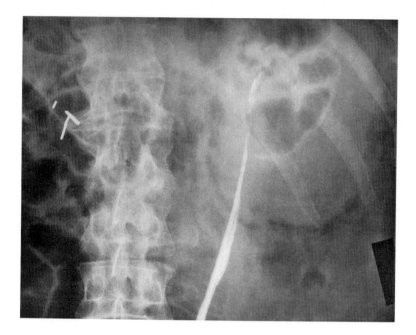

Figure 8-1

34. Which *one* of the following is the MOST likely diagnosis?

   (A) Arterial occlusion
   (B) Subcapsular hematoma
   (C) Failure to use a ureteral stent
   (D) Renal vein thrombosis
   (E) Steinstrasse

QUESTIONS 35 THROUGH 37: MARK YOUR ANSWER SHEET TRUE (T) OR FALSE (F) FOR EACH OF THE RESPONSE CHOICES.

35. Concerning subcapsular hematomas after ESWL,

   (A) Page kidney occasionally results
   (B) they are more common with calyceal calculi
   (C) preexisting hypertension is a risk factor
   (D) surgical evacuation is the treatment of choice
   (E) bleeding is from the capsular arteries

36. Concerning ureteral stents in ESWL,

   (A) insertion prior to the procedure is recommended for calculi larger than 2 cm
   (B) they provide a lumen for passage of the calculus fragments
   (C) they allow vesicoureteral reflux
   (D) they cause steinstrasse

37. Concerning ESWL,

   (A) new stones will form in up to 8% of patients by 1 year after treatment
   (B) associated hematuria is primarily due to ureteral passage of stone fragments
   (C) persistent hypertension is a complication in 15% of patients
   (D) it has virtually eliminated percutaneous nephrostolithotomy for staghorn calculi

CASE 8 (Cont'd)

For each of the calculi listed below (Questions 38 through 41), select the *one* lettered therapeutic approach (A, B, C, D, or E) that is MOST effective. Each lettered therapy may be used once, more than once, or not at all.

38. A 4-cm uric acid calculus in the renal pelvis
39. A 4-cm struvite calculus in the renal pelvis
40. A 2-mm calcium phosphate ureteral calculus
41. A 4-cm calcium oxalate calculus in the renal pelvis

    (A) Stent, then ESWL
    (B) Ureteroscopy
    (C) Sodium bicarbonate
    (D) No intervention
    (E) Antibiotics, stent, then ESWL

CASE 9: Questions 42 through 44

This 40-year-old man with diabetes mellitus presented with left flank pain and fever. You are shown two contrast-enhanced CT scans (Figures 9-1 and 9-2).

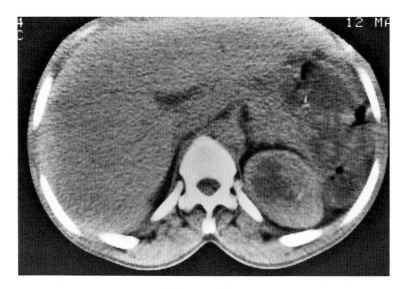

Figure 9-1

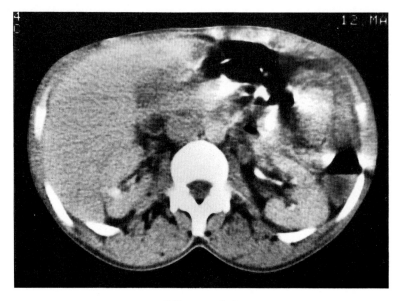

Figure 9-2

42. Which *one* of the following is the MOST likely diagnosis?

   (A) Necrotic renal cell carcinoma
   (B) Focal acute pyelonephritis
   (C) Abscess
   (D) Segmental infarction
   (E) Focal xanthogranulomatous pyelonephritis

QUESTIONS 43 AND 44: MARK YOUR ANSWER SHEET TRUE (T) OR FALSE (F) FOR EACH OF THE RESPONSE CHOICES.

43. Concerning renal abscess,

   (A) percutaneous drainage is effective in about 60% of cases
   (B) when it is associated with struvite calculi, *Klebsiella pneumoniae* is the most common organism
   (C) it is a hematogenous infection in most patients
   (D) perinephric involvement is present in fewer than 10% of cases

44. Concerning xanthogranulomatous pyelonephritis,

   (A) it usually occurs in the presence of calculi and obstruction
   (B) a common predisposing organism is *Proteus mirabilis*
   (C) perinephric extension is common
   (D) the tumefactive variety is the most common form

CASE 10: Questions 45 through 49

This 35-year-old woman has hematuria. You are shown a contrast-enhanced abdominal CT scan (Figure 10-1).

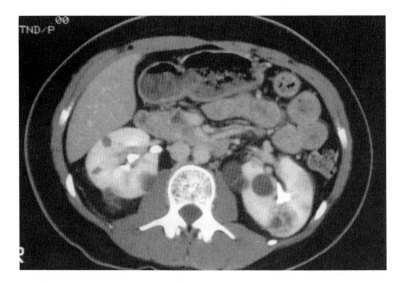

Figure 10-1

45. Which *one* of the following is the MOST likely diagnosis?

   (A) Autosomal dominant polycystic kidney disease
   (B) Acquired cystic kidney disease
   (C) von Hippel-Lindau disease
   (D) Tuberous sclerosis
   (E) Multilocular cystic nephroma

CASE 10 (Cont'd)

QUESTIONS 46 THROUGH 49: MARK YOUR ANSWER SHEET TRUE (T) OR FALSE (F) FOR EACH OF THE RESPONSE CHOICES.

46. Patients with autosomal dominant polycystic kidney disease have an increased incidence of:

   (A) hypertension
   (B) renal infection
   (C) renal adenocarcinoma
   (D) berry aneurysms
   (E) hepatic fibrosis

47. Findings associated with von Hippel-Lindau disease include:

   (A) retinal angiomas
   (B) adenoma sebaceum
   (C) pancreatic cysts
   (D) pheochromocytoma
   (E) hemihypertrophy

48. Findings associated with tuberous sclerosis include:

   (A) cerebellar hemangioblastoma
   (B) retinal phakomas
   (C) hypertension
   (D) renal adenocarcinomas
   (E) periungual fibromas

49. Concerning multilocular cystic nephroma,

   (A) it is often malignant
   (B) it occasionally herniates into the renal pelvis
   (C) most patients have hypertension
   (D) in adults, it is more common in women than in men
   (E) it is most accurately diagnosed by arteriography

CASE 11: Questions 50 through 55

Four patients underwent urethrography after sustaining blunt pelvic trauma. You are shown a retrograde urethrogram from each patient (Figures 11-1 through 11-4). For each patient's retrograde urethrogram (Questions 50 through 53), select the *one* lettered condition (A, B, C, D, or E) that BEST corresponds to that image. Each condition may be used once, more than once, or not at all.

50. Figure 11-1
51. Figure 11-2
52. Figure 11-3
53. Figure 11-4

 (A) Complete Type II urethral injury
 (B) Partial Type III urethral injury
 (C) Complete Type III urethral rupture
 (D) Straddle injury
 (E) Extraperitoneal bladder rupture

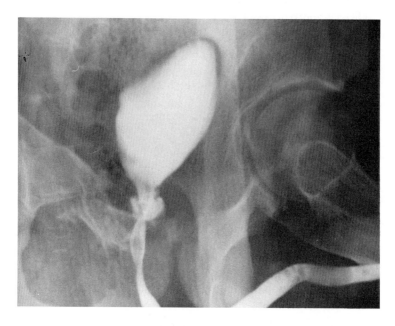

Figure 11-1

CASE 11 (Cont'd)

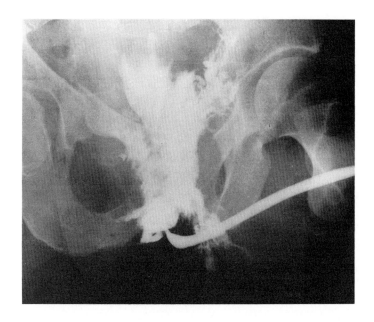

Figure 11-2

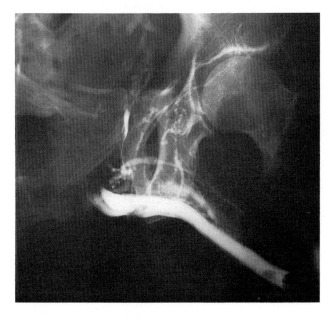

Figure 11-3

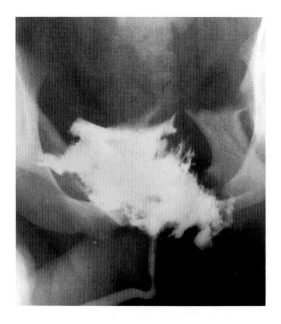

Figure 11-4

QUESTIONS 54 AND 55: MARK YOUR ANSWER SHEET TRUE (T) OR FALSE (F) FOR EACH OF THE RESPONSE CHOICES.

54. Concerning posterior urethral injuries from blunt pelvic trauma,

   (A) a pelvic fracture is generally present
   (B) they are caused by laceration of the prostatic urethra by a bone spicule
   (C) they are generally classified by their relationship to the urogenital diaphragm
   (D) on urethrography, the urogenital diaphragm prevents contrast material leakage from extending into the perineum in the majority of cases
   (E) the puboprostatic ligaments are generally ruptured

CASE 11 (Cont'd)

55. Concerning blunt anterior urethral injuries,

   (A) a pelvic fracture is generally present
   (B) they result when the bulbous urethra is crushed against the inferior aspect of the symphysis pubis
   (C) on urethrography, venous intravasation of contrast material generally indicates rupture of the corpus cavernosum
   (D) a normal retrograde urethrogram generally excludes anterior urethral contusion
   (E) leakage of contrast material into the scrotum or perineum indicates disruption of Buck's fascia

CASE 12: Questions 56 through 63

This 43-year-old man has bilateral nonpalpable testes. You are shown left parasagittal (A) and coronal (B) T1-weighted MR images and a transverse T2-weighted MR image (C) (1.0 T) of the pelvis (Figure 12-1). For each of the numbered arrows (Questions 56 through 60), select the *one* lettered structure (A, B, C, D, or E) that is MOST closely associated with it. Each lettered structure may be used once, more than once, or not at all.

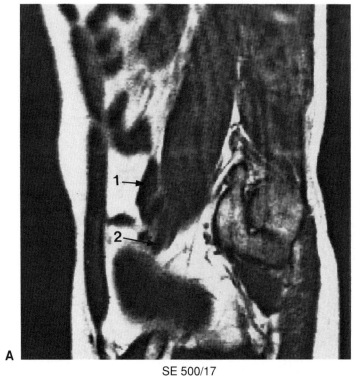

SE 500/17

Figure 12-1

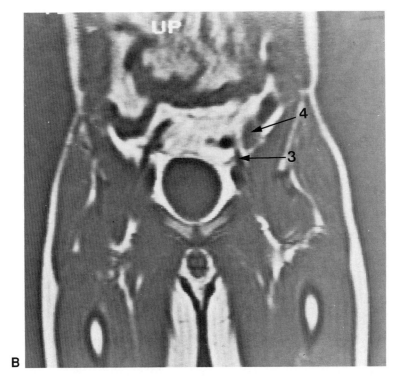

SE 700/28

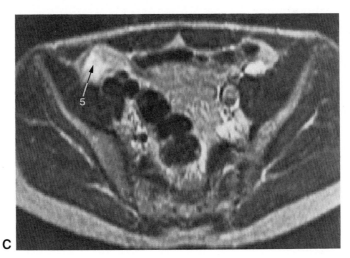

SE 1,500/90

56. Arrow 1
57. Arrow 2
58. Arrow 3
59. Arrow 4
60. Arrow 5

    (A) Undescended testis
    (B) Iliac vein
    (C) Iliac artery
    (D) Bowel loop
    (E) Lymph node

QUESTIONS 61 AND 62: MARK YOUR ANSWER SHEET TRUE (T) OR FALSE (F) FOR EACH OF THE RESPONSE CHOICES.

61. Concerning undescended testes,

    (A) the frequency in full-term neonates is about 10%
    (B) 10 to 12% of patients with testicular cancer have an undescended testis
    (C) those within the pelvis are found in the adventitia of the bladder
    (D) 80% are below the internal inguinal ring

62. Concerning imaging of undescended testes,

    (A) ultrasonography is more accurate than CT for detection of this condition
    (B) the signal intensity of testes on T1-weighted MR images is similar to that of muscle
    (C) lymph nodes are less echogenic than undescended testes on ultrasonography
    (D) identification of the internal inguinal ring is crucial for differentiating intra-abdominal from intracanalicular testes
    (E) most intra-abdominal testes are found at the aortic bifurcation

63. Which *one* of the following is MOST likely to be associated with an undescended testis?

   (A) Seminoma
   (B) Infertility
   (C) Inguinal hernia
   (D) Prune belly syndrome
   (E) Intersex disorders

CASE 13: Questions 64 through 72

Urographic images were obtained from five separate patients (Figures 13-1 through 13-5). For each numbered image (Questions 64 through 68), select the *one* lettered diagnosis (A, B, C, D, or E) that is MOST likely. Each lettered diagnosis may be used once, more than once, or not at all.

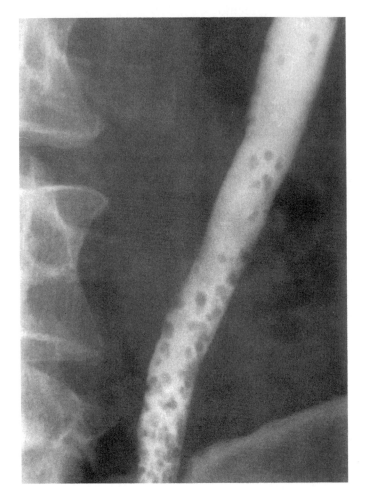

Figure 13-1

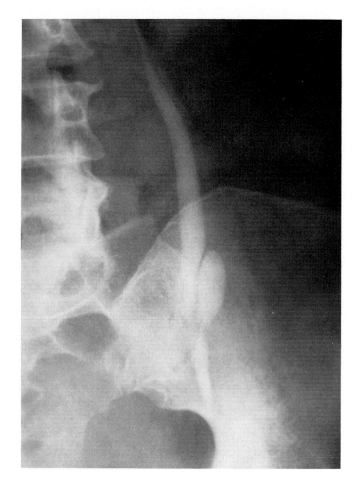

Figure 13-2

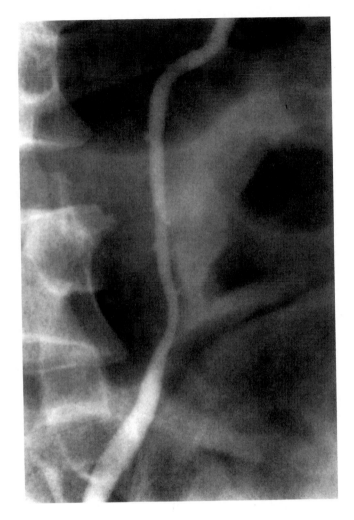

Figure 13-3

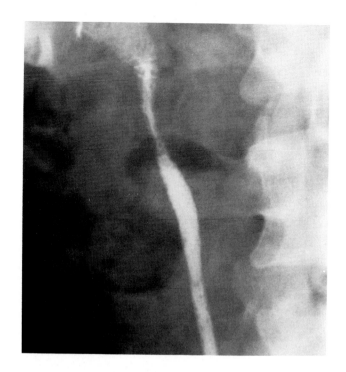

Figure 13-4

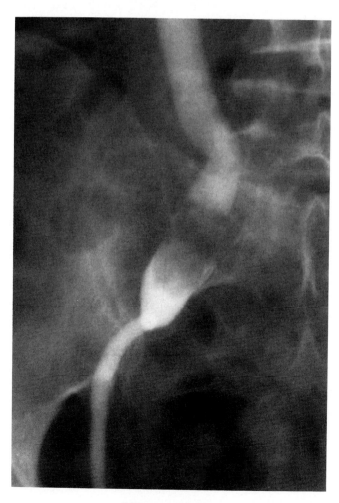

Figure 13-5

64. Figure 13-1
65. Figure 13-2
66. Figure 13-3
67. Figure 13-4
68. Figure 13-5

(A) Ureteritis cystica
(B) Transitional cell carcinoma
(C) Pseudodiverticulosis
(D) Mucosal edema
(E) Blind-ending ureteral bud

QUESTIONS 69 THROUGH 72: MARK YOUR ANSWER SHEET TRUE (T) OR FALSE (F) FOR EACH OF THE RESPONSE CHOICES.

69. Concerning ureteritis cystica,

(A) multiple small, contrast-filled diverticula project from the ureteral wall
(B) most patients have a history of chronic urinary tract infections
(C) it is more common in the proximal than the distal ureter
(D) it often involves the renal pelvis and bladder
(E) it is associated with transitional cell carcinoma

CASE 13 (Cont'd)

70. Concerning transitional cell carcinoma,

    (A) the frequency of occurrence in the renal pelvis, ureter, bladder, and urethra is proportional to the surface area of the urothelium in these structures
    (B) a negative urinary cytologic test makes it an unlikely diagnosis
    (C) obstruction of the collecting system is rare
    (D) dilatation of the ureter distal to a filling defect is much more commonly seen with this condition than with a ureteral stone
    (E) the risk of spreading the tumor along the catheter tract contraindicates percutaneous nephrostomy for tumor in the upper urinary tract

71. Concerning pseudodiverticulosis,

    (A) it is due to a series of congenital defects in the ureteral wall
    (B) most patients have a history of chronic urinary tract infections
    (C) it is most common in the upper and middle portions of the ureter
    (D) radiographically it is indistinguishable from ureteritis cystica
    (E) it is associated with an increased incidence of transitional cell carcinoma

72. Concerning a blind-ending ureteral bud,

    (A) it may arise from the ureter or the bladder
    (B) a common sheath surrounds both the ureter and the bud
    (C) the blind-ending ureter fills by retrograde peristalsis
    (D) most patients present with symptoms of urinary tract infection
    (E) it is more common in men than in women

CASE 14: Questions 73 through 77

This 32-year-old woman presented with flank pain and hematuria. You are shown a 1-hour radiograph from an excretory urogram (A) and a selective right renal arteriogram (B) (Figure 14-1).

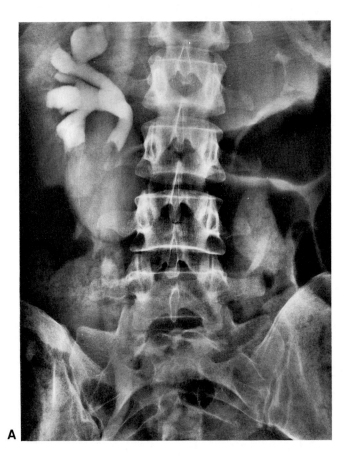

Figure 14-1

73. Which *one* of the following is the MOST likely diagnosis?

    (A) Renal cell carcinoma
    (B) "Nutcracker" phenomenon
    (C) Vascular malformation
    (D) Transitional cell carcinoma
    (E) Substance abuse

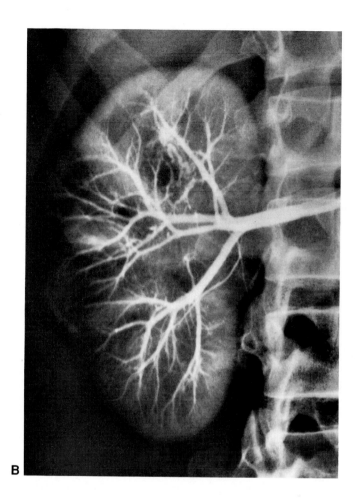

B

QUESTIONS 74 AND 75: MARK YOUR ANSWER SHEET TRUE (T) OR FALSE (F) FOR EACH OF THE RESPONSE CHOICES.

74. Concerning renal cell carcinoma,

(A) embolotherapy is not indicated for small tumors

(B) sonography is preferred for staging

(C) alcohol embolization should be performed through a balloon-occlusion catheter

(D) the 5-year survival rate with renal vein involvement is 10%

(E) 50% of patients have renal vein involvement at presentation

75. Concerning the "nutcracker" phenomenon,

    (A) the frequency of right and left renal involvement is the same
    (B) it causes hematuria
    (C) a pressure gradient exists in the renal vein
    (D) embolization is the treatment of choice

76. Which *one* of the following is MOST important in embolizing a renal vascular malformation?

    (A) Occluding the nidus
    (B) Occluding all visible feeding vessels
    (C) Eliminating the arteriovenous shunting
    (D) Use of a permanent coil
    (E) Use of a balloon-occlusion catheter

QUESTION 77: MARK YOUR ANSWER SHEET TRUE (T) OR FALSE (F) FOR EACH OF THE RESPONSE CHOICES.

77. Concerning renal vascular disease associated with substance abuse,

    (A) methamphetamine is a cause
    (B) LSD is a cause
    (C) microaneurysms are a typical feature
    (D) hypertension is a common feature
    (E) associated gastrointestinal vascular lesions are rare

CASE 15: Questions 78 through 80

This 20-year-old man was involved in a motor vehicle accident and sustained a pelvic fracture. You are shown a radiograph from a cystogram performed through a percutaneously placed suprapubic catheter (Figure 15-1).

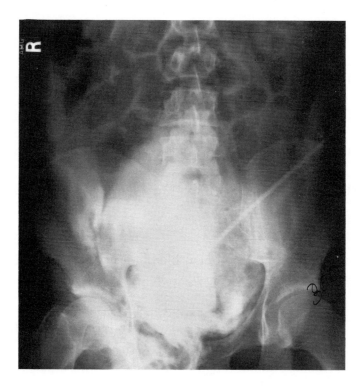

Figure 15-1

78. Which *one* of the following is the MOST likely diagnosis?

    (A) Intraperitoneal bladder rupture
    (B) Extraperitoneal bladder rupture
    (C) Combined intraperitoneal and extraperitoneal bladder rupture
    (D) Combined intraperitoneal bladder and urethral rupture

CASE 15 (Cont'd)

QUESTIONS 79 AND 80: MARK YOUR ANSWER SHEET TRUE (T) OR FALSE (F) FOR EACH OF THE RESPONSE CHOICES.

79. Concerning intraperitoneal bladder rupture following blunt trauma,

    (A) the mechanism of injury is secondary to a laceration of the dome of the bladder by a bone spicule
    (B) it is the most common form of major bladder injury in children
    (C) it generally occurs in patients with a distended bladder at the time of injury
    (D) contrast-enhanced CT is the diagnostic procedure of choice
    (E) return of urine through a Foley catheter usually excludes the diagnosis

80. Concerning extraperitoneal bladder rupture following blunt trauma,

    (A) on cystography, leakage of contrast material beyond the pelvic extraperitoneal space in men generally indicates an associated urethral injury
    (B) the bladder injury is most often found adjacent to the area of pelvic fracture
    (C) most cases can be managed nonoperatively
    (D) a false-negative cystogram occurs in at least 25% of cases

CASE 16: Questions 81 through 85

This 27-year-old woman presented with acute flank pain. You are shown a contrast-enhanced abdominal CT scan (Figure 16-1).

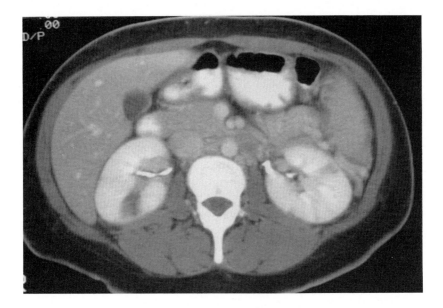

Figure 16-1

81. Which *one* of the following is the MOST likely diagnosis?

    (A) Acute tubular necrosis
    (B) Renal infarction
    (C) Acute bacterial pyelonephritis
    (D) Lymphoma
    (E) Renal vein thrombosis

QUESTIONS 82 THROUGH 85: MARK YOUR ANSWER SHEET TRUE (T) OR FALSE (F) FOR EACH OF THE RESPONSE CHOICES.

82. Concerning acute tubular necrosis,

  (A) it is less likely to occur after the use of a nonionic than of an ionic contrast agent
  (B) it is usually reversible
  (C) the nephrogram is diminished in intensity
  (D) sonography can distinguish it from obstruction
  (E) recovery is hastened by diuretic therapy

83. Concerning renal infarction,

  (A) the initial reaction of the kidney to occlusion of the renal artery is a decrease in size
  (B) the combination of a normal nephrogram with no contrast excretion is typical
  (C) calyceal blunting is not seen
  (D) a patent main renal artery excludes this diagnosis
  (E) segmental renal infarction usually causes cortical scarring

84. Concerning the radiologic features of acute bacterial pyelonephritis,

  (A) the nephrogram is diminished
  (B) the collecting system is attenuated
  (C) the kidney appears normal on sonography
  (D) a striated nephrogram is often seen on CT
  (E) perfusion of the periphery of the kidney by capsular vessels is more common with pyelonephritis than with infarction

85. Concerning renal vein thrombosis,

    (A) infants of diabetic mothers are predisposed to it

    (B) membranous glomerulonephritis is a common etiology in adults

    (C) marked proteinuria is nearly always present

    (D) right-sided involvement is easier to visualize on sonography than left-sided involvement

    (E) it responds well to systemic anticoagulation

This 64-year-old man has prostatic carcinoma. You are shown transverse T2-weighted MR images at the level of the mid-prostate (A) and above the level of the prostate (B) (Figure 17-1).

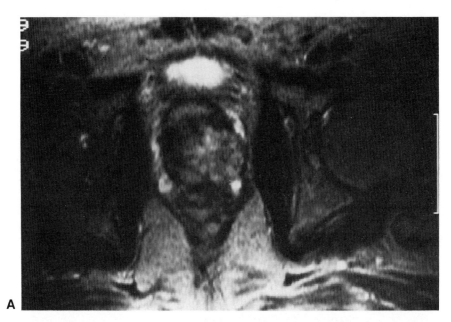

A

SE 2,500/90

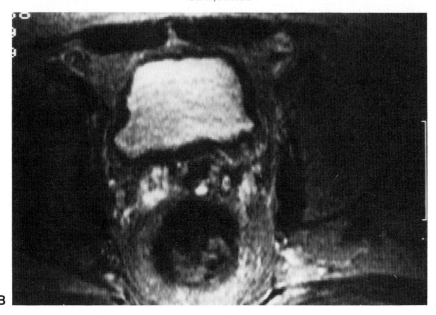

B

SE 2,500/90

Figure 17-1

86. Based on these images, which *one* of the following is the CORRECT stage of the tumor?

    (A) Stage A
    (B) Stage B
    (C) Stage C1
    (D) Stage C2
    (E) Stage D

For each of the following conditions related to prostatic carcinoma (Questions 87 through 91), select the *one* lettered stage (A, B, C, D, or E) that BEST describes it. Each lettered stage may be used once, more than once, or not at all.

87. Palpable nodule that is >1.5 cm on one side
88. Nonpalpable diffuse glandular involvement
89. Neurovascular bundle involvement
90. Metastasis to bone
91. Metastasis to pelvic lymph nodes

    (A) Stage A
    (B) Stage B
    (C) Stage C
    (D) Stage D1
    (E) Stage D2

QUESTIONS 92 AND 93: MARK YOUR ANSWER SHEET TRUE (T) OR FALSE (F) FOR EACH OF THE RESPONSE CHOICES.

92. Concerning imaging of prostatic carcinoma,

   (A) CT is more specific than MRI for detecting stage C disease
   (B) on T2-weighted MR images, the signal intensity of tumor is low compared with that of the peripheral zone
   (C) inguinal nodes are generally involved with metastasis before iliac nodes
   (D) on transrectal ultrasonography, more than 50% of hypoechoic lesions are malignant
   (E) MRI and transrectal ultrasonography have equal specificity for evaluating seminal vesicle invasion

93. Concerning prostatic carcinoma,

   (A) it occurs in about 30% of men over the age of 50 years
   (B) it rarely metastasizes until the primary tumor exceeds 1 cm^3 in volume
   (C) elevated prostate-specific antigen values are specific for the diagnosis
   (D) it arises in the peripheral zone in more than 90% of patients
   (E) it occurs as often in the anterior half of the prostate as in the posterior half

CASE 18: Questions 94 through 97

This 50-year-old woman developed persistent urine leakage from an abdominal drain 1 week after a hysterectomy and lymph node dissection for carcinoma of the cervix. You are shown a nephrostogram (Figure 18-1).

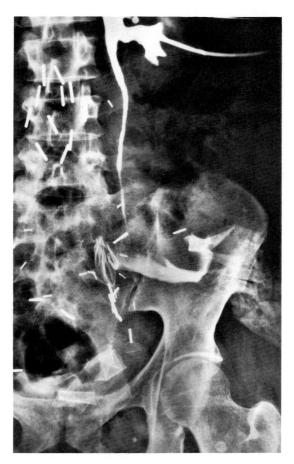

Figure 18-1

94. Which *one* of the following is the BEST course of action?

    (A) Immediate ureteral reimplantation
    (B) Transureteroureterostomy
    (C) Nephrectomy
    (D) Continued nephrostomy drainage
    (E) Ureteral stent placement

CASE 18 (Cont'd)

QUESTIONS 95 THROUGH 97: MARK YOUR ANSWER SHEET TRUE (T) OR FALSE (F) FOR EACH OF THE RESPONSE CHOICES.

95. Ureteral reimplantation with a short ureter is facilitated by:

    (A) psoas hitch
    (B) ileal interposition
    (C) Boari flap
    (D) autotransplantation

96. Concerning percutaneous nephrostomy,

    (A) the transcortical route is preferred
    (B) gas is a useful contrast agent
    (C) at least a 10-French catheter is needed for adequate drainage
    (D) major bleeding occurs in about 10% of patients
    (E) entering a lower-pole calyx facilitates subsequent ureteral stenting

97. Concerning stenting of ureteral fistulas,

    (A) the injured segment should be balloon dilated first
    (B) a 6-French stent is the largest that should be used
    (C) stents draining into an ileal conduit frequently occlude
    (D) the stent should be removed within 14 days

CASE 19: Questions 98 through 103

This 15-year-old girl presented with vague abdominal complaints. You are shown an enhanced CT scan (Figure 19-1).

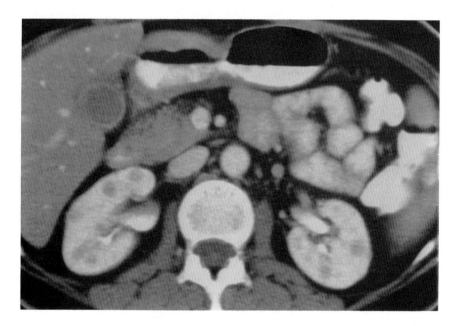

Figure 19-1

98. Which *one* of the following is the MOST likely diagnosis?

    (A) Burkitt's lymphoma
    (B) Candidiasis
    (C) Medullary cystic disease
    (D) Renal metastases
    (E) Leukemia

CASE 19 (Cont'd)

QUESTIONS 99 THROUGH 103: MARK YOUR ANSWER SHEET TRUE (T) OR FALSE (F) FOR EACH OF THE RESPONSE CHOICES.

99. Concerning renal lymphoma,

   (A) it is seen more often with Hodgkin's disease than with non-Hodgkin's lymphoma
   (B) it is seldom seen with Burkitt's lymphoma
   (C) renal failure is common
   (D) lymphomatous masses are usually homogeneous on CT
   (E) there is often other retroperitoneal tumor

100. Concerning medullary cystic disease,

   (A) in children, ophthalmologic abnormalities are common
   (B) in adults, renal function is seldom affected
   (C) the medullary cysts communicate freely with the renal tubules
   (D) many patients have accompanying nephrolithiasis
   (E) ultrasonography demonstrates increased parenchymal echogenicity

101. Concerning metastases to the kidneys,

   (A) the kidneys are sites for metastatic disease in fewer than 5% of patients with cancer
   (B) there are usually multiple lesions
   (C) they are usually asymptomatic
   (D) a solitary metastasis cannot be distinguished radiographically from a primary renal adenocarcinoma
   (E) they seldom demonstrate tumor necrosis

102. Concerning leukemia,

    (A) the kidneys are rarely involved at autopsy

    (B) patients seldom have symptoms due to renal involvement

    (C) solid masses composed of poorly differentiated cells may occur with acute myeloblastic leukemia

    (D) accompanying retroperitoneal lymphadenopathy is seldom present

    (E) hemorrhage (intrarenal, subcapsular, or perinephric) is common

103. Concerning candidiasis,

    (A) *Candida albicans* is seldom a pathogen in an immunocompetent host

    (B) multiple small parenchymal abscesses are a feature of renal involvement

    (C) papillary necrosis is rare unless the patient has underlying diabetes mellitus

    (D) extension into the renal pelvis may result in a mycetoma

    (E) fungus balls in the renal pelvis cannot be distinguished from tumor or blood clot by ultrasonography

History withheld. You are shown a scout radiograph (Figure 20-1), a 10-minute radiograph from an excretory urogram (Figure 20-2), and a coned view of the left ureter (Figure 20-3).

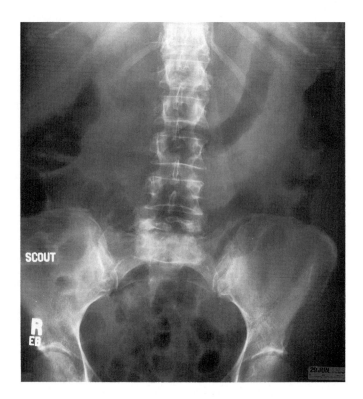

Figure 20-1

104. Which *one* of the following is the MOST likely diagnosis?

    (A) Renal artery stenosis
    (B) Endometriosis
    (C) Metastatic disease
    (D) Primary urothelial tumor
    (E) Suburothelial hemorrhage

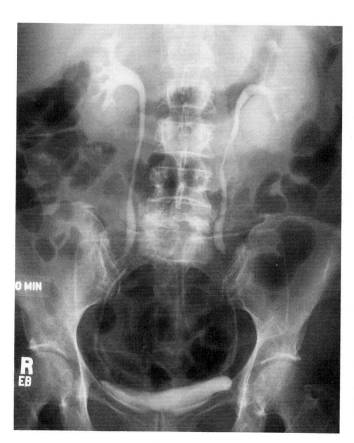

Figure 20-2

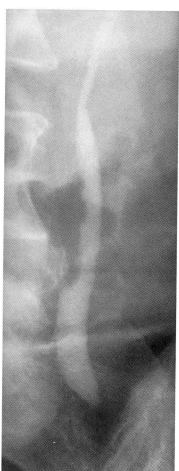

Figure 20-3

QUESTIONS 105 THROUGH 107: MARK YOUR ANSWER SHEET TRUE (T) OR FALSE (F) FOR EACH OF THE RESPONSE CHOICES.

105. Concerning vascular "notching" of the ureter,

   (A) when it accompanies renal artery stenosis, it is usually the result of hypertrophy of the ureteral artery
   (B) when it involves the proximal one-third of the ureter, it is usually arterial
   (C) when it is secondary to varices of the broad ligament, it involves the right ureter more commonly than the left
   (D) it occurs with occlusion of either the superior or inferior vena cava

106. Concerning ureteral endometriosis,

   (A) the typical radiographic appearance is that of extrinsic compression
   (B) the lesion is usually located just above the level of the sacroiliac joint
   (C) CT is the imaging study of choice to assess the extent of ureteral involvement
   (D) nearly all patients also have endometrial implants involving the sigmoid colon

107. Concerning primary ureteral neoplasms,

   (A) about 75% are found in the proximal one-third of the ureter
   (B) between 5 and 10% of patients with transitional cell carcinoma of the ureter have a concurrent or antecedent transitional cell tumor of the bladder
   (C) between 5 and 10% of patients with a primary transitional cell tumor of the bladder will develop transitional cell carcinoma of the ureter
   (D) they are twice as common in men as in women

108. Which *one* of the following is MOST closely associated with suburothelial hemorrhage?

    (A) Analgesic abuse
    (B) Hemophilia
    (C) Collagen vascular disease
    (D) Trauma
    (E) Anticoagulant therapy

You are shown a coronal MR image of the abdomen of a 2-week-old boy who became symptomatic at home following an uncomplicated birth (Figure 21-1). Additional history withheld.

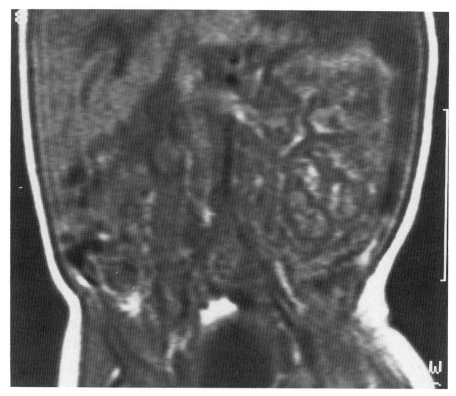

SE 500/17

Figure 21-1

109. Which *one* of the following is the MOST likely diagnosis?

    (A) Hydronephrosis
    (B) Renal vein thrombosis
    (C) Mesoblastic nephroma
    (D) Renal infarction
    (E) Multicystic dysplastic kidney

CASE 21 (Cont'd)

QUESTIONS 110 AND 111: MARK YOUR ANSWER SHEET TRUE (T) OR FALSE (F) FOR EACH OF THE RESPONSE CHOICES.

110. Concerning hydronephrosis,

(A) pelvic pressure measurements are normal after several weeks

(B) the glomerular filtration rate declines as a result of preglomerular vasoconstriction

(C) there is reduced renal blood flow in long-standing obstruction

(D) dilated ducts of Bellini are seen with chronic obstruction

(E) diuresis renography effectively separates obstruction from nonobstructive dilatation

(F) highly compliant upper tracts yield false-negative Whitaker test results

111. Concerning imaging of renal vein thrombosis,

(A) the characteristic finding on duplex Doppler sonography is reversed arterial diastolic flow

(B) early sonographic changes include decreased renal echogenicity

(C) a high intraluminal vascular signal on spin-echo MR images is specific for thrombosis

(D) narrow-flip-angle MR images are of little value in identifying thrombosis

(E) the intensity of contrast enhancement on CT depends on the adequacy of collateral flow

This 52-year-old man presented with weakness, lethargy, hypotension, and hyponatremia. You are shown an enhanced abdominal CT scan at the level of the adrenal glands (Figure 22-1).

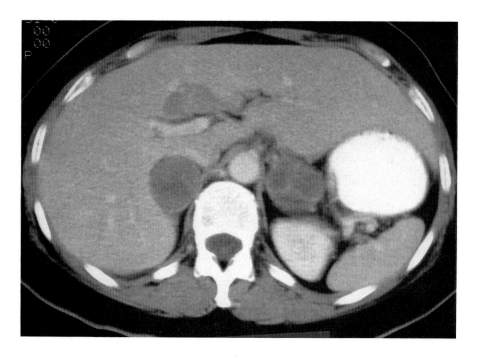

Figure 22-1

112. Which *one* of the following is the LEAST likely diagnosis?

    (A) Tuberculosis
    (B) Adrenal hemorrhage
    (C) Autoimmune adrenal insufficiency
    (D) Adrenal metastases
    (E) Histoplasmosis

QUESTIONS 113 THROUGH 116: MARK YOUR ANSWER SHEET TRUE (T) OR FALSE (F) FOR EACH OF THE RESPONSE CHOICES.

113. Concerning adrenal tuberculosis,

  (A) it is the most common cause of Addison's disease
  (B) it is often due to direct spread from the kidneys
  (C) it is usually bilateral
  (D) its appearance on CT is similar to that of an adrenal adenoma
  (E) proving the tuberculous etiology of Addison's disease is often difficult

114. Concerning adrenal hemorrhage,

  (A) it is commonly seen in newborn infants
  (B) it is unlikely to occur after trauma unless there are associated rib or spine fractures
  (C) in blunt trauma the left adrenal gland is affected more often than the right
  (D) in the absence of trauma, systemic anticoagulation is a common cause
  (E) a recent hematoma is recognized on CT as a soft tissue mass of increased density

115. Concerning autoimmune adrenal insufficiency,

  (A) it is more common among women than men
  (B) patients present at an older age than those with tuberculous destruction of the adrenal glands
  (C) the adrenal glands appear diffusely and symmetrically enlarged
  (D) it is commonly associated with other endocrine or autoimmune diseases

116. Concerning adrenal metastases,

    (A) they are common
    (B) they can often be distinguished from benign adenomas by MRI
    (C) they are a common cause of Addison's disease
    (D) Hodgkin's disease more commonly involves the adrenal glands than does non-Hodgkin's lymphoma
    (E) Addison's disease is not seen with lymphomatous infiltration of the adrenal glands

CASE 23: Questions 117 through 122

This 48-year-old man presented with impotence. Following clinical evaluation, he was referred for corpora cavernosometry and cavernosography. You are shown a corpora cavernosogram following intracorporeal administration of 60 mg of papaverine and 1 mg of phentolamine (Figure 23-1).

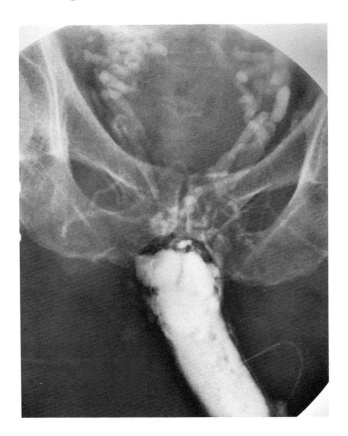

Figure 23-1

117. Which *one* of the following is the MOST likely diagnosis?

    (A) Veno-occlusive incompetence
    (B) Peyronie's disease
    (C) Psychogenic impotence
    (D) Penile artery disease
    (E) Multiple sclerosis

QUESTIONS 118 THROUGH 122: MARK YOUR ANSWER SHEET TRUE (T) OR FALSE (F) FOR EACH OF THE RESPONSE CHOICES.

118. Concerning duplex and color-flow Doppler ultrasonography of the deep penile arteries after intracavernosal papaverine administration,

    (A) the mean peak systolic velocity in the deep penile artery is normally 15 to 25 cm/second
    (B) cavernosal arteries are constricted by the drug
    (C) detectable dorsal vein flow is present during all phases of erection
    (D) normally, diastolic velocity decreases below 5 cm/second as the intracavernosal pressure increases

119. Concerning penile arteriography,

    (A) the vessels are best studied with the penis in the flaccid state
    (B) opacification of the spongiosal artery is associated with a vascular stain
    (C) helicine branches arise from the dorsal artery
    (D) bilateral internal pudendal arteriography is sufficient for a complete evaluation of arterial disease
    (E) a single cavernosal artery indicates arteriogenic impotence

120. Concerning corpora cavernosography,

    (A) both corpora should be injected
    (B) it should be performed after cavernosometry
    (C) the saphenous vein is a potential route of penile venous drainage
    (D) opacification of the glans is abnormal

121. Concerning veno-occlusive incompetence,

    (A) it is rarely associated with arterial disease
    (B) ligation of the deep dorsal vein is a highly effective form of treatment
    (C) it is due to testosterone deficiency
    (D) self-administration of papaverine is beneficial

122. Concerning Peyronie's disease,

    (A) it is a fibrous cavernositis
    (B) it is associated with Dupuytren's contracture
    (C) it most often begins laterally in the corpora cavernosa
    (D) the corpus spongiosum is often involved
    (E) calcification is common

CASE 24: Questions 123 through 127

This 64-year-old man developed swelling of the right leg 2 weeks after a prostatectomy for adenocarcinoma. You are shown a venogram of the right leg (Figure 24-1).

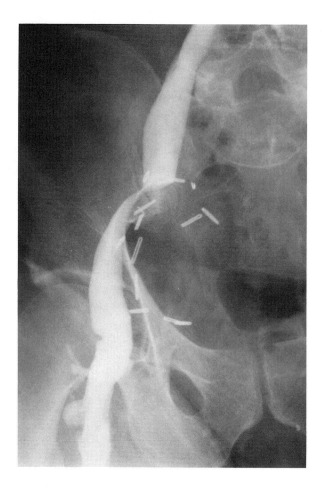

Figure 24-1

QUESTION 123: MARK YOUR ANSWER SHEET TRUE (T) OR FALSE (F) FOR EACH OF THE RESPONSE CHOICES.

123. Likely diagnoses include:

    (A) thrombosis of the iliac vein
    (B) extrinsic compression of the iliac vein by metastatic prostatic carcinoma
    (C) lymphocele
    (D) pelvic lipomatosis
    (E) pelvic hematoma

124. Which *one* of the following is the MOST appropriate examination for this patient after the venogram?

    (A) Retrograde pyelography
    (B) Ultrasonography
    (C) CT
    (D) MRI
    (E) Arteriography

QUESTIONS 125 THROUGH 127: MARK YOUR ANSWER SHEET TRUE (T) OR FALSE (F) FOR EACH OF THE RESPONSE CHOICES.

125. Concerning lymphoceles,

    (A) they occur after disruption of the lymphatic system
    (B) septations are commonly seen on ultrasonography
    (C) the diagnosis is confirmed by visual inspection of the aspirated fluid
    (D) the lymphatic etiology of the cyst can be predicted by MRI
    (E) they are readily cured by percutaneous aspiration

126. Concerning pelvic lipomatosis,

   (A) it is most commonly seen in black men
   (B) it is associated with chronic urinary tract infection
   (C) large amounts of benign adipose tissue compress the bladder and rectum
   (D) ureteral obstruction is a common problem among older men
   (E) it is associated with transitional cell carcinoma

127. Concerning pelvic hematoma,

   (A) it is uncommon in the absence of pelvic trauma
   (B) an acute hemorrhage can be diagnosed on CT by its high density
   (C) ultrasonography may reveal either an anechoic or an echogenic mass
   (D) the MR appearance is a function of the iron content
   (E) it rarely causes venous obstruction

This 4-year-old girl has left flank pain and fever. You are shown coronal T1-weighted (A) and gradient-recalled-echo (B) MR images (Figure 25-1).

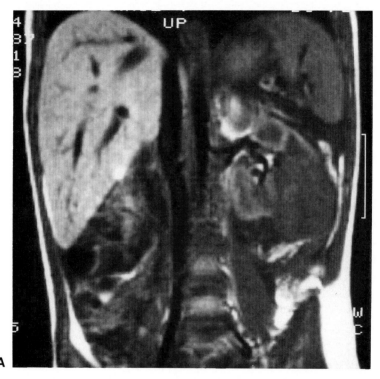

SE 500/17

Figure 25-1

128. Which *one* of the following is the MOST likely diagnosis?

    (A) Traumatic subcapsular hematoma
    (B) Mesoblastic nephroma
    (C) Burkitt's lymphoma
    (D) Wilms' tumor
    (E) Renal abscess

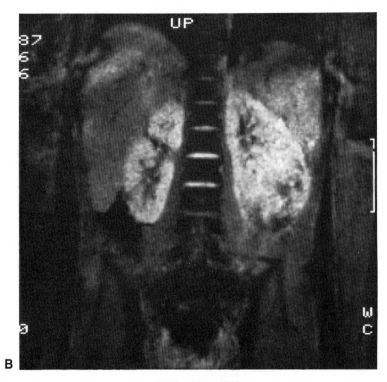

GRE 300/30/20°

QUESTIONS 129 THROUGH 131: MARK YOUR ANSWER SHEET TRUE (T) OR FALSE (F) FOR EACH OF THE RESPONSE CHOICES.

129. Concerning the MR appearance of hemorrhage,

    (A) it is determined partially by the pulse sequences

    (B) the age of the hemorrhage influences the signal intensity

    (C) narrow-flip-angle images are more sensitive for detection of hemorrhage than are standard spin-echo images

    (D) a bright signal on short-TR/short-TE images is specific for hemorrhage

    (E) hemorrhage can be differentiated from proteinaceous fluid on narrow-flip-angle GRE images

130. Concerning mesoblastic nephroma,

   (A) it is the most common intrarenal tumor in neonates
   (B) it is occasionally associated with nephroblastomatosis
   (C) calcification is common
   (D) it is considered premalignant

131. Concerning Wilms' tumor,

   (A) about 80% are diagnosed in patients less than 6 years old
   (B) it is composed of tubular, epithelial, and stromal tissue
   (C) aniridia is an associated feature
   (D) cell type is a better predictor of long-term prognosis than is the stage at presentation
   (E) nonfunction of the affected kidney is typical

This 46-year-old man presented with a palpable mass in the scrotum. You are shown coronal T1-weighted (A) and T2-weighted (B) MR images (Figure 26-1).

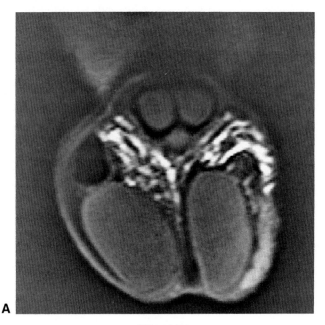

SE 500/26

Figure 26-1

132. Which *one* of the following is the MOST likely diagnosis?

    (A) Varicocele
    (B) Spermatocele
    (C) Epididymal cyst
    (D) Epididymitis
    (E) Embryonal cell carcinoma

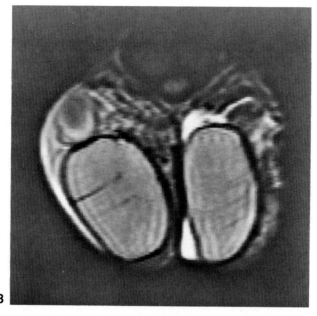

SE 2,500/80

QUESTIONS 133 THROUGH 135: MARK YOUR ANSWER SHEET TRUE (T) OR FALSE (F) FOR EACH OF THE RESPONSE CHOICES.

133. Concerning spermatoceles,

    (A) they are located in the head of the epididymis
    (B) typical components include lymphocytes and fat
    (C) they are often confused with sperm granulomas
    (D) they are incorporated within the tunica albuginea

134. Concerning epididymal cysts,

    (A) they occur anywhere along the course of the epididymis
    (B) the MR characteristics are those of a simple cyst
    (C) they are often confused with varicoceles on MR imaging
    (D) they are usually secondary to infection
    (E) they are associated with adenomatoid extratesticular tumors

135. Concerning imaging of the scrotum,

    (A) on T2-weighted MR images, the normal epididymis has low signal intensity
    (B) ultrasonography is the modality of choice for differentiating intratesticular from extratesticular masses
    (C) diffuse bilateral testicular involvement by leukemia is better detected by MRI than by ultrasonography
    (D) MRI is the best method for diagnosing a varicocele
    (E) tumor and abscess are reliably differentiated by signal characteristics on T2-weighted MR images

CASE 27: Questions 136 through 138

This 33-year-old hypertensive woman with normal renal function underwent Tc-99m DTPA renal scintigraphy before (Figure 27-1) and after (Figure 27-2) the oral administration of captopril.

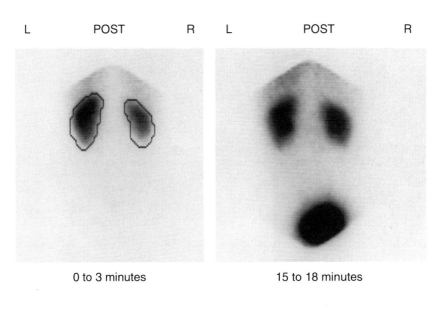

0 to 3 minutes   15 to 18 minutes

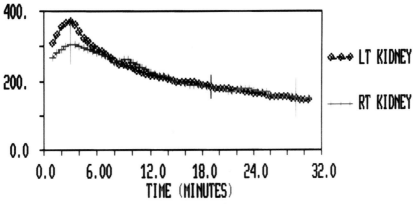

Figure 27-1

CASE 27 (Cont'd)

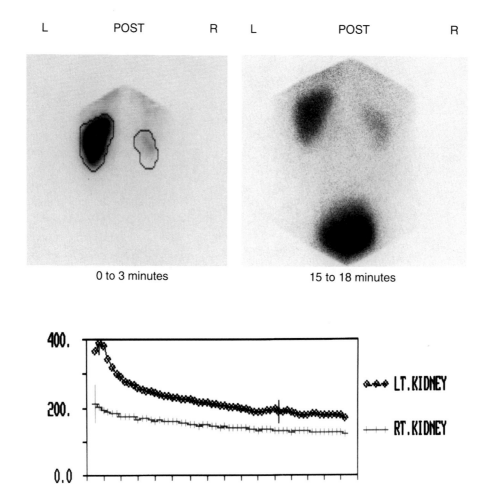

Figure 27-2

QUESTIONS 136 THROUGH 138: MARK YOUR ANSWER SHEET TRUE (T) OR FALSE (F) FOR EACH OF THE RESPONSE CHOICES.

136. Concerning the test patient,

    (A) left renal artery stenosis is likely to be present

    (B) a greater discrepancy in relative tracer accumulation after captopril administration would have been present if I-131 *o*-iodohippurate had been used instead of Tc-99m DTPA

    (C) the changes seen after captopril administration are secondary to efferent arteriolar vasodilatation

    (D) a satisfactory blood pressure response to renal revascularization is likely

137. Regarding renovascular hypertension,

    (A) if there is no lateralization of renal vein renin activity, revascularization is unlikely to be beneficial

    (B) intravenous digital subtraction angiography has poor sensitivity for detecting fibromuscular dysplasia

    (C) the results of intravenous digital subtraction angiography correlate well with those of conventional arteriography for detecting atheromatous disease in the renal artery

    (D) peripheral plasma renin measurements are unreliable for its exclusion

138. Regarding captopril,

   (A) it is an angiotensin-converting enzyme inhibitor
   (B) it is the antihypertensive agent of choice in patients with bilateral renal artery stenosis
   (C) in a kidney with renal artery stenosis, its primary effect is to increase glomerular filtration
   (D) it occasionally produces a profound hypotensive response
   (E) captopril scintigraphy with Tc-99m DTPA is effective in assessing for renovascular hypertension in patients with poor renal function

History withheld. You are shown CT scans (Figure 28-1) made at the level of the upper pole of the left kidney (A) and through the midportion of both kidneys (B) following an excretory urogram.

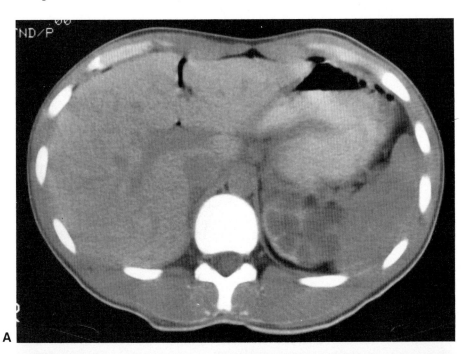

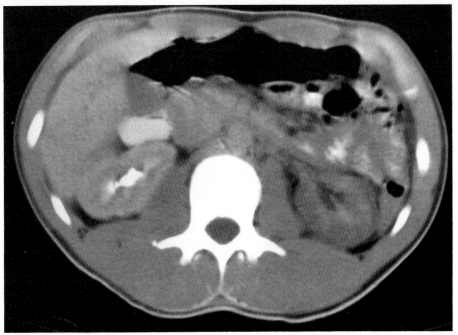

Figure 28-1

139. Which *one* of the following is the MOST likely diagnosis?

    (A) Acute ureteral obstruction
    (B) Renal vein thrombosis
    (C) Acute cortical necrosis
    (D) Acute pyelonephritis
    (E) Acute renal infarction

QUESTIONS 140 THROUGH 143: MARK YOUR ANSWER SHEET TRUE (T) OR FALSE (F) FOR EACH OF THE RESPONSE CHOICES.

140. Concerning acute ureteral obstruction,

    (A) a significant irreversible loss of renal function occurs after as little as 48 hours of complete ureteral obstruction
    (B) backflow mechanisms (e.g., pyelolymphatic, pyelosinus, pyelotubular, and pyelovenous backflow) allow continued glomerular filtration in the early phase
    (C) increased enhancement of both the renal cortex and medulla is evident on CT
    (D) the "obstructive nephrogram" occurs principally because of leakage of contrast material into the renal interstitium
    (E) the most sensitive urographic sign is dilatation of the pyelocalyceal system

141. Concerning acute cortical necrosis,

    (A) it generally occurs as a complication of pregnancy
    (B) CT will demonstrate a thin zone of enhancement adjacent to the renal capsule
    (C) radiographs demonstrate a characteristic pattern of tramlike cortical calcifications
    (D) sonography in the early phase generally demonstrates a hyperechoic renal cortex
    (E) bilateral involvement is invariable

142. Concerning acute pyelonephritis,

    (A) CT or ultrasonography is generally required for diagnosis
    (B) vesicoureteral reflux is commonly demonstrated in adult patients
    (C) in adults, inadequately treated acute infection is the major cause of chronic pyelonephritis
    (D) complicating abscesses most commonly occur in patients with altered host defense mechanisms

143. Concerning acute renal infarction,

    (A) the most common cause is embolism
    (B) the CT appearance is characteristic
    (C) when it is secondary to trauma, hematuria is frequently absent
    (D) hypertension is a common late complication

This 33-year-old man presented with pain and marked scrotal swelling. You are shown a retrograde urethrogram (Figure 29-1).

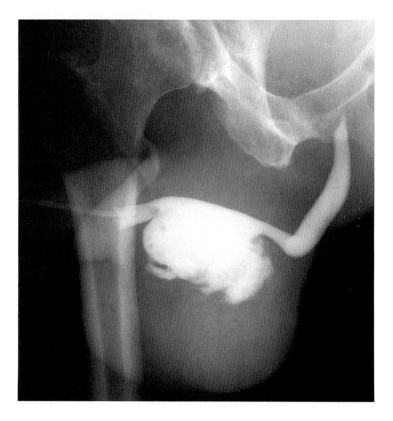

Figure 29-1

144. Which *one* of the following is the MOST likely diagnosis?

   (A) Periurethral abscess
   (B) Carcinoma of the anterior urethra
   (C) Megalourethra
   (D) Congenital saccular urethral diverticulum
   (E) Cowper's duct cyst

QUESTION 145: MARK YOUR ANSWER SHEET TRUE (T) OR FALSE (F) FOR EACH OF THE RESPONSE CHOICES.

145. Concerning carcinoma of the urethra,

    (A) the bulbous urethra is the most common site in men
    (B) the most common cell type is adenocarcinoma
    (C) when it involves the anterior urethra in men, it generally is associated with underlying stricture disease
    (D) it is more common in women than in men
    (E) the most common presenting complaint is voiding difficulty

146. Which *one* of the following is MOST closely associated with megalourethra?

    (A) Seminal vesicle cyst
    (B) Congenital megacalyces
    (C) Prune-belly syndrome
    (D) Megacystis-microcolon syndrome
    (E) Hirschsprung's disease

QUESTION 147: MARK YOUR ANSWER SHEET TRUE (T) OR FALSE (F) FOR EACH OF THE RESPONSE CHOICES.

147. Concerning Cowper's duct cyst,

    (A) it most commonly presents in childhood
    (B) post-voiding dribbling is the most common presenting complaint
    (C) it appears as a filling defect in the bulbous urethra
    (D) urethral obstruction is uncommon

DEMOGRAPHIC DATA QUESTIONS

Please answer all of the questions below. The data you provide will be used to supply information that will allow you to compare your performance on the examination with that of others at similar levels of training and with similar backgrounds, and for purposes of planning continuing education projects. Please answer each question as accurately and as objectively as possible. Please mark the *one* BEST response for each question. Recall, of course, that we do *not* want individual names. Our analyses will reflect only categories and groups; everything will remain completely anonymous and no attempt will be made to identify any specific individual.

148. The ACR will be evaluating the questions in this examination to determine their degree of difficulty and to determine the success of the examination as an instrument of self-evaluation and continuing education. To assist the ACR, please indicate in which of the following ways you took this examination.

    (A) Used reference materials or read the syllabus portion of this book to assist in answering some portion of the examination
    (B) Did not use reference materials and did not read the syllabus portion of this book while taking the examination

149. How much residency and fellowship training in Diagnostic Radiology have you completed as of December 1992?

    (A) None
    (B) Less than 1 year
    (C) 1 year
    (D) 2 years
    (E) 3 years
    (F) 4 or more years

150. When did you finish your residency training in Radiology?

    (A) Prior to 1982
    (B) 1982–1986
    (C) 1987–1991
    (D) 1992
    (E) Not yet completed
    (F) Radiology is not my specialty

151. Have you been certified by the American Board of Radiology in Diagnostic Radiology?

    (A) Yes
    (B) No

152. Which one of the categories listed below BEST describes the setting of your practice in the immediate past 3 years? (For residents and fellows, in which one did you or will you spend the major portion of your residency or fellowship?)

    (A) Community or general hospital—less than 200 beds
    (B) Community or general hospital—200 to 499 beds
    (C) Community or general hospital—500 or more beds
    (D) University-affiliated hospital
    (E) Office practice

153. In which one of the following general areas of Radiology do you consider yourself MOST expert?

    (A) Chest radiology
    (B) Bone radiology
    (C) Gastrointestinal radiology
    (D) Genitourinary radiology
    (E) Head and neck radiology
    (F) Neuroradiology
    (G) Pediatric radiology
    (H) Cardiovascular radiology
    (I) Other

154. In which one of the following radiologic modalities do you consider yourself MOST expert?

(A) General angiography
(B) Interventional radiology
(C) Magnetic resonance imaging
(D) Nuclear radiology
(E) Ultrasonography
(F) Computed tomography
(G) Radiation therapy
(H) Other

Genitourinary Tract Disease
(Fourth Series)

Table of Contents

The Table of Contents is placed in this unusual location so that the reader will not be distracted by the answers before completeing the test. A detailed index of the areas considered in this syllabus is provided (beginning on p. 519) for further reference.

Genitourinary Tract Disease (Fourth Series) Syllabus

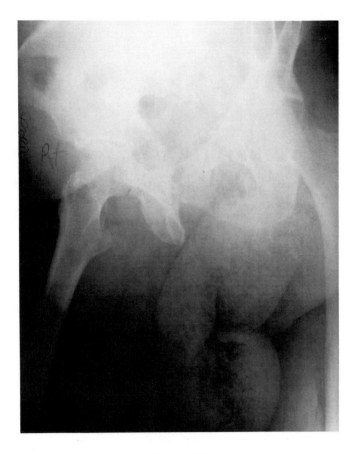

Figure 1-1
Figures 1-1 and 1-2. History withheld. You are shown a radiograph
(Figure 1-1) centered at the symphysis pubis of a 25-year-old man. You
are also shown a urethrogram (Figure 1-2).

Case 1: Fournier's Gas Gangrene

Question 1

Which *one* of the following is the MOST likely diagnosis?

(A) Scrotal hernia
(B) Torsion of the testis
(C) Epididymo-orchitis
(D) Scrotal gangrene
(E) Decompression sickness

Careful analysis of the radiograph (Figure 1-1) demonstrates extensive fine gas bubbles within a distended scrotum. These bubbles extend under Scarpa's fascia behind the symphysis pubis. The retrograde urethrogram (Figure 1-2) shows a normal intact bulbous and penile urethra, as well as the scrotal gas. The findings are typical of scrotal gangrene (Fournier's gangrene), with its characteristic necrosis and infection caused by gas-forming organisms **(Option (D) is correct).**

Scrotal hernia (Option (A)) is characterized by gas-containing bowel in the scrotum (Figure 1-3). The presence of valvulae conniventes of the small bowel or the haustral pattern of the large bowel should be identifiable and permits the distinction between this condition and gangrene.

Torsion of the testis (Option (B)) is one of the acute scrotal disorders seen in young patients. Although testicular necrosis will occur without treatment in cases of torsion, scrotal gas would not be a common finding. Patients with infections of the epididymis or testes (Option (C)) often present with acute pain and fever. However, gas in the scrotum is a rare radiographic finding. On conventional radiographic studies, the only expected finding with either torsion or epididymo-orchitis would be scrotal swelling.

Decompression sickness (Option (E)), or caisson disease, is caused by the release of nitrogen bubbles in body tissues or fluids. Symptoms relate to the site of gas formation and are classically described as the "bends." Other complaints include itching of the skin, chest pain, and coughing.

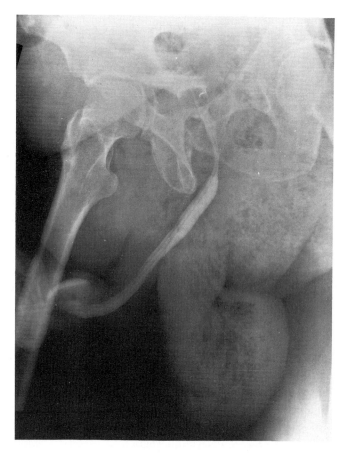

Figure 1-2

Decompression sickness would not present with the localized findings in the test case.

Other causes of scrotal air that are encountered in current clinical practice include pulmonary barotrauma in mechanically ventilated patients, colonic perforation secondary to colonoscopy, and air leaking and dissecting from faulty chest tube positioning. A gas-containing scrotal abscess secondary to Crohn's disease with fistula formation can mimic a scrotal hernia (Figure 1-4). As clearly described by Grant and Mitchell-Heggs, gas secondary to rectal perforations dissects along the deeper planes rather than along the superficial planes as seen in Fournier's gangrene. With rectal perforation, the gas dissects along the iliopsoas, pyriformis, and obturator internus muscles and vertically down into the thigh or buttocks.

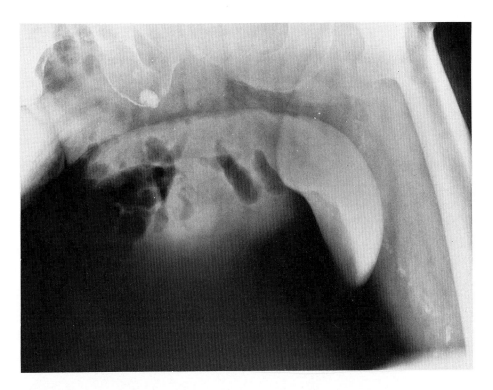

Figure 1-3. Scrotal hernia. Radiograph shows that the gas pattern of the bowel is quite different from that in Fournier's gangrene.

Fournier's gangrene was named for Jean Alfred Fournier, who described it in 1883. It is an aggressive process with a reported mortality rate approaching 50%. It often occurs in healthy patients below the age of 50 but is also found in debilitated elderly persons, patients with diabetes mellitus or alcoholism, and patients with measles. Although, as in this case, the cause is often unknown, trauma, insect bites, burns, and circumcision are reported causes in children. The causative organisms can be aerobic bacteria, anaerobic bacteria, or a combination of both, as proved to be the situation in the test case. The pathogenesis is unclear, but it has been suggested that the process is an obliterative endarteritis of the small scrotal cutaneous arteries, with subsequent spread of bacteria from the periurethral glands. This is followed by a spread of the infection from the corpus spongiosum through the tunica albuginea to Buck's fascia and the dartos muscle. From there, the infection extends under Colles' fascia to reach the anterior abdominal wall, where it is limited by the inguinal ligament. It does not routinely dissect deep to the inguinal ligament into the leg. If the patient's condition permits, CT (Figure 1-5) can be used to localize the spread of air preoperatively.

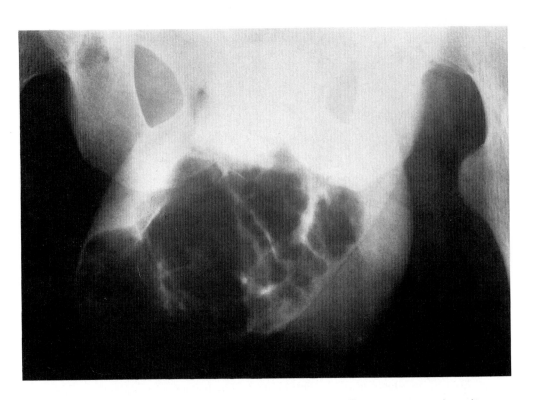

Figure 1-4. Scrotal abscess in a 17-year-old boy. The gas pattern is quite similar to that seen in Figure 1-2. No actual haustra are seen. The patient is known to have had Crohn's disease for many years. The abscesses were initially drained percutaneously, but surgery was ultimately required. (Case courtesy of Harold Mitty, M.D., Mount Sinai School of Medicine, New York, N.Y.)

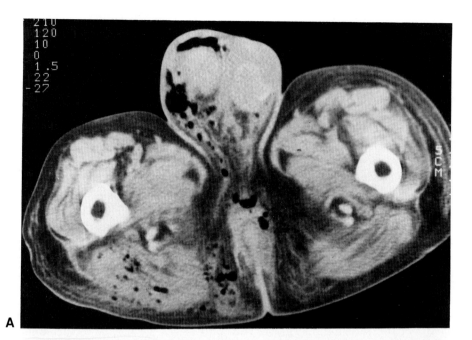

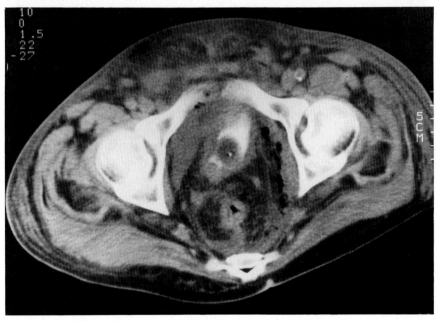

Figure 1-5. Scrotal gangrene in a 46-year-old man. (A) CT of the scrotum shows extensive amounts of soft tissue gas predominantly surrounding the right testis and in the right buttock, as well as the gluteus muscles. (B) At the level of the acetabula, the air is seen dissecting along the iliopsoas muscle. (Case courtesy of Mallinckrodt Institute of Radiology, St. Louis, Mo.)

Question 2

On gray-scale ultrasonography of the scrotum, a scrotal hernia is MOST likely to be confused with which *one* of the following?

(A) Hydrocele
(B) Varicocele
(C) Spermatocele
(D) Sperm granuloma
(E) Adenomatoid tumor of the epididymis

Gray-scale ultrasonography is an important tool for assessing intra-scrotal pathology. Although it may not confirm a particular pathologic diagnosis, it usually provides excellent anatomic detail, allowing exact localization of the pathologic process. Thus, intratesticular disease can usually be distinguished from extratesticular processes.

A varicocele consists of dilated veins or varicosities of the pampiniform plexus of the internal spermatic vein and arises secondary to incompe-tence of the valves of the internal spermatic vein. Varicoceles are a frequent, correctable cause of oligospermia, which results in infertility in males. Ninety-eight percent of varicoceles are on the left near the head of the epididymis and behind the testis. In general, the left spermatic vein empties into the left renal vein, whereas the right spermatic vein drains directly into the inferior vena cava. In the upright position the left renal vein is compressed by the superior mesenteric artery, and this causes retrograde flow in the left testicular vein. On gray-scale ultra-sonography, the varicocele often mimics a scrotal hernia because the distended veins may approach 5 to 6 mm in caliber instead of the normal 1 to 1.5 mm **(Option (B) is correct).** Careful analysis, however, will reveal that the varicosities appear different from the one or two bowel loops in a hernia. Doppler ultrasonography should readily differentiate these entities because it can demonstrate venous flow within the varicoceles (Figure 1-6).

One of the more common extratesticular findings noted on ultrasonog-raphy is an intrascrotal fluid collection. The most common such blind collection is a hydrocele (Option (A)), a collection of serous fluid between the two layers of tunica vaginalis (Figure 1-7). This fluid may be a nonspecific response to trauma, inflammation, or tumor. Most hydroceles are idiopathic. Ultrasonographically, the fluid in a hydrocele should be totally anechoic. Although fluid-filled loops of bowel within the scrotum may resemble a hydrocele on first inspection, careful attention to detail will demonstrate peristalsis as well as valvulae conniventes or haustra.

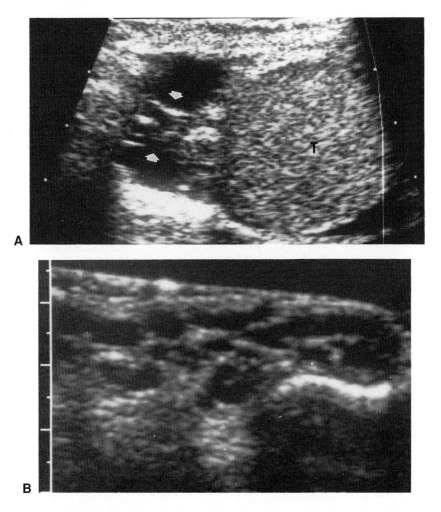

Figure 1-6. Two cases of varicocele. (A) Case 1. An incidental right vari-cocele is identified on a longitudinal sonogram in an 80-year-old man with hematuria. Arrows point to the dilated veins. T = testis. (B to D) Case 2. (B) A left varicocele is demonstrated on a longitudinal gray-scale sonogram made during a Valsalva maneuver; the dilated veins are readily identified. (C) This was confirmed by Doppler ultrasonography (transverse scan during Valsalva maneuver); this image documents a continuous-flow venous waveform in one of the dilated veins. (D) Ultra-sonography performed at the level of the left renal vein (lrv) shows that this vein is narrowed between the aorta (a) and spine (s). There is secondary dilatation of the proximal renal vein; this is the cause of the varicocele. (Case 2 courtesy of Sheila Sheth, M.D., Johns Hopkins University, Baltimore, Md.)

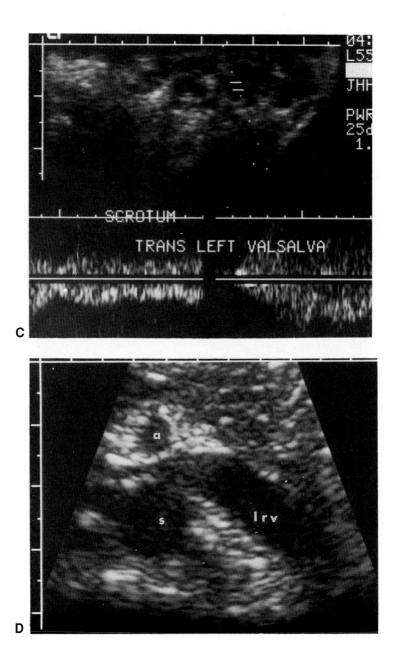

C

D

Furthermore, the accompanying mesenteric fat is echogenic. Thus, a hydrocele should not be confused with scrotal hernia.

A spermatocele (Option (C)) is a cyst that contains spermatozoa and is found in the globus major in the rete testis of the epididymis. Ultrasonographically, spermatoceles are fluid-containing masses ranging

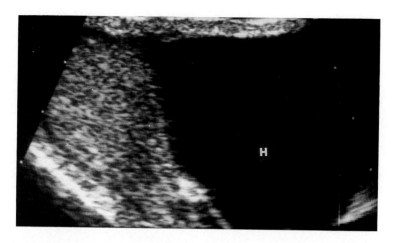

Figure 1-7. Incidental left hydrocele. A typical anechoic fluid collection (H) is seen above the testis.

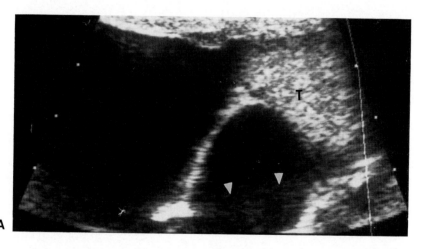

Figure 1-8. Two examples of spermatoceles on ultrasonography. (A) Case 1. The sediment is seen within the spermatocele (arrowheads). (B and C) Case 2. Longitudinal (B) and transverse (C) views show septations (arrowheads) within the cephalad and posteriorly located spermatocele. T = testis. (Case 2 courtesy of Sheila Sheth, M.D.)

in size from a few millimeters to several centimeters in diameter (Figure 1-8A). They may be simple or septated, separated from the testis, or within the epididymis itself. They can be differentiated from hydroceles because they are cephalad or posterior rather than anterior to the testis. It can be difficult to differentiate a spermatocele from a varicocele.

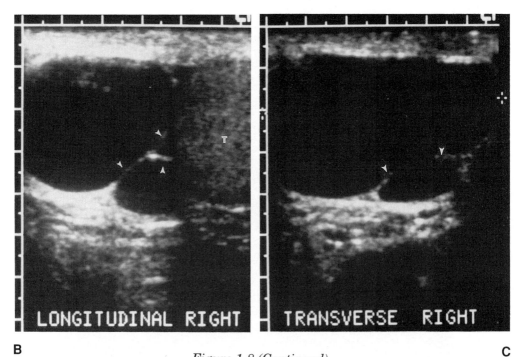

B

Figure 1-8 (Continued)

C

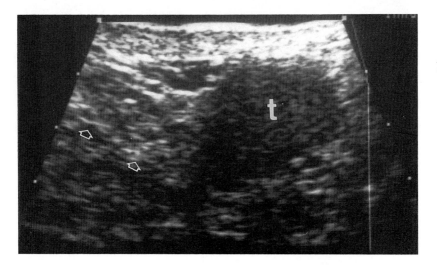

Figure 1-9. Scrotal hernia in a 20-year-old man. Arrows point to a collection of linear structures mimicking a varicocele. The pattern is not characteristic of the bowel. There is also no hyperreflection due to fat or gas. The bowel was probably filled with fluid. Doppler ultrasonography showed no blood flow. t = testis.

However, unlike varicoceles, spermatoceles do not enter the inguinal canal. Moreover, sediment representing spermatozoa, lymphocytes, fat globules, or cellular debris can usually be identified within the spermatocele; this will help differentiate it from a varicocele or a scrotal hernia (Figure 1-8B).

Extravasation of sperm into the surrounding tissue may lead to granuloma formation (Option (D)). These scrotal masses are painless and can be found both inside and outside the testicle. Ultrasonographically, a sperm granuloma is hypoechoic and solid and is not likely to be confused with a hernia.

An adenomatoid tumor of the epididymis (also called benign mesothelioma, lymphangioma, adenomyoma, or grade 1 adenocarcinoma) (Option (E)) is the most common benign epididymal tumor. It is seen most often in Caucasian men 30 to 50 years of age. It is usually unilateral and most often arises in the globus minor. Adenomatoid tumors are generally painless, but some discomfort or tenderness can be present. Occasionally, they mimic epididymitis. They grow slowly and are usually about 2 cm in diameter, although lesions as large as 5 cm have been encountered. They are solid tumors with a grossly whorled appearance and have internal echoes and poor through transmission on ultrasonography.

Thus, as described above, bowel herniation into the scrotum (Figures 1-9 and 1-10) can be confused with the dilated veins of a varicocele or, less likely, with the septations in a spermatocele. Other ultrasonographic clues to the correct diagnosis of hernia include the observation that the bowel gas and the fat surrounding the bowel are often hyperechoic. Careful monitoring will demonstrate bowel peristalsis.

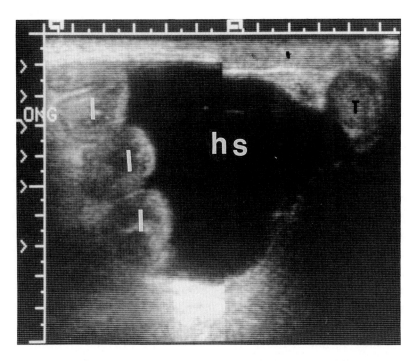

Figure 1-10. Scrotal hernia. Note the fluid-filled loops (l) within the hernial sac (hs). T = testis. (Case courtesy of Sheila Sheth, M.D.)

Question 3

Concerning testicular torsion,

F (A) at 6 hours, a peritesticular rim of intensely increased activity is usually seen on scintigraphy

F (B) it is most often seen in men in their late twenties

T (C) color-flow Doppler ultrasonography reliably distinguishes it from epididymitis

F (D) after 24 hours the likelihood of testicular salvage is approximately 50%

F (E) gray-scale ultrasonography reliably differentiates it from contusion

Acute testicular torsion is one of the true genitourinary emergencies. Patients present with abrupt, excrutiating pain, often accompanied by nausea, vomiting, and inability to walk. The peak incidence occurs around puberty; there is a second small peak in early childhood, but torsion can be seen in the elderly as well **(Option (B) is false).** Unfortunately, the classic clinical presentation is absent in up to one-third of the patients. These patients have a gradual onset of pain or even no pain at all. The need for urgent treatment of testicular torsion is determined by the marked dependency of the salvage rate on the time since the onset of torsion. Salvageability is almost 100% if detorsion occurs within 4 hours but decreases to 50% or less at 24 hours. After that, it is virtually zero **(Option (D) is false).**

Although color-flow Doppler ultrasonography appears to have at least an equivalent role and magnetic resonance imaging (MRI) looms on the horizon, radioisotopic scintigraphy currently remains readily available for evaluating the acute scrotum in most institutions. However, color-flow Doppler ultrasonography is gradually replacing scrotal scintigraphy in such cases.

With acute torsion (Figure 1-11), the arterial supply to the cord and testis is not seen during the radionuclide angiographic phase of testicular scintigraphy. The pathognomonic (although infrequently seen) "nubbin" sign represents increased activity in the testicular artery up to the torsion site. On the later angiographic images and on the static images, there is no activity in the testis. This pattern usually lasts for 4 to 6 hours. After that time, the involved hemiscrotum gradually becomes more and more hyperemic via collateral circulation through the pudendal and other pelvic arteries, which are unaffected by the testicular torsion. This is reflected by the initial development of mildly increased peritesticular activity on testicular scintigraphy performed after about 6 hours (Figure 1-12). The rim of increased activity around the ischemic testicle ("bull's-eye" pattern) progressively increases in intensity after 6 hours **(Option (A) is false).** Chen et al. report that if this scrotal wall activity is less than that of the femoral arteries, salvageability is excellent, whereas if the scrotal wall activity is the same as that of the femoral arteries, testicular salvageability is poor. With epididymo-orchitis (Figure 1-13), there is increased flow during the vascular phase with marked hyperemia on the static images.

There are many reports of the utility of gray-scale ultrasonography in evaluating the acute scrotum. However, gray-scale ultrasonography really shows only secondary morphologic changes; these include swelling and the loss of the normal homogeneous texture of the testis. The epididymis may become swollen, and a reactive hydrocele may develop. As such, the findings may be late in developing and nonspecific, and differentiation from epididymo-orchitis, tumor, or trauma may be difficult or impossible **(Option (E) is false).**

With the development of high-resolution color-flow Doppler ultrasonography (Figure 1-14), direct sonographic demonstration of absent testicular flow is now possible. Burks et al. successfully diagnosed six of seven

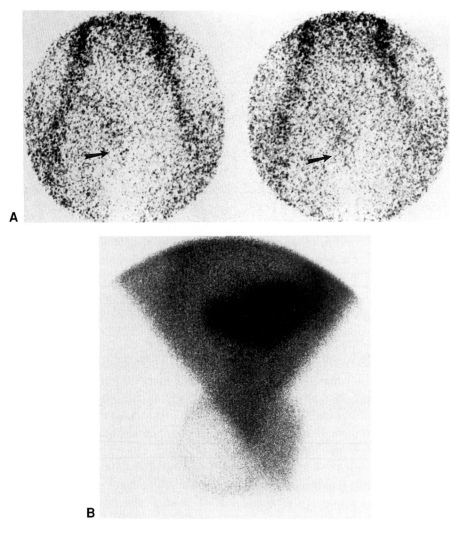

Figure 1-11. Acute testicular torsion. (A) Two radionuclide angiographic images show increased flow in the right internal iliac and spermatic cord vessels with a relatively sharp cutoff (arrows), the "nubbin" sign. (B) A delayed image with lead shielding behind the scrotum shows normal activity on the left but absent testicular activity on the right. There is some hyperemia in the right scrotal soft tissues. (Case courtesy of Lawrence E. Holder, M.D., Union Memorial Hospital, Baltimore, Md.)

cases of proven torsion by using color-flow Doppler ultrasonography. They believe that the failure was in a patient who developed complete torsion after the scan. Ralls et al. report that color-flow Doppler ultrasonography almost always shows increased flow to the epididymis

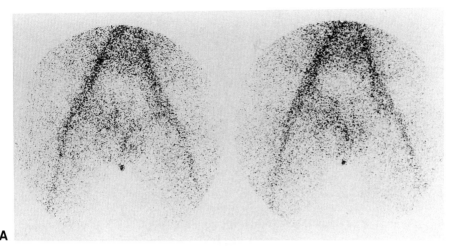

A

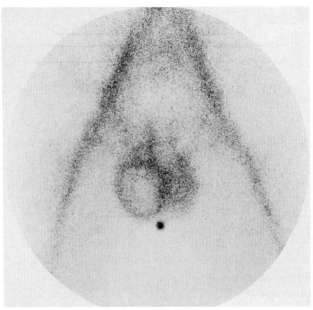

B

Figure 1-12. Late torsion of right testis in a 20-year-old man. (A) Flow studies show increased flow to the right paratesticular area. (B) The static image shows normal activity on the left. On the right, the testis is photon deficient, and there is a rim of hyperactivity in the surrounding soft tissues.

in acute epididymitis. In a recent prospective comparison of color-flow Doppler ultrasonography and testicular scintigraphy, Middleton et al. found sonography to be at least as accurate as scintigraphy in distinguishing torsion from inflammatory disease. In their study, one of seven

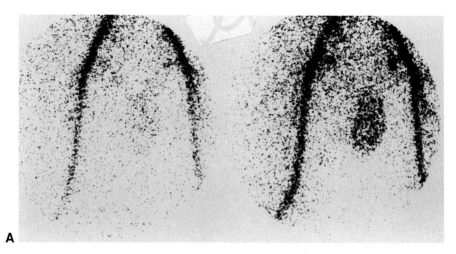

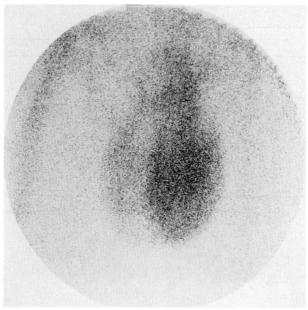

Figure 1-13. Left epididymo-orchitis in a 32-year-old man. The dynamic images (A) clearly show increased flow on the left, which persists on the static image (B).

patients with torsion had a false-negative scintigraphic study, but there were no false-negative sonographic results **(Option (C) is true).**

The role of MRI in testicular torsion is not yet known. Tzika et al. report the use of P-31 MRI in assessing testicular viability after inducing torsion in rats. Similarly, Landa et al. report a spiral distortion of the

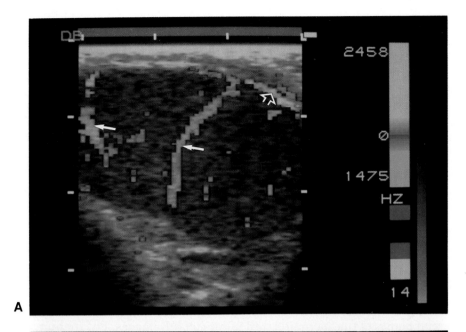

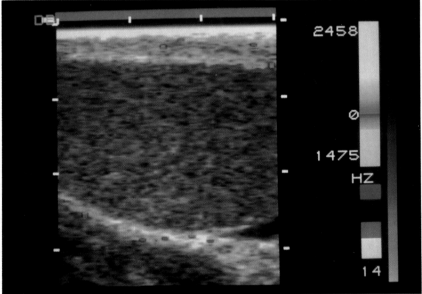

Figure 1-14. Color-flow Doppler ultrasonography of the scrotum. (A) Normal right testis showing multiple centripetal arteries (arrows) and a capsular artery (open arrow). (B) Left testis with complete testicular torsion demonstrating complete absence of flow. (C) Static scintigram shows absence of uptake in the left testis (arrow). (Reprinted with permission from Middleton et al. [14].)

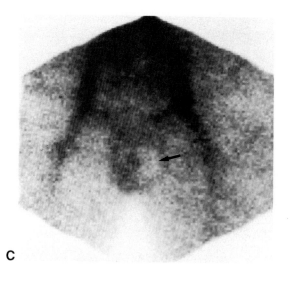

C

fascial planes of the spermatic cord in rats on MR images. Future human studies will be necessary to determine the clinical usefulness of MRI.

Question 4

Concerning scrotal gangrene,

F (A) mortality exceeds 60%
F (B) cultures most commonly contain *Clostridium welchii*
F (C) the infection is most common in elderly diabetic patients
T (D) the testes are rarely involved
T (E) effective treatment requires both antibiotics and extensive debridement

Fournier's gas gangrene can be rapidly fatal if not recognized and treated early. Grant and Mitchell-Heggs emphasized that for the cases reported in the literature before 1981, mortality approached 50%. More recently, Adams et al. reported a drop from 23 to 9% in children. This may reflect increased awareness, earlier intervention, or the development of more-potent antibiotics **(Option (A) is false).**

Cultures of the affected areas usually reveal a mixed flora. Both aerobic and anaerobic organisms are causative agents; they include *Escherichia coli, Bacillus puriformis*, microaerophilic and nonhemolytic *Streptococcus faecalis, Pseudomonas aeruginosa,* and various *Proteus* and *Klebsiella* species. While *Clostridium welchii* can cause scrotal gangrene, it is a rare cause **(Option (B) is false)**.

Although elderly diabetic patients can develop scrotal gangrene, most patients with this disorder are between 20 and 50 years of age and have either no underlying medical conditions or a variety of debilitating conditions **(Option (C) is false)**.

Scrotal gangrene is really a superficial cellulitis and fasciitis. The testes themselves are rarely involved. Even when the gangrene is caused by gas-forming organisms, the testes themselves appear uninvolved **(Option (D) is true)**.

Because of the severity of this process, immediate wide incisional drainage and debridement are necessary. This treatment must be accompanied by appropriate intravenous antibiotic therapy **(Option (E) is true)**.

Stanford M. Goldman, M.D.

SUGGESTED READINGS

FOURNIER'S GAS GANGRENE

1. Adams JR Jr, Mata JA, Venable DD, Culkin DJ, Bocchini JA Jr. Fournier's gangrene in children. Urology 1990; 35:439–441
2. Grant RW, Mitchell-Heggs P. Radiological features of Fournier gangrene. Radiology 1981; 140:641–643

ACUTE SCROTUM

3. Bird K, Rosenfield AT, Taylor KJ. Ultrasonography in testicular torsion. Radiology 1983; 147:527–534
4. Burks DD, Markey BJ, Burkhard TK, Balsara ZN, Haluszka MM, Canning DA. Suspected testicular torsion and ischemia: evaluation with color Doppler sonography. Radiology 1990; 175:815–821
5. Chen DC, Holder LE, Melloul M. Radionuclide scrotal imaging: further experience with 210 patients. J Nucl Med 1983; 24:735–742, 841–853
6. Dunn EK, Macchia RJ, Solomon NA. Scintigraphic pattern in missed testicular torsion. Radiology 1981; 139:175–180
7. Eshghi M, Silver L, Smith AD. Technetium 99m scan in acute scrotal lesions. Urology 1987; 30:586–593
8. Hill GJ. Adenomatoid tumor of the epididymis. In: Hill GJ (ed), Uropathology. New York: Churchill Livingstone; 1989:1146–1150
9. Horstman WG, Middleton WD, Melson GL. Scrotal inflammatory disease: color Doppler US findings. Radiology 1991; 179:55–59

10. Landa HM, Gylys-Morin V, Mattery RF, et al. Detection of testicular torsion by magnetic resonance imaging in a rat model. J Urol 1988; 140:1178–1180
11. Lerner RM, Mevorach RA, Hulbert WC, Rabinowitz R. Color Doppler US in the evaluation of acute scrotal disease. Radiology 1990; 176:355–358
12. Lutzker LG, Zuckier LS. Testicular scanning and other applications of radio-nuclide imaging of the genital tract. Semin Nucl Med 1990; 20:159–188
13. Martin B, Conte J. Ultrasonography of the acute scrotum. JCU 1987; 15:37–44
14. Middleton WD, Siegel BA, Melson GL, Yates CK, Andriole GL. Acute scrotal disorders: prospective comparison of color Doppler US and testicular scintigraphy. Radiology 1990; 177:177–181
15. Ralls PW, Jensen MC, Lee KP, Mayekawa DS, Johnson MB, Halls JM. Color Doppler sonography in acute epididymitis and orchitis. JCU 1990; 18:383–386
16. Rodríguez DD, Rodríguez WC, Rivera JJ, Rodríguez S, Oterro AA. Doppler ultrasound versus testicular scanning in the evaluation of the acute scrotum. J Urol 1981; 125:343–346
17. Sanders LM, Premkumar A, Amis ES Jr, Cohen M, Newhouse JH. Trauma-induced testicular torsion: ultrasonographic features and pathologic correlation. JCU 1989; 17:538–541
18. Trambert MA, Mattery RF, Levine D, Berthoty DP. Subacute scrotal pain: evaluation of torsion versus epididymitis with MR imaging. Radiology 1990; 175:53–56
19. Tzika AA, Vigneron DB, Hricak H, Moseley ME, James TL, Kogan BA. P-31 MR spectroscopy in assessing testicular torsion: rat model. Radiology 1989; 172:753–757

SCROTAL ULTRASONOGRAPHY

20. Fleischer AC. Renal and urological sonography. In: Fleischer AC, James AE Jr (eds), Diagnostic sonography. Principles and clinical applications. Philadelphia: WB Saunders; 1989:433–513
21. Krone KD, Carroll BA. Scrotal ultrasound. Radiol Clin North Am 1985; 23:121–139
22. Middleton WD, Thorne DA, Melson GL. Color Doppler ultrasound of the normal testis. AJR 1989; 152:293–297
23. Subramanyam BR, Balthazar EJ, Raghavendra BN, Horii SC, Hilton S. Sonographic diagnosis of scrotal hernia. AJR 1982; 139:535–538

SCROTAL MRI

24. Mattrey R. MRI of the male genitalia: testes, seminal vesicles, and urethra. In: Goldman SM, Gatewood OMB (eds), CT and MRI of the genitourinary tract. New York: Churchill Livingstone; 1990:245–286

Notes

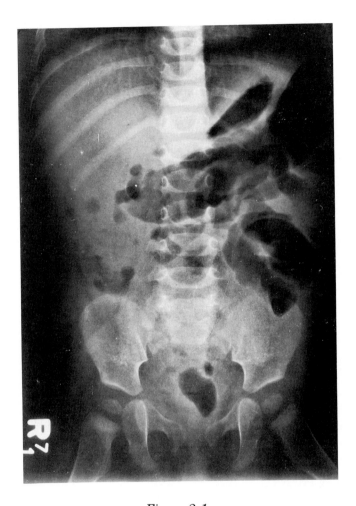

Figure 2-1
Figures 2-1 and 2-2. This 6-month-old boy presented with difficulty in voiding. You are shown an abdominal radiograph (Figure 2-1) and a cystogram (Figure 2-2).

Case 2: Rhabdomyosarcoma

Question 5

Which *one* of the following is the MOST likely diagnosis?

(A) Sacrococcygeal teratoma
(B) Lymphoma
(C) Rhabdomyosarcoma
(D) Neurofibromatosis
(E) Neuroblastoma

The radiograph (Figure 2-1) reveals displacement of bowel by a large pelvic mass (arrowheads, Figure 2-3). In a 6-month-old boy, an enlarged bladder or a retroperitoneal mass would be suspected. The sacrum is intact, and the sacral foramina are normal. The cystogram (Figure 2-2) clearly demonstrates that the mass seen on the radiograph is the bladder. The bladder is slightly trabeculated. Most important is that the base of the bladder is elevated by an irregular, multilobulated mass (arrowheads, Figure 2-4). There is no evidence of calcification in the mass. The findings are characteristic of a rhabdomyosarcoma of either the bladder or the prostate **(Option (C) is correct).**

In the newborn and in the young child, a large variety of pelvic masses can arise from the sacrum or presacral space. Most of these are sacrococcygeal dermoids or teratomas (Option (A)). Although dermoids and teratomas were originally considered to be distinct, it is now clear that most of these tumors do possess all three dermal layers and should be referred to as teratomas. Other lesions arising in the presacral area and sacrum include anterior meningocele, neuroblastoma, and chordoma. Sacrococcygeal teratomas are four times more common in girls, whereas the test patient is a boy. They are calcified 60% of the time. They may cause deformity of the sacrum (Figure 2-5A). Although they may displace the bladder anteriorly and compress it (Figure 2-5B), they do not cause a mass that displaces the bladder floor, such as that seen in Figure 2-2.

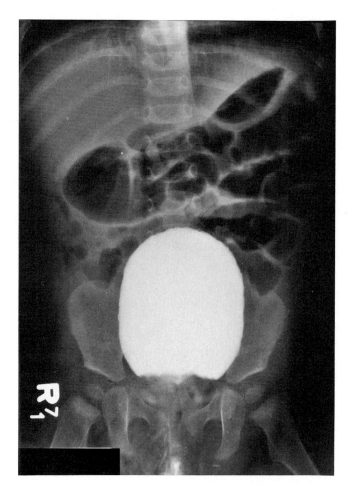

Figure 2-2

Lymphoma (Option (B)) (Figure 2-6), especially non-Hodgkin's lymphoma, arising in the pelvis will involve the retroperitoneal lymph nodes, which are adjacent to the iliac artery and vein. In the retroperitoneum, the normal lymph nodes have an inverted-Y configuration, with the arms of the Y hugging the pelvic brim laterally. When these nodes are enlarged, they typically compress the bladder from the side rather than inferiorly. Additionally, lymphoma would be quite uncommon at 6 months of age; it most often affects children older than 5 years.

Neurofibromatosis (Option (D)) in the pelvis (Figure 2-7) most commonly presents either as single or multiple retroperitoneal neurofibromas or sarcomas pushing on the bladder from behind or as a sharply defined solitary mass within the bladder itself. Neurofibromas are often associ-

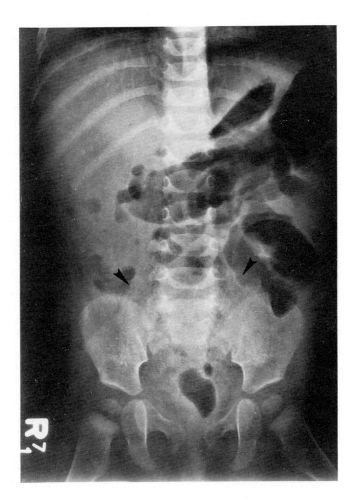

Figure 2-3
Figures 2-3 and 2-4 (Same as Figures 2-1 and 2-2). Rhabdomyosarcoma
of the bladder. The radiograph (Figure 2-3) shows an enlarged bladder
(arrowheads). The sacrum appears normal. The cystogram (Figure 2-4)
shows the bladder elevated by a lobular mass (arrowheads). There is no
calcification evident within the mass.

ated with sacral anomalies; there is no evidence for sacral abnormality
in the test patient. Although there is a possible association of neurofibromatosis with rhabdomyosarcomas of the prostate or uterus, the neurofibromas themselves would not present as a multinodular mass lifting up
the bladder.

Neuroblastoma (Option (E)) in children arises most often in the adrenal
but can develop in the presacral space or wherever neural crest tissue is

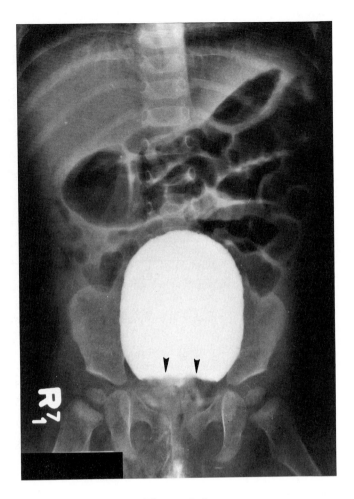

Figure 2-4

present (Figure 2-8). A pelvic neuroblastoma would most commonly present as a posterior pelvic mass pushing the bladder forward and usually contains coarse calcification.

A sonogram (Figure 2-9A) of the test patient reveals a lobulated echogenic mass filling most of the inferior aspect of the bladder. The sonogram shows that the mass is largely intraluminal. This appearance suggests that the rhabdomyosarcoma in this patient arose from within the bladder rather than from the prostatic bed. An enhanced CT scan (Figure 2-9B) also shows the solid bladder mass, although the site of origin of the mass is less clear than on the sonogram.

MRI can also be especially helpful in this kind of case because of its ability to obtain coronal and sagittal images in addition to the axial

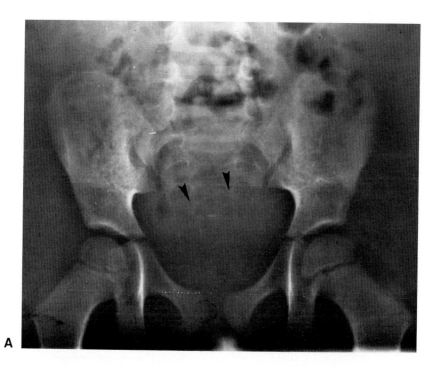

A

Figure 2-5. Sacrococcygeal tumor. (A) The radiograph shows destruction of the left side and caudal aspect of the sacrum (arrowheads). (B) The intravenous urogram shows that the tumor compresses the bladder from behind and above (arrowhead).

views. Figure 2-10 is an example of an MR study in another patient with rhabdomyosarcoma and shows a mass lifting and compressing the bladder. This pattern of tumor development in a young child is most characteristic of a rhabdomyosarcoma arising from the prostate.

Rhabdomyosarcomas do not evolve from mature muscle cells but from totipotent mesenchymal cells. They are the most common soft tissue sarcomas of childhood and most commonly originate at sites in the head and neck. Rhabdomyosarcomas are the most common lower genitourinary tract tumors found in the first 20 years of life. They usually occur in early childhood but are occasionally seen in patients in their late twenties. As noted above, they appear to be more common in patients with neuro-fibromatosis. Boys are affected more frequently than girls. Affected children usually present with symptoms of bladder outlet obstruction or urinary retention. Rhabdomyosarcomas are highly aggressive neoplasms. In the past, they were almost invariably incurable as a result of local invasion and both lymphatic and hematogenous spread, but modern

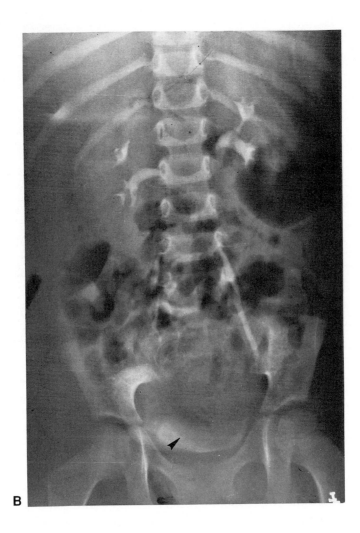

therapeutic strategies have led to a much-improved prognosis (see below).

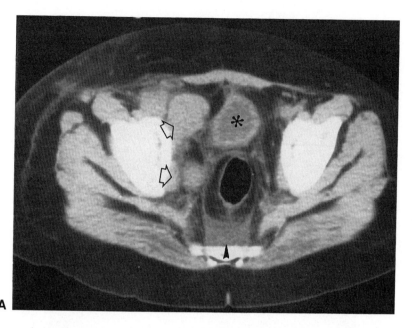

A

Figure 2-6. Two examples of lymphoma within the pelvis. (A) CT scan of a 16-year-old boy with a presacral mass (arrowhead) and enlarged right iliac lymph nodes (open arrows). Neither the presacral mass nor the enlarged right iliac nodes are in a position to elevate the bladder (*). (B) Intravenous urogram of an elderly man with extensive abdominal and pelvic lymphoma. There is bilateral compression of the bladder by the iliac nodes, but the bladder is not elevated. There is also marked lateral deviation of the ureters as a result of para-aortic adenopathy. (Figure 2-6A is provided courtesy of Marilyn J. Siegel, M.D., Mallinckrodt Institute of Radiology, St. Louis, Mo.)

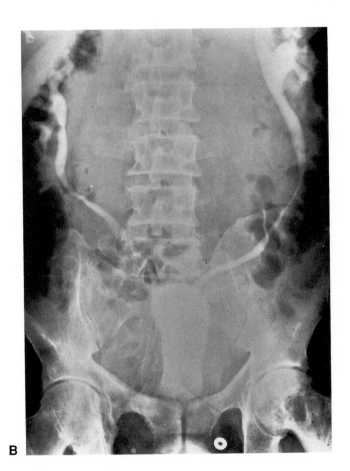

B

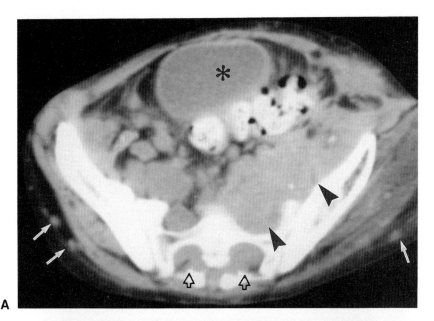

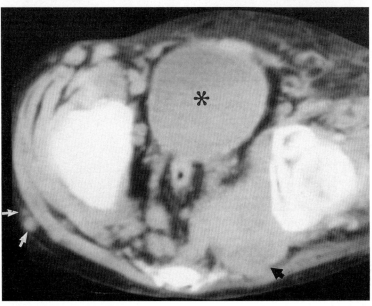

Figure 2-7. Neurofibromatosis with sarcomatous degeneration. (A) CT scan at the level of the sacroiliac joints. Note the large tumor extending along the medial aspect of the left iliac wing (arrowheads). A few specks of calcification are seen in the tumor. Also note the enlarged sacral foramina (open arrows) (* = bladder). (B) CT scan at the level of the ischiorectal fossa. The tumor is seen to extend out of the pelvis (arrow). There are also multiple neurofibromas in the soft tissues of the buttocks (white arrows) and along the right sacral nerve plexus. Despite the extensive tumors, the bladder (*) is hardly affected. (Case courtesy of Marilyn J. Siegel, M.D.)

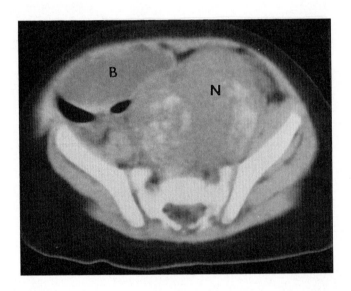

Figure 2-8. Calcified pelvic neuroblastoma (N) in a 10-month-old boy. The bladder (B) is pushed laterally by the tumor but is not lifted upward from below.

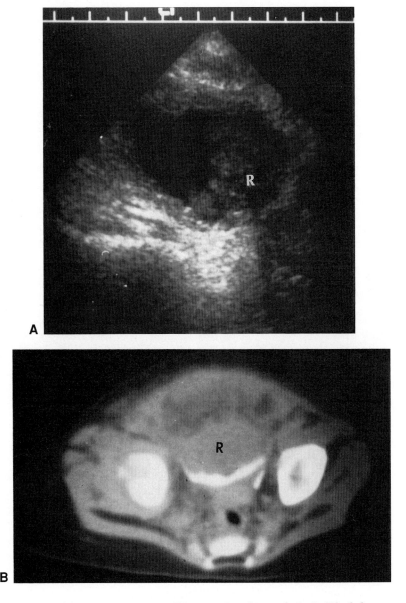

Figure 2-9 (Same patient as in Figures 2-1 through 2-4). Rhabdomyosar-coma of the bladder. (A) The sonogram of the test patient reveals the intracystic, echogenic rhabdomyosarcoma (R). (B) The CT scan also demonstrates the nodular rhabdomyosarcoma (R) within the contrast-filled bladder.

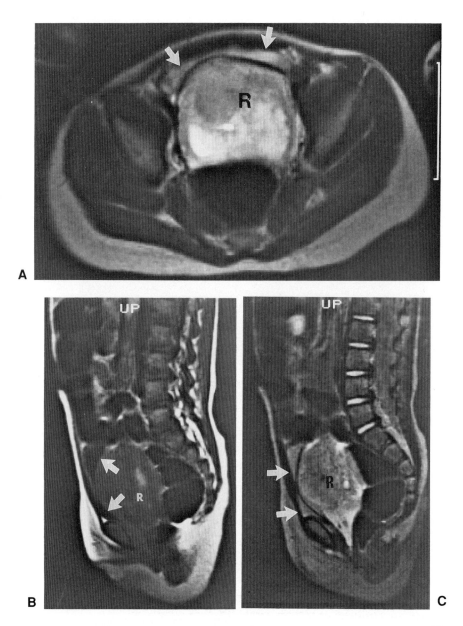

Figure 2-10. Rhabdomyosarcoma of the prostate in a young man. The T2-weighted axial MR image (A) reveals the rhabdomyosarcoma (R) to be inhomogeneous, compressing the bladder (arrows). The T1-weighted (B) and T2-weighted (C) sagittal MR images show that the rhabdomyosarcoma (R) compresses the bladder (arrows) against the anterior abdominal wall. (Case courtesy of Peggy Fritzsche, M.D., Loma Linda University, Loma Linda, Calif.)

Question 6

Concerning pelvic lymphoma in children,

F (A) it is most common in children under 2 years of age
F (B) hematuria is a common presenting feature
F (C) it usually arises in the pelvic floor
F (D) multiple filling defects in the bladder are typical on cystography
T (E) non-Hodgkin's lymphomas predominate

Lymphoma is the third most common cancer in childhood but is rarely seen before the age of 5 years **(Option (A) is false).** Approximately 40% of childhood lymphomas are of the Hodgkin's type and 60% are non-Hodgkin's lymphomas **(Option (E) is true).** Non-Hodgkin's lymphoma is approximately three times more common in boys than in girls. Boys are also more commonly affected by Hodgkin's disease when this develops before puberty.

Hodgkin's lymphoma is divided into several types. The lymphocyte-predominant and the nodular-sclerosing varieties have the best prognosis and are more common in girls. The mixed-cellularity and lymphocyte-depleted forms have the poorest prognosis. Non-Hodgkin's lymphoma is classified according to the architecture (nodular or diffuse) and the type of cells present (lymphocytic, histiocytic, etc.). Luke's classification (T cell, B cell, and U cell) is also used.

Patients with Hodgkin's lymphoma almost uniformly show contiguous intranodal involvement, whereas non-Hodgkin's lymphoma is more aggressive and is more likely to be extranodal. Half of all children and adults with non-Hodgkin's lymphoma have retroperitoneal and pelvic lymph node involvement. The bladder is commonly compressed by the iliac lymph nodes that are lateral to it. It is not often lifted by involved pelvic floor lymph nodes **(Option (C) is false).** Lymphoma is the second most common nonepithelial tumor of the bladder and is most often seen in the fourth to sixth decades. Hematuria is not a common presenting feature in children **(Option (B) is false);** when present, it is a late finding. Multiple nodular filling defects in the bladder are more commonly seen with leukemia and would not be seen with typical pelvic lymphoma, which causes predominantly smooth bladder compression secondary to extravesical iliac node enlargement **(Option (D) is false).**

Question 7

Concerning rhabdomyosarcomas,

(A) they are the most common tumors affecting the bladder in the first decade of life
(B) in childhood, they most commonly arise in the bladder and prostate
(C) those of the prostate characteristically cause elongation of the prostatic urethra
(D) those of the bladder typically arise in the dome
(E) radiation therapy is the treatment of choice for those of the bladder and prostate

Rhabdomyosarcomas represent between 5 and 15% of all malignant tumors in childhood. The most common location of these tumors in childhood is the head and neck region (about 40% of cases). About 20% arise in the genitourinary tract **(Option (B) is false).** As mentioned above, rhabdomyosarcoma is the most common lower genitourinary childhood neoplasm **(Option (A) is true).** In a series of 18 pelvic rhabdomyosarcomas of children reported by Geoffray et al., 12 involved the bladder, prostate, or uterus. Almost invariably, bladder and prostatic rhabdomyosarcomas affect the base of the bladder, so that it is often difficult to determine the exact site of origin in boys and young adult males. MRI studies performed in the coronal and sagittal planes may be helpful in this regard. These tumors do not typically arise in the bladder dome **(Option (D) is false).**

On intravenous urography, there is usually evidence of an obstructive uropathy with hydroureter. The bladder base shows an irregular multinodular mass; this appearance is typical of the sarcoma botryoides variant of embryonal rhabdomyosarcoma, which grossly resembles a bunch of grapes and most often occurs when there is mucosal-surface involvement of a hollow structure, such as the bladder or vagina. Prostatic rhabdomyosarcomas elevate the entire bladder, and the prostatic urethra is elongated **(Option (C) is true).** On ultrasonography, the intravesical portion of the tumor is clearly defined against the anechoic urine (Figure 2-9A). It is nodular and usually moderately echogenic. Ultrasonography can be used to monitor the response of the tumor to treatment but is less reliable than CT for lymph node evaluation. On a contrast-enhanced CT scan, the bulging nodular mass can be seen against the contrast-filled bladder (Figure 2-9B). CT will show the extravesical component of the tumor, but staging is more difficult in children than in adults because of the paucity of extravesical fat. CT is important both for lymph node evaluation and for monitoring the response to treatment. Lymphangiography is rarely used in the management of these tumors.

In the past, radiation and surgery were the only available modalities of treatment. In general, the results were poor. In recent years, aggressive chemotherapy has been strongly advocated and has led to a significant improvement in outcome **(Option (E) is false).** Five-year survival rates for stage II disease have increased from 31% to 53%. Drugs used include vincristine, dactinomycin, cyclophosphamide, doxorubicin, cisplatin, methotrexate, and melphalan. Pizzo et al. report an overall survival rate of 70 to 75%. Bladder salvage is now possible in 35% of patients. Radiation and surgery are now adjuvants to chemotherapy.

Question 8

Genitourinary tract findings in patients with neurofibromatosis include:

(A) clitoral hypertrophy
(B) renal artery stenosis
(C) extrinsic masses deforming the floor of the bladder
(D) polypoid filling defect in the membranous urethra

Two genetically distinct forms of neurofibromatosis exist. Both are autosomal dominant disorders, the but genetic abnormality for neurofibromatosis 1 (NF-1) resides on chromosome 17, whereas that for neurofibromatosis 2 (NF-2) is on chromosome 22. The most common form is NF-1, commonly known as von Recklinghausen's disease. It consists of two or more of the following: six or more café-au-lait spots, two or more neurofibromas or one plexiform neurofibroma, freckling in the axillary or inguinal regions, optic glioma, two or more iris hamartomas, distinctive bone lesions, and a first-degree relative with the characteristics mentioned above. The second form, NF-2, is recognized by and limited to bilateral acoustic neuromas or a first-degree relative with NF-2 and evidence of either a unilateral eighth nerve tumor or two neurofibromas, meningiomas, gliomas, schwannomas, or juvenile posterior subcapsular, lenticular opacities.

Although neurofibromas in NF-1 develop throughout the body, urinary tract involvement is uncommon. Individual case reports of neurofibromas of the renal pelvis, the renal capsule, and the ureter have been reported. Retroperitoneal neurofibromas arising in the bony pelvis or the lumbosacral spine will sometimes cause extrinsic compression or deviation of the ureter, bladder, or kidney. There are, however, two significant aspects of urinary involvement in NF-1: hypertension and bladder neurofibroma-tosis.

Hypertension in NF-1 can be caused by the presence of a pheochro-mocytoma; this is the most common cause of hypertension in adults. There is also a definite association between NF-1 and von Hippel-Lindau disease. Renal artery stenosis is the most common cause of hypertension in patients under 18 years of age with NF-1 **(Option (B) is true),** except for an occasional pheochromocytoma between 12 and 18 years. The renal artery stenosis is at the orifice in 50% of cases and bilateral in 40%. When unilateral, the left side is much more commonly involved and is frequently associated with aortic coarctation. The stenosis may actually be due to an encircling neurofibroma itself or may be caused by intimal proliferation of endoneural cells with destruction of the media and the internal elastic lamina.

Slightly fewer than 40 cases of neurofibroma of the bladder have been reported, with only three having undergone malignant degeneration. About half have been found in children, more commonly in girls. Between 40 and 75% have been associated with NF-1. The bladder neurofibroma may secondarily extend into the urethra, seminal vesicles, spermatic cord, etc. Patients may present with hematuria, frequency, urgency, and abdominal, pelvic, and genital pain.

In his classic review of neurofibromatosis in children, Holt reported approximately 20 cases in which neurofibromas presented as isolated intravesical masses. In his review, at least nine patients had clitoral hypertrophy and three had penile enlargement **(Option (A) is true).** A few cases of rhabdomyosarcomas of the uterus or prostate have been found in patients with neurofibromatosis. These can be clearly differenti-ated histologically from the benign, solitary neurofibroma arising in the bladder.

In the pelvis, neurofibromas are often associated with sacral anoma-lies. These tumors may degenerate into frank sarcomas. When these masses affect the bladder, they usually do so by extrinsically compressing the posterior aspect of the bladder **(Option (C) is true).** These tumors often present in young adults and should not be confused with rhab-domyosarcoma of the bladder or prostate.

In children and young adults, fibrous polyps and even bladder diver-ticula may be seen in the prostatic urethra. However, neurofibromas do not develop in the membranous urethra or present as polypoid urethral filling defects **(Option (D) is false).**

Stanford M. Goldman, M.D.

SUGGESTED READINGS

RHABDOMYOSARCOMA OF THE BLADDER AND PROSTATE

1. Bahnson RR, Zaontz MR, Maizels M, Shkolnik AA, Firlit CF. Ultrasonography and diagnosis of pediatric genitourinary rhabdomyosarcoma. Urology 1989; 33:64–68

2. Flamant F, Hill C. The improvement in survival associated with combined chemotherapy in childhood rhabdomyosarcoma. A historical comparison of 345 patients in the same center. Cancer 1984; 53:2417–2421

3. Geoffray A, Couanet D, Montagne JP, Leclère J, Flamant F. Ultrasonography and computed tomography for diagnosis and follow-up of pelvic rhabdomyosarcomas in children. Pediatr Radiol 1987; 17:132–136

4. Grosfeld JL, Weber TR, Weetman RM, Baehner RL. Rhabdomyosarcoma in childhood: analysis of survival in 98 cases. J Pediatr Surg 1983; 18:141–146

5. Hays DM, Raney RB Jr, Lawrence W Jr, et al. Primary chemotherapy in the treatment of children with bladder–prostate tumors in the Intergroup Rhabdomyosarcoma Study (IRS-II). J Pediatr Surg 1982; 17:812–820

6. Kaplan WE, Firlit CF, Berger RM. Genitourinary rhabdomyosarcoma. J Urol 1983; 130:116–119

7. Ortega JA. A therapeutic approach to childhood pelvic rhabdomyosarcoma without pelvic exenteration. J Pediatr 1979; 94:205–209

8. Pizzo PA, Horowitz ME, Poplack DG, Hays DM, Kun LE. Solid tumors of childhood. In: DeVita VT Jr, Hellman S, Rosenberg SA (eds), Cancer. Principles and practice of oncology, 3rd ed. Philadelphia: JB Lippincott; 1989:1612–1670

SACROCOCCYGEAL TUMORS

9. Grosfeld JL, Billmire DF. Teratomas in infancy and childhood. Curr Probl Cancer 1985; 9:1–53

10. Schey WL, Shkolnik A, White H. Clinical and radiographic considerations of sacrococcygeal teratomas: an analysis of 26 new cases and review of the literature. Radiology 1977; 125:189–195

11. Sheth S, Nussbaum AR, Sanders RC, Hamper UM, Davidson AJ. Prenatal diagnosis of sacrococcygeal teratoma: sonographic-pathologic correlation. Radiology 1988; 169:131–136

12. Swischuk LE (ed). Imaging of the newborn, infant and young child, 3rd ed. Baltimore: Williams & Wilkins; 1989:1024–1027

LYMPHOMA

13. Cohen MD, Siddiqui A, Weetman R, Provisor A, Coates T. Hodgkin disease and non-Hodgkin lymphomas in children: utilization of radiological modalities. Radiology 1986; 158:499–505

14. Patel S. Retroperitoneal tumors and cysts. In: Pollack HP (ed), Clinical urography. Philadelphia: WB Saunders; 1990:2443–2452

15. Poplack DG, Kun LE, Cassady JR, Pizzo PA. Leukemias and lymphomas of childhood. In: DeVita VT Jr, Hellman S, Rosenberg SA (eds), Cancer.

Principles and practice of oncology, 3rd ed. Philadelphia: JB Lippincott; 1989:1671–1695

NEUROFIBROMATOSIS

16. Biondetti PR, Vigo M, Fiore D, De Faveri D, Ravasini R, Benedetti L. CT appearance of generalized von Recklinghausen neurofibromatosis. J Comput Assist Tomogr 1983; 7:866–869
17. Blum MD, Bahnson RR, Carter MF. Urologic manifestation of von Recklinghausen neurofibromatosis. Urology 1985; 26:209–217
18. Coleman BG, Arger PH, Dalinka MK, Obringer AC, Raney BR, Meadows AT. CT of sarcomatous degeneration in neurofibromatosis. AJR 1983; 140:383–387
19. Daneman A, Grattan-Smith P. Neurofibromatosis involving the lower urinary tract in children. A report of three cases and a review of the literature. Pediatr Radiol 1976; 4:161–166
20. Haller JO, Klein J. Neurofibromatosis. In: Sumner TE (ed), Pediatric disease (third series) test and syllabus. Reston, VA: American College of Radiology; 1989:365–379
21. Halpern M, Currarino G. Vascular lesions causing hypertension in neurofibromatosis. N Engl J Med 1965; 273:248–252
22. Holt JF. Edward B.D. Neuhauser lecture: neurofibromatosis in children. AJR 1978; 130:615–639
23. Klatte EC, Franken EA, Smith JA. The radiographic spectrum in neurofibromatosis. Semin Roentgenol 1976; 11:17–33
24. Le Cheong L, Khan AN, Bisset RA. Sonographic features of a renal pelvic neurofibroma. JCU 1990; 18:129–131
25. McKeen EA, Bodurtha J, Meadows AT, Douglass EC, Mulvihill JJ. Rhabdomyosarcoma complicating multiple neurofibromatosis. J Pediatr 1978; 93:992–993
26. Mena E, Bookstein JJ, Holt JF, Fry WJ. Neurofibromatosis and renovascular hypertension in children. AJR 1973; 118:39–45
27. Mulvihill JJ, Parry DM. Introduction: symposium on linkage of von Recklinghausen neurofibromatosis (NF-1). Genomics 1987; 1:337–339
28. Myerson D, Rosenfield AT, Itzchak Y. Renal capsular tumors: the angiographic features. J Urol 1979; 121:238–241
29. National Institutes of Health Consensus Development. Neurofibromatosis. Arch Neurol 1988; 45:575–578
30. Patel YD, Morehouse HT. Neurofibrosarcomas in neurofibromatosis: role of CT scanning and angiography. Clin Radiol 1982; 33:555–560
31. Salyer WR, Salyer DC. The vascular lesions of neurofibromatosis. Angiology 1974; 25:510–519
32. Shapeero LG, Vordermark JS. Bladder neurofibromatosis in childhood: noninvasive imaging. J Ultrasound Med 1990; 9:177–180
33. Tilford DL, Kelsch RC. Renal artery stenosis in childhood neurofibromatosis. Am J Dis Child 1973; 26:665–668

Notes

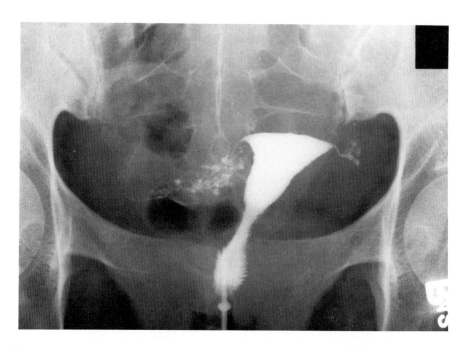

Figure 3-1. This 33-year-old woman was evaluated for infertility. Her pelvic sonogram was normal. You are shown a hysterosalpingogram.

Case 3: Salpingitis Isthmica Nodosa

Question 9

Which *one* of the following is the MOST likely diagnosis?

(A) Tuberculosis
(B) Endometriosis
(C) Salpingitis isthmica nodosa
(D) Maternal exposure to diethylstilbestrol
(E) Pelvic inflammatory disease

The hysterosalpingogram (HSG) (Figure 3-1) reveals the uterine cavity to be completely normal. However, the proximal portions of both fallopian tubes demonstrate the presence of extensive small outpouchings or diverticula (arrowheads, Figure 3-2). This pattern is characteristic for salpingitis isthmica nodosa (SIN) **(Option (C) is correct).** Other patterns less commonly seen include large nodular areas or linear tracts, as demonstrated by Creasy et al.

During the 1950s and 1960s, diethylstilbestrol (DES) was used in treating threatened abortions (Option (D)). Evaluation of the female offspring of these mothers revealed an increased frequency of clear cell adenocarcinoma of the cervix and vagina, cervical ectropion, and vaginal adenosis. In addition, HSGs of affected patients show a characteristic small T-shaped uterus (Figure 3-3), often with synechiae and polypoid defects. There may be widening of the oviducts, but this is not usually associated with fallopian tube "diverticula." The presence of a T-shaped uterus is suggestive of DES exposure even without a definitive history of such exposure. Such patients should be carefully monitored because of an increased frequency of ectopia, spontaneous abortions, and, most importantly, neoplasia. In the male offspring of DES-exposed mothers, there is an increased prevalence of semen abnormalities, epididymal cysts, hypoplastic testes, and cryptorchidism.

The HSG findings in patients with pelvic inflammatory disease (PID) (Option (E)) have been well known for years. Before antibiotics were

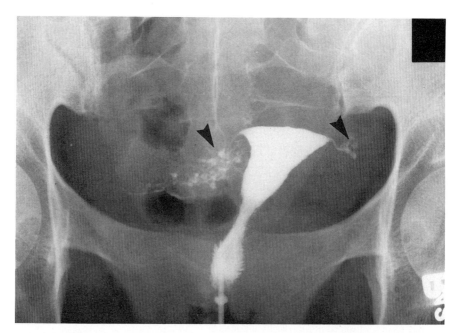

Figure 3-2 (Same as Figure 3-1).   Salpingitis isthmica nodosa. The hysterosalpingogram shows typical outpouchings or diverticula (arrowheads) in the proximal portions of the fallopian tubes bilaterally.

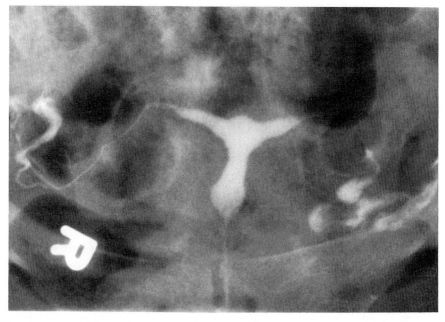

Figure 3-3.   Effect of *in utero* diethylstilbestrol exposure. A T-shaped uterus in an infertile 34-year-old woman whose mother, when pregnant with the patient, was treated with DES to prevent spontaneous abortion.

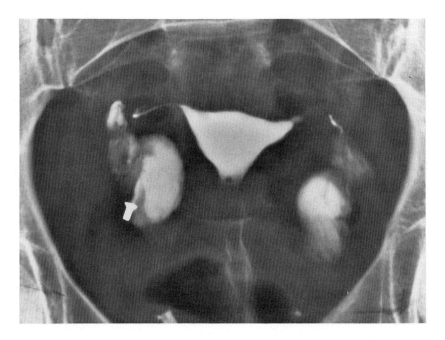

Figure 3-4. Pelvic inflammatory disease in a 32-year-old woman. The proximal portions of the fallopian tubes are relatively normal. The distal parts of both tubes are markedly widened, characteristic of hydrosalpinx, and there is absence of free peritoneal spillage.

available, gonorrhea was the cause of 30% of tubal occlusions. On HSG, PID is reflected variously by a thickened and widened tube, a hydro-salpinx or pyosalpinx, tubal occlusion, or tubal adhesions (Figure 3-4). Even when an affected tube is patent, the contrast material does not spill freely because of peritoneal adhesions. This HSG pattern is clearly different from that seen with SIN.

Genitourinary tuberculosis (Option (A)) can occasionally be recognized on radiographs by the presence of calcified lymph nodes or calcified fallopian tubes (Figure 3-5). Genital tuberculosis is characterized by the same type of pathologic processes seen with tuberculous involvement of other body organs, i.e., fibrosis, ulceration, cavity (abscess) formation, fistulization, and granuloma formation. This is translated on the HSG (Figure 3-6) into the findings of an irregular or jagged outline of the uterine cavity, an appearance similar to that of Asherman's syndrome. (Asherman originally described the development of intrauterine adhesions secondary to curettage, but the term is used for the presence of synechiae due to multiple causes, including idiopathic ones.) The uterine

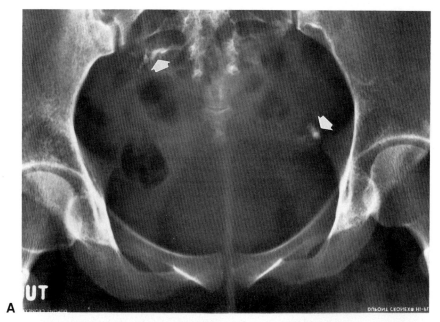

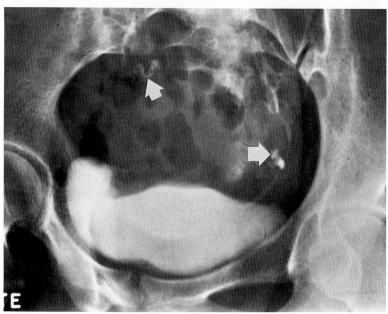

Figure 3-5. Genitourinary tuberculosis. Calcified fallopian tubes in a 24-year-old woman with genitourinary tuberculosis. Arrows point to the calcified tubes on the anteroposterior radiograph (A) and oblique urogram film (B).

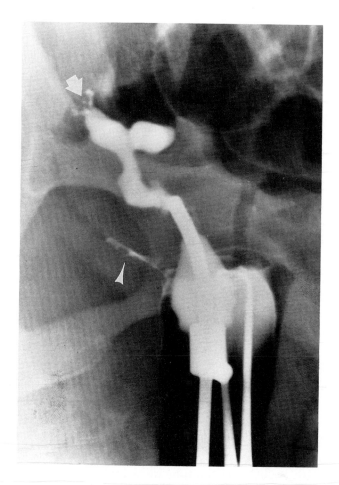

Figure 3-6. Genitourinary tuberculosis. HSG of a patient with genitourinary tuberculosis. Note the shrunken "Mickey Mouse" uterus with adnexal fistulae (arrow) and a vaginal-cutaneous fistula (arrowhead).

cavity may become quite small and mimic the T-shaped uterus characteristic of *in utero* DES exposure or can be deformed and look like "Mickey Mouse ears." These changes can be best understood as the marked fibrotic response by the host in an attempt to isolate the mycobacterial organisms. Uterolymphatic and uterovenous intravasation is not uncommon, especially in the fibrosed scarred tuberculous uterus. Fistulae to the peritoneum, adnexae, vagina, or skin may be identified. These can be understood as the result of a breakdown in the host defense mechanism. When the fallopian tubes are involved, the tubes may not fill at all or may be partially patent because of fibrotic strictures at the isthmus or elsewhere along their length. Between the strictures the tubes may be dilated, mimicking a hydrosalpinx or pyosalpinx, with occlusion of the fimbriated end of the tubes. Occasionally, tuberculosis of the fallopian tubes can be indistinguishable on HSG from SIN. Patients with a pattern of SIN on HSG should be carefully evaluated for tuberculosis. However, tuberculosis is uncommon in the United States, and isolated tuberculosis mimicking SIN without additional abnormalities of the fallopian tubes or uterus is not likely.

Endometriosis (Option (B)) is defined as the presence of ectopic endometrial tissue, which frequently forms cysts, often filled with blood. These endometrial implants primarily affect the ovary, fallopian tubes, parametrium, peritoneum, and bowel. Pathologically, the endometrium may appear normal and the tubes may appear patent, despite extensive peritubal and periovarian adhesions. Occasionally, foci of endometriosis involve the serosa of the tubes, causing endosalpingiosis, which mimics SIN on HSG. Creasy et al. even suggest that tubal adenomyosis is "in all probability an identical condition to SIN"; according to some, endometriosis may cause SIN. Tubal endometriosis is not usually isolated to the endosalpinx but, as Rozin states, is "part of the more general picture of pelvic endometriosis in a fairly large number of cases." Primary tubal endometriosis is rare, and tubal involvement is more often due to extrinsic invasion. On HSG there is no characteristic pattern (Figure 3-7). Although it may mimic or even cause SIN, endometriosis more commonly shows evidence of pelvic adhesions, occlusion of the fimbriated end, complete occlusion of the tube in its midportion, or deviation of the tube by large endometriomas on HSG. The sonogram of a patient with endometriosis that exhibits a SIN-like pattern would probably show extratubal disease and would not have been normal. Therefore, endometriosis is not the most likely diagnosis in the test case.

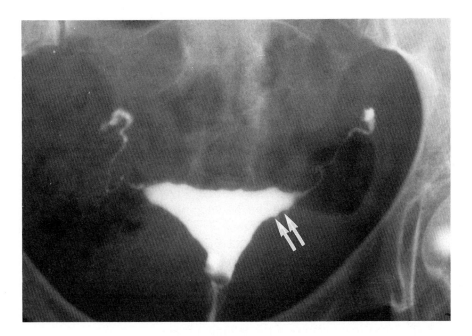

Figure 3-7. Endometriosis. Hysterosalpingogram of a 31-year-old woman with proven adenomyosis and endometriosis reveals a few focal outpouchings (arrows) near the left adnexa, as seen with adenomyosis. The proximal tubes appear normal on this early film despite extensive adhesions due to endometrial implants seen at laparoscopy.

Question 10

Concerning tuberculosis of the female genital tract,

F (A) it is usually spread via periureteric and periuterine lymphatics
F (B) it is associated with an increased incidence of tubal neoplasms
F (C) it is most commonly caused by *Mycobacterium bovis*
F (D) fistulization to the bladder is common
T (E) adnexal calcification suggests the diagnosis

    Female genital tuberculosis is rare in the United States; it was found in only 8 of more than 1,160 HSGs performed prior to 1955. The incidence is currently even lower in the United States because of the decreasing prevalence of active tuberculosis. Tubal involvement is almost always secondary to a focus elsewhere. It is most often spread hematogenously from the lung. The kidneys or the lymphatics are less commonly the source of tuberculous spread to the genital tract **(Option (A) is false).**

This is in contradistinction to tuberculous cystitis, which is invariably of renal origin.

Although *Mycobacterium bovis* was a cause of tuberculosis at the turn of the century, pasteurization of milk has all but eliminated this organism as a cause of tuberculosis in the United States. Today, almost all cases are caused by *Mycobacterium tuberculosis* **(Option (C) is false).**

Calcification in lymph nodes or along the fallopian tube on radiography is suggestive of tuberculosis. Calcifications in the fallopian tube are small, measuring 1 to 2 mm. They may be straight, bent, or curvilinear and usually follow the course of the tubes. When this pattern is present, the diagnosis of tuberculosis can be suggested **(Option (E) is true).** Because of their characteristic pattern of calcification, phleboliths should not be confused with tuberculous calcifications. Ovarian dermoid calcification is more laterally located and often is recognizable as a formed tooth or as bone. The presence of fatty material is also often recognizable in dermoids. Uterine artery calcifications can mimic tubal calcifications but tend to run in a straight lateral line toward the iliac vessels as compared with the curvilinear course of the fallopian tube.

Fistulization to the parametrium can occur, as can a fistula from the uterus to the skin. However, a fistula to the bladder is mentioned only twice by Siegler in his extensive studies of genital tuberculosis **(Option (D) is false).** Similarly, there is no known increase in the incidence of tubal neoplasms associated with tuberculosis **(Option (B) is false).**

Question 11

Concerning endometriosis,

F (A) the ultrasonographic pattern is specific
F (B) there is a correlation between the extent of the disease and the severity of symptoms
T (C) MRI appears to be more sensitive than ultrasonography in detecting diffuse endometriosis
T (D) it is discovered in about 20% of patients undergoing gynecologic laparotomy
F (E) it is more common in Caucasian than in non-Caucasian patients

At present, gray-scale ultrasonography is the imaging study most commonly used for the evaluation of endometriosis (Figure 3-8). Sandler and Karo divide the sonographic appearance into three patterns: cystic, mixed, and solid. In the cystic form, the cysts usually measure 2 to 5 cm in diameter, although cysts up to 20 cm have been reported. They are

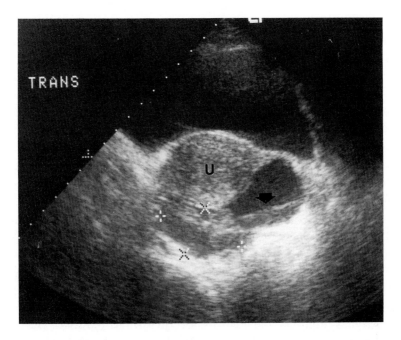

Figure 3-8. Endometriosis. Ultrasonogram in a patient with endometriosis. Note a fluid-fluid level (arrow) in one endometrioma. Another endometrioma is delineated by the markers. U = uterus.

frequently septated and may be multiple. Bilaterality is common, with the cysts being found behind the uterus and in the pouch of Douglas. Not infrequently, the cyst walls are shaggy and irregularly thickened. Fluid-fluid levels or layered debris consisting of fibrous tissue, lipids, and hemosiderin pigment may be identified within them. Actual clots are occasionally present. The rare solid form is indistinguishable from a tumor.

From the description given above, it is clear that the sonographic pattern is nonspecific and can be confused with those of tubo-ovarian abscesses, ectopic pregnancies, ovarian cysts, polycystic ovaries, and ovarian carcinoma, among others **(Option (A) is false)**.

Clinically, endometriosis cases can be divided into two subgroups. One, usually called adenomyosis or endometriosis interna, is confined to the uterus and is found in multiparous women, usually in their fifth decade. The other group consists of patients with the more commonly recognized syndrome of endometriosis. Such women have predominantly extrauterine implants, and this form is called endometriosis externa. It is classically identified in young infertile women with dysmenorrhea. It was long believed that this form was more common in Caucasians. However, Kitchin and Nunley believe that this merely reflects medical care availability and that the actual incidence is probably the same in non-Caucasians **(Option (E) is false).** This finding is supported by diagnostic laparoscopy, which has shown a 21% frequency in blacks. In descending order, endometrial involvement will affect the ovary, the serosa of the uterus, the uterosacral ligament, and the cul-de-sac.

Endometriosis is found in about 17 to 20% of gynecologic laparotomies **(Option (D) is true).** It is thought to be present in 5% of women seen in gynecological practice. Sandler et al. reported that 40 to 50% of women with endometriosis are infertile; in 6 to 15% of these women, endometriosis is the single known causative factor for the infertility. According to Kitchin and Nunley, prior to laparotomy about one-third of patients with endometriosis were misdiagnosed as suffering from PID. Symptoms correlate more with the location of the disease than with its extent. Thus, these authors report patients with extensive and widespread endometriosis with no symptoms and vice versa **(Option (B) is false).** Dysmenorrhea in one form or another is the classic symptom. The pelvic pain is often poorly localized and may be described as merely a "bearing-down" sensation, a "low backache," or "rectal pressure." This is the second most common complaint after infertility. The degree of pain may be related to the growth rate of the endometriosis. Abnormal uterine bleeding is the third most common symptom. Other symptoms include dyspareunia, dyschezia, and infertility.

The CT pattern of endometriosis has been reported by Fishman et al., but CT is not routinely used in evaluation of this condition. This reflects the ready availability and lower cost of diagnostic ultrasonography. Recent articles have described the MR patterns of endometriosis and adenomyosis (Figure 3-9). Using T1-weighted and T2-weighted images variously performed on high- and mid-field-strength magnets, Nishimura et al. described a variety of findings, including (1) evidence of adhesions to surrounding organs, as noted by a loss of sharp definition of the uterine margin or tethering of the rectum; (2) a low-intensity zone of fibrous tissue surrounding the endometriomas on both T1-weighted and T2-weighted images; (3) hemorrhagic cysts, as evidenced by T1 shortening and T2 prolongation; and (4) "cysts" with a low-intensity internal signal on T2-weighted images. However, it is clear from the work of Arrivé et al. and Zawin et al. that MRI cannot substitute for definitive laparoscopy, even though MRI does occasionally demonstrate lesions not seen at laparoscopy. MRI may be helpful in identifying presacral lesions that are difficult to evaluate either by ultrasonography or clinically. MRI also

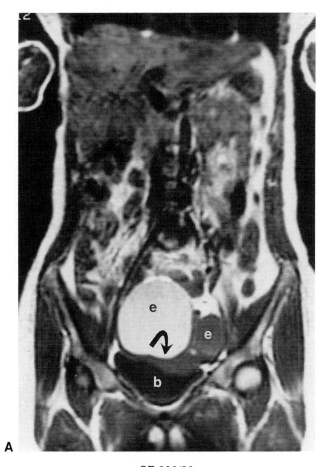

SE 600/20

Figure 3-9. MRI of endometriosis. Coronal T1-weighted (A) and sagittal proton-density (B) views of the uterus and adnexa in a 31-year-old woman with extensive endometriosis. (A) The T1-weighted image shows endometriomas (e) of different signal intensities, reflecting the different amounts and ages of the breakdown by-products of blood within the "chocolate cysts" (b = bladder; curved arrow = uterus). (B) The proton-density image shows higher signal intensity in three endometriomas (e), indicative of higher protein content (i.e., blood by-products) in their fluid compared with the urine in the bladder (b). Note the exquisite anatomic detail of the uterus (curved arrow).

seems to be more sensitive than ultrasonography in demonstrating diffuse endometriosis (64 and 11% sensitivity, respectively) **(Option (C) is true).** It may also be the method of choice in monitoring the response to treatment by obviating some follow-up laparoscopies.

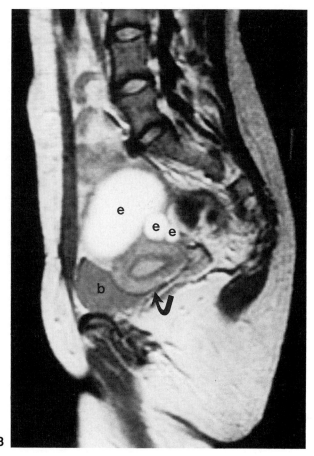

B

SE 2,500/30

Question 12

Concerning salpingitis isthmica nodosa,

T (A) it is commonly associated with tubal obstruction
F (B) the ultrasonographic findings are characteristic
F (C) it represents congenital Wolffian rests
T (D) it is associated with an increased frequency of ectopic pregnancies
F (E) it is not associated with primary infertility

SIN was first described in 1887 by Chiari, who observed epithelium-lined cystic spaces within the hypertrophied muscular portion of the tubal wall. SIN can involve the entire tube but most commonly involves only the proximal two-thirds. In a study of 1,194 HSGs, Creasy et al. found a 4% incidence of SIN. In the past, SIN was variously thought to be secondary to congenital (i.e., diverticulosis), postinflammatory, or acquired causes. Von Recklinghausen was the first to propose a congenital etiology for SIN. He believed that the diverticula were due to Wolffian rests. This was refuted by Creasy et al., who showed an 89% frequency of associated inflammation based on studies of 70 involved tubes **(Option (C) is false)**. They also showed a 37.5% rate of primary infertility among patients with SIN **(Option (E) is false)** and a significant rate of ectopic pregnancies (9.4%) **(Option (D) is true)**. The diagnosis of SIN is made by HSG; there are no known reliable ultrasonographic criteria for the diagnosis **(Option (B) is false)**. Tubal occlusion is common in patients with SIN **(Option (A) is true)**. In the series of Creasy et al., HSG showed absence of spill or loculation in 49 of 70 tubes (70%). This may reflect the now accepted inflammatory etiology of SIN.

Question 13

Concerning pelvic inflammatory disease,

T (A) ectopic pregnancy is a common complication
F (B) it is commonly seen in patients with a bicornuate uterus
F (C) it usually can be differentiated from endometriosis on ultrasonography
F (D) its development can be prevented by the use of an intrauterine device
F (E) transuterine fallopian tube recanalization is an effective mode of therapy for associated infertility

According to Curran, almost a million American women suffer from PID or its sequelae each year. Most PID is venereal in origin, affecting the tubes via the ascending route. Although *Neisseria gonorrhoeae* is usually considered the most common cause of PID, there is a great deal of evidence that *Chlamydia trachomatis* may now be as important in the development of PID. Both microorganisms are clearly significant factors in infertility. Although *N. gonorrhoeae* is usually the initiating cause of PID, a mixed group of aerobic and anaerobic bacteria are the more usual cause of its progression.

The intrauterine device (IUD), so well known for its birth control capabilities, is, in fact, a major factor in the development of PID (increasing the relative risk by a factor of 2 to 4 compared with that in women not using IUDs), possibly as a result of an adverse effect of the

IUD on uterine defense mechanisms **(Option (D) is false).** The IUD-associated increase in the relative risk of PID is higher for middle- and high-income individuals than for the low-income group. The high- and middle-income patient is very likely to present with a nongonorrheal infection and be nulliparous.

Besides the pain and known fertility problems, the scarring that occurs from PID is a major cause of ectopic pregnancies. The result is that 30 to 50% of ectopic pregnancies are found in patients with a history of salpingitis **(Option (A) is true).**

Congenital anomalies of the female genital tract clearly have important implications for sterility, repeated abortions, premature labor, abnormal fetal presentation, and possibly fetal anomalies. The bicornuate uterus is one of the most frequent of these anomalies. There is, however, no significant relationship between this anomaly and the development of PID **(Option (B) is false).**

Ultrasonography plays a major role in the diagnosis of PID. It permits visualization of the obliteration of the margins between uterine and adnexal structures. The common tubo-ovarian abscess is recognized as a dilated cystic structure that is often narrowed at the uterotubal junction. Septation, intracystic debris, and irregular walls may all be present. Evidence of spread to the cul-de-sac and elsewhere is also often present. However, these findings are nonspecific. As stated above, the ultrasonographic patterns of PID and endometriosis may be indistinguishable **(Option (C) is false).**

Transuterine fallopian tube recanalization has recently been developed, predominantly by Thurmond et al., as an effective means of opening short segments of tubal occlusion. This technique has been especially effective when the obstruction has been limited to the uterotubal junction. In these patients, viable pregnancies have resulted. Unfortunately, in the majority of patients with PID, the disease is not confined entirely to a short segment of tube. In these situations, the technique has usually failed or has led to an undesirable ectopic pregnancy **(Option (E) is false).**

Stanford M. Goldman, M.D.

SUGGESTED READINGS

SALPINGITIS ISTHMICA NODOSA

1. Creasy JL, Clark RL, Cuttino JT, Groff TR. Salpingitis isthmica nodosa: radiologic and clinical correlates. Radiology 1985; 154:597–600
2. McComb PF, Rowe TC. Salpingitis isthmica nodosa: evidence that it is a progressive disease. Fertil Steril 1989; 51:542–545
3. Siegler AM. Hysterosalpingography. New York: Medcom; 1974:171–178

TUBERCULOSIS

4. Gilinsky NH, Marks IN, Kottler RE, Price SK. Abdominal tuberculosis: a 10-year review. S Afr Med J 1983:849–857
5. Siegler AM. Hysterosalpingography. New York: Medcom; 1974:159–170
6. Silva PD, Richmond JA, Lobo RA. Diagrams and management of a tuberculous tuboappendiceal fistula. Am J Obstet Gynecol 1988; 159:440–441
7. Walzer A, Koenigsberg M. Ultrasonographic demonstration of pelvic tuberculosis. J Ultrasound Med 1983; 2:139–140

ENDOMETRIOSIS

8. Arrivé L, Hricak H, Martin MC. Pelvic endometriosis: MR imaging. Radiology 1989; 171:687–692
9. Coleman BG, Arger PH, Mulhern CB Jr. Endometriosis: clinical and ultrasonic correlation. AJR 1979; 132:747–749
10. Fishman EK, Scatarige JC, Saksouk FA, Rosenshein NB, Siegelman SS. Computed tomography of endometriosis. J Comput Assist Tomogr 1983; 7:257–264
11. Friedman H, Vogelzang R, Mendelson EB, Neiman HL, Cohen M. Endometriosis detection by US with laparoscopic correlation. Radiology 1985; 157:217–220
12. Grimes EM, Richardson MR. Management of the infertile couple. In: Sciarra JJ (ed), Gynecology and obstetrics, vol 5. Philadelphia: JB Lippincott; 1990:1–21
13. Kitchin JD III, Nunley WC Jr. Endometriosis. In: Sciarra JJ (ed), Gynecology and obstetrics, vol 1. Philadelphia: JB Lippincott; 1990:1–28
14. Mark AS, Hricak H, Heinrichs LW, et al. Adenomyosis and leiomyoma: differential diagnosis with MR imaging. Radiology 1987; 163:527–529
15. Nishimura K, Togashi K, Itoh K, et al. Endometrial cysts of the ovary: MR imaging. Radiology 1987; 162:315–318
16. Sanders RC, James AE Jr. The principles and practice of ultrasonography in obstetrics and gynecology, 3rd ed. Norwalk, CT: Appleton-Century-Crofts; 1985:484, 582–596
17. Sandler MA, Karo JJ. The spectrum of ultrasonic findings in endometriosis. Radiology 1978; 127:229–231
18. Siedler D, Laing FC, Jeffrey RB Jr, Wing VW. Uterine adenomyosis. A difficult sonographic diagnosis. J Ultrasound Med 1987; 6:345–349
19. Togashi K, Nishimura K, Itoh K, et al. Adenomyosis: diagnosis with MR imaging. Radiology 1988; 166:111–114

20. Walsh JW, Taylor KJ, Rosenfield AT. Gray scale ultrasonography in the diagnosis of endometriosis and adenomyosis. AJR 1979; 132:87–90
21. Zawin M, McCarthy S, Scoutt L, Comite F. Endometriosis: appearance and detection at MR imaging. Radiology 1989; 171:693–696

DIETHYLSTILBESTROL EXPOSURE

22. Kaufman RH, Binder L, Gray PM Jr, Adam E. Upper genital tract changes associated with exposure in utero to diethylstilbestrol. Am J Obstet Gynecol 1977; 128:51–59
23. Rennell CL. T-shaped uterus in diethylstilbestrol (DES) exposure. AJR 1979; 132:979–980

PELVIC INFLAMMATORY DISEASE

24. Curran JW. Economic consequences of pelvic inflammatory disease in the United States. Am J Obstet Gynecol 1980; 138:848–851
25. Eschenbach DA. Acute pelvic inflammatory disease. In: Sciarra JJ (ed), Gynecology and obstetrics, vol 1. Philadelphia: JB Lippincott; 1986:1–20
26. Hall DA, Hann LE. Gynecologic radiology: benign disorders. In: Taveras JM, Ferrucci JT (eds), Radiology. Diagnosis—imaging—intervention. Philadelphia: JB Lippincott; 1988; 4; 87:1–17
27. Keith L, Berger GS, Brown ER. Female pelvic infection and contraception. In: Sciarra JJ (ed), Gynecology and obstetrics, vol 1. Philadelphia: JB Lippincott; 1985:1–9
28. Laing FC. Ectopic pregnancy. In: Taveras JM, Ferrucci JT (eds), Radiology. Diagnosis—imaging—intervention. Philadelphia: JB Lippincott; 1988; 4; 87A:1–7
29. Novy MJ, Eschenbach DA. Infections as a cause of infertility. In: Sciarra JJ (ed), Gynecology and obstetrics, vol 5. Philadelphia: JB Lippincott; 1989:1–18
30. Rösch J, Thurmond AS, Uchida BT, Sovak M. Selective transcervical fallopian tube catheterization: technique update. Radiology 1988; 168:1–5
31. Rozin S. Uterosalpingography in gynecology. Springfield, IL: Charles C Thomas; 1965:109–146, 287–329
32. Schwartz RH. The treatment of major gynecologic sepsis. In: Sciarra JJ (ed), Gynecology and obstetrics, vol 1. Philadelphia: JB Lippincott; 1990:1–12
33. Thurmond AS, Novy M, Uchida BT, Rösch J. Fallopian tube obstruction: selective salpingography and recanalization. Work in progress. Radiology 1987; 163:511–514

HYSTEROSALPINGOGRAPHY

34. Rozin S. Uterosalpingography in gynecology. Springfield, IL: Charles C Thomas; 1965
35. Siegler AM. Hysterosalpingography. New York: Medcom; 1974
36. Winfield A. Diagnostic imaging of infertility, 1st ed. Baltimore: Williams & Wilkins; 1986

Notes

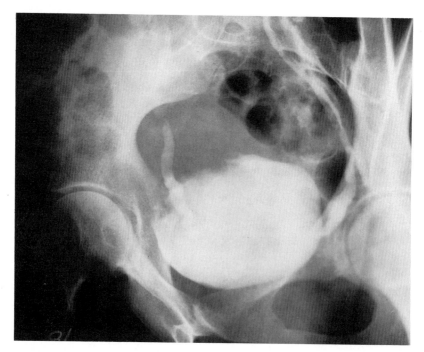

Figure 4-1

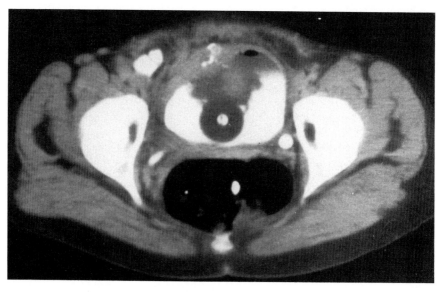

Figure 4-2
Figures 4-1 and 4-2. This 54-year-old woman presented with hematuria. You are shown a bladder image from an excretory urogram (Figure 4-1) and a CT scan (Figure 4-2).

Case 4: Urachal Carcinoma

Question 14

Which *one* of the following is the MOST likely diagnosis?

(A) Transitional cell carcinoma of the bladder
(B) Crohn's disease
(C) Squamous cell carcinoma of the bladder
(D) Schistosomiasis
(E) Urachal carcinoma

Analysis of the oblique coned-down view of the bladder from the excretory urogram (Figure 4-1) reveals a multilobular destructive mass of the dome of the bladder (Figure 4-3, arrows). This is confirmed on the CT scan (Figure 4-2), which shows a low-density irregular mass (Figure 4-4, arrows) within the bladder. In addition, there is a more solid, well-defined mass with central coarse calcifications (arrowhead) slightly to the right of the midline next to the bladder below the rectus abdominis muscles. This is the course of the urachal remnant. The most likely diagnosis is therefore a urachal carcinoma **(Option (E) is correct).**

The urachus, a vestigial remnant of the fetal genitourinary tract, is a midline tubular structure that runs from the anterior dome of the bladder in the space of Retzius to the umbilicus. It is the remnant of the cloaca and the allantois. Urachal carcinomas develop as predominantly extra-vesical masses with a tendency to invade the bladder. As a result, they may appear similar to primary bladder dome lesions.

This rare tumor clearly must be differentiated from the far more common transitional cell carcinoma (TCC) of the bladder (Option (A)), which is the fifth most common cause of cancer deaths in men over 75 years old. Development of bladder TCC has been causally related to occupational exposure to a variety of chemicals, cigarette smoking, coffee drinking, analgesic abuse, bacterial and parasitic infections, bladder calculi, pelvic irradiation, exposure to cytotoxic drugs, and ingestion of saccharin (in experiments with mice). Since these carcinogens generally

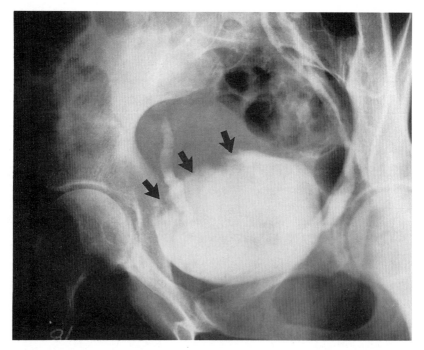

Figure 4-3

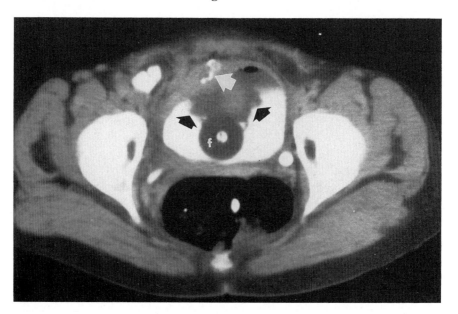

Figure 4-4
Figures 4-3 and 4-4 (Same as Figures 4-1 and 4-2, respectively). Urachal carcinoma. The intravenous urogram (Figure 4-3) shows an irregular, nodular tumor of the bladder dome (arrows). The CT scan (Figure 4-4) shows the tumor to have an intracystic component (arrows). In addition, there is a more solid dome component containing calcification (arrowhead). f = Foley catheter balloon.

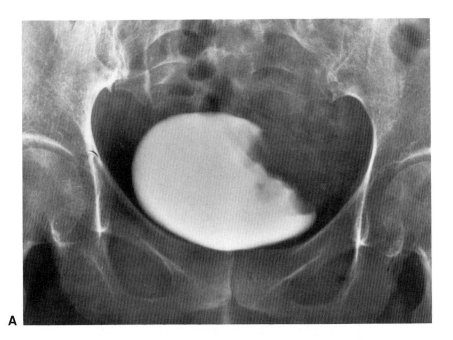

A

Figure 4-5. Squamous cell carcinoma of the bladder. (A) An intravenous urogram of a 72-year-old man shows a lobular tumor of the left lateral wall of the bladder. No calcification is noted. (B) A CT scan of a 70-year-old man shows a nodular mass of the right lateral wall (arrowheads).

affect the entire bladder mucosa, bladder TCC can be multifocal or may develop anywhere in the bladder. TCCs are mucosal in origin, whereas urachal cancer invades from outside the bladder and then secondarily involves the bladder wall. Calcification in TCC is rare, occurring in fewer than 1% of cancers. The frequency of calcification in urachal carcinoma is 50 to 70% as reported by Brick et al.

Squamous cell carcinoma (SCC) of the bladder (Option (C)) (Figure 4-5) is relatively rare in the United States (1.6 to 7% of bladder cancers). It results from metaplastic changes to the normal transitional cell mucosa of the bladder. Just as with TCC, there is an association with such insults as chronic infection and bladder calculi. There is also a definite relationship between SCC and schistosomiasis. The lesion can be found anywhere in the bladder. SCC lesions are often bulky with ulceration and necrosis. Calcification is not a prominent feature of SCC or TCC except in patients with schistosomiasis. However, schistosomal calcifications are linear. They are found in the bladder and ureter and represent calcification in trapped degenerated ova. There is no known relationship between the

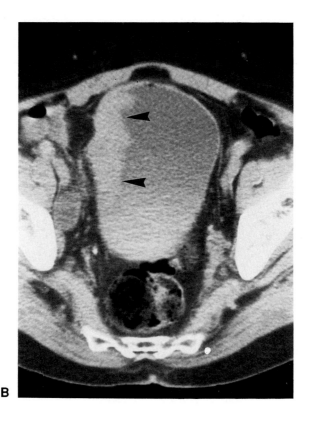

B

SCC itself and the calcification (see below). On occasion, SCC of the bladder can be suggested because of its marked tendency for infiltration. Narumi et al. (1989) suggested that SCC of the bladder tends to have almost equal extra- and intraluminal growth or predominantly extraluminal growth with no intraluminal extension. In contradistinction, bladder TCC usually has at least some intraluminal component.

Schistosomiasis of the bladder (Option (D)) is caused by *Schistosoma haematobium*, a parasite found in the Near East and Africa. The parasite penetrates the skin of humans in contact with infested water. The larvae enter the lymphatics and venous system and migrate to the liver, where they mature and copulate. The smaller female then migrates through the inferior mesenteric vein to the bladder, where the eggs are deposited in the bladder wall. Those that do not penetrate the bladder mucosa die and undergo calcification in the bladder wall. Schistosomal calcification (Figure 4-6A) is usually linear in a distended bladder and involves the bladder and often the distal ureter. This calcification is best seen on CT and, according to Lautin et al., is present in at least 50% of cases. There

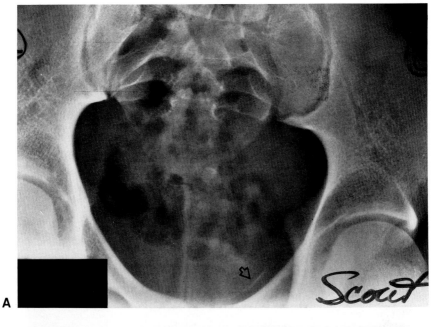

A

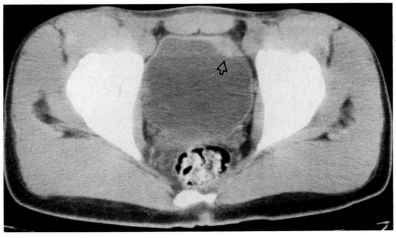

B

Figure 4-6. Schistosomiasis of the bladder in a 21-year-old man who moved to the United States from Nigeria at 5 years of age. (A) Radiograph of the pelvis shows typical linear mural calcification in the left lower aspect of the bladder (arrow). (B) CT scan of the bladder shows a schistosomoma (arrow) of the bladder.

may also be calcification in the seminal vesicles and the vas deferens. So-called bladder "tumors" are commonly associated with schistosomiasis. These "tumors" merely represent schistosomomas (Figure 4-6B). More importantly, development of an SCC of the bladder is a significant

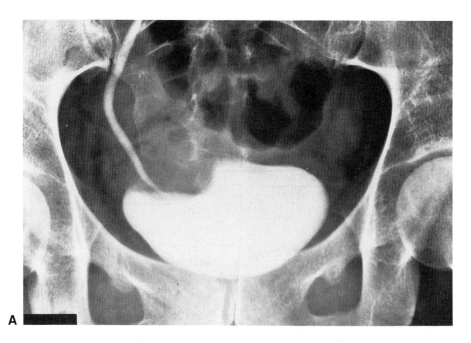

A

Figure 4-7. Crohn's disease of the bladder in a 24-year-old woman. (A) The intravenous urogram shows an inflammatory mass involving the right superior wall of the bladder. (B) The CT scan shows the inflammatory mass (arrow) in the typical location, involving the right upper aspect of the bladder near the terminal ileum. (C) A view of the terminal ileum from a small bowel series shows the characteristic changes of Crohn's disease extending into the pelvis near the bladder. (Panel B is reprinted with permission from Goldman et al. [22].)

complication, with a 16% mortality rate. Jorulf and Lindstedt stress the importance of CT in diagnosing and staging these SCCs. The CT shown in Figure 4-5B shows no linear calcifications within the bladder wall. The calcification seen in Figures 4-2 and 4-4 is within an extracystic mass.

Crohn's disease (Option (B)) (Figure 4-7) is the most common cause of a vesicoenteric fistula from the small bowel. Crohn's disease most commonly develops in the terminal ileum. The resultant abscesses are often found in the right lower quadrant. Crohn's disease first affects the bladder by causing extrinsic pressure on its right lateral aspect, giving the so-called "herald" sign. Further involvement leads to a bladder wall mass. Finally, fistulization through the mucosa leads to intracystic air and pneumaturia. On CT, Crohn's disease is most likely to involve the bladder from the right anterior wall near the site of the terminal ileum, not the midline. The inflammatory mass does not usually calcify, and intracystic air may be present.

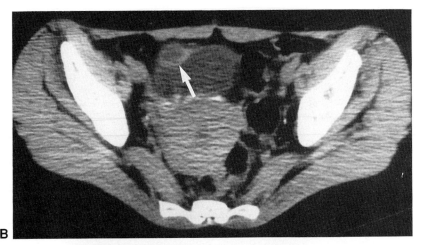

B

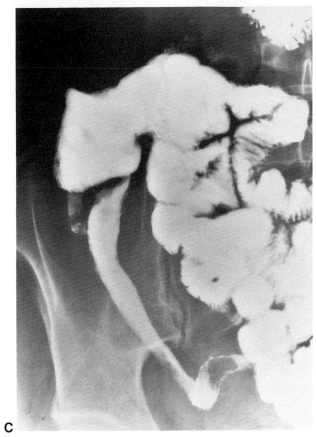

C

Question 15

Factors predisposing to the development of transitional cell carcinoma of the bladder include:

T (A) exposure to aniline dyes
T (B) cigarette smoking
F (C) exstrophy of the bladder
F (D) schistosomiasis
F (E) malakoplakia

The transitional cell mucosa of the bladder is known to be susceptible to cancer induction by chemical carcinogens. As early as 1895, the role of aniline and fuchsin dyes in the development of TCCs was recognized. There is now a well-documented clinical and experimental association between TCC and aromatic amines such as 2-naphthylamine, 4-aminodiphenyl, and 4,4-diaminobiphenyl (benzidine) fuchsin, to mention just a few. Occupational exposure to such agents may be a factor in one-quarter to one-third of patients with TCC, with a latent period of 40 to 50 years **(Option (A) is true).**

The relationship of TCC to cigarette smoking is also well established (see the review by Catalona) **(Option (B) is true).** The incidence of TCC in smokers is four times that in nonsmokers. There is a correlation between the incidence of TCC and the number of cigarettes smoked, the duration of smoking, and the depth of inhalation. More than one-third of TCCs may be related to smoking. The causative agent may be 2-naphthylamine, nitrosamines, or tryptophan metabolites.

Exstrophy of the bladder and epispadias represent opposite ends of the spectrum of anterior abdominal wall defects. Exstrophy occurs in 1 in 30,000 live births. The exposed bladder mucosa may be normal or ulcerated. It may undergo squamous metaplasia, cystitis glandularis, or polyp formation. There is a 200-fold-increased incidence of bladder cancer in untreated patients, but 90% of these cancers are low-grade adenocarcinomas rather than TCCs **(Option (C) is false).**

As discussed above, up to 50% of patients with schistosomiasis develop SCC, not TCC **(Option (D) is false).**

"Malakoplakia" means soft plaque. These lesions are most commonly associated with recurrent urinary tract infections, usually in women. Classically, Michaelis-Gutmann bodies are found on tissue specimens stained with hematoxylin and eosin. These are round or oval inclusion bodies in the histiocyte or the macrophage. On electron microscopy, these inclusion bodies represent ingested bacterial particles within the lysosomes of the macrophage. Malakoplakia is clearly an inflammatory lesion. There is no proven correlation between malakoplakia and cancer other than a relationship between infection and tumor formation **(Option (E) is false).**

Question 16

Concerning Crohn's disease,

F (A) the most common type of associated calculus is struvite
T (B) it is the most common cause of a fistula between the small bowel and the bladder
F (C) the bladder is the most common site of urinary tract involvement
F (D) the right and left ureters are affected with equal frequency
F (E) it most commonly involves the mid-ureter

Involvement of the urinary tract in Crohn's disease occurs by two mechanisms: direct extension and development of a metabolic disorder causing urolithiasis. Direct urinary tract involvement is a consequence of the spread of the inflammation from the terminal ileum into the surrounding retroperitoneum. Right lower quadrant phlegmon and frank abscess formation develop. These inflammatory masses may obstruct the right ureter. They may also extrinsically compress the bladder; however, with time, actual bladder wall involvement with ultimate fistulization to the bladder lumen may develop.

Stone formation is a common complication of Crohn's disease, with reported frequencies of 9 and 18% in patients without and with ileostomies, respectively; it is the result of the diarrhea and of the shortened gut (if surgery has been performed). The most commonly found stones are composed of either uric acid or calcium oxalate. There is almost a direct relationship between stone formation, the amount of distal small bowel disease, and the degree of malabsorption. It is thought that stone formation results from two major types of metabolic derangement: (1) dehydration, acidic urine, and increased urate excretion in the ileostomy patients; and (2) malabsorption of fat, leading to calcium oxalate stones. One explanation for the oxalate stones is that the excess soaps and fatty acids formed in the gut lumen combine with calcium ions. This results in fewer calcium ions available to combine with intraluminal oxalate to form insoluble calcium oxalate. Excessive absorption of dietary oxalate results, which in turn leads to hyperoxaluria and the precipitation of calcium oxalate in the urine. Another cause of stones is diarrhea, which causes dehydration, bicarbonate loss, and volume depletion. The low-pH hyperconcentrated urine that results favors uric acid stone formation. Struvite (magnesium ammonium phosphate) stones are most often secondary to infection with urea-splitting bacteria and are not the stones commonly associated with Crohn's disease **(Option (A) is false).**

Although most enterovesical fistulas are secondary to diverticulitis or, less commonly, colonic cancer, small bowel-bladder fistulas are usually secondary to Crohn's disease **(Option (B) is true).** They are seen in 2 to 7.7% of cases. For diagnostic evaluation of a suspected enterovesical fistula, CT is the simplest method of demonstrating air in the bladder and the presence or absence of an associated abscess. In patients with diverticulitis, the abscesses develop behind or to the left of the bladder (i.e., the area of the sigmoid colon). Appendicitis and Crohn's disease involve the bladder from the right and the front (i.e., the area of the terminal ileum). Recently, the MRI findings of fistulization have been described; the fistulous tracts appear as high-intensity linear streaks on T2-weighted images.

Since the terminal ileum is the most common site of Crohn's disease, there is no doubt that the secondary abscesses are more likely to involve the right (7 to 27% of cases) rather than the left ureter **(Option (D) is false).** For the same reason, the distal rather than middle one-third of this ureter is more likely to be affected **(Option (E) is false).** The bladder is less commonly affected than the right ureter **(Option (C) is false).**

Question 17

Concerning urachal carcinoma,

T (A) the bulk of the tumor is extravesical
T (B) it is more common in men than in women
T (C) it is most commonly an adenocarcinoma
T (D) calcification is common
F (E) it has a 5-year survival rate similar to that of transitional cell carcinoma of the bladder
T (F) voided urine often contains mucus

Urachal carcinomas (Figure 4-8) represent only 0.01% of all adult cancers. However, with the advent of CT, recognition of these tumors has become more and more common. They are found most often in patients in the fourth through seventh decades of life. According to Brick et al.

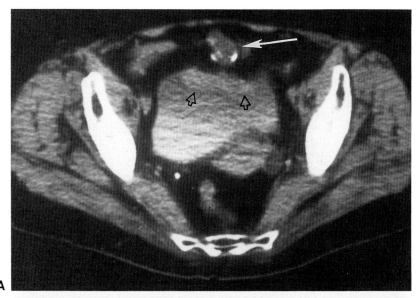

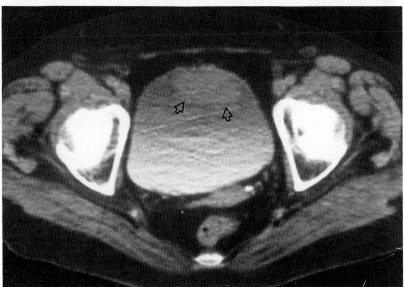

Figure 4-8. Urachal carcinoma in a 68-year-old woman. (A) The CT scan shows the typical calcified urachal component (solid arrow), as well as the intracystic component (open arrows). (B) A lower section shows only the intracystic component (open arrows) involving the superior aspect of the bladder. (Reprinted with permission from Brick et al. [2].)

(1988), 65 to 75% of urachal carcinomas are found in men **(Option (B) is true)**. Signs and symptoms are often nonspecific and include hematuria (71%), suprapubic mass, abdominal pain, and dysuria. A bloody, purulent, or mucinous umbilical discharge may be present. One characteristic finding is the voiding of mucus in about 25% of cases **(Option (F) is true)**.

According to Hill, almost all urachal tumors are adenocarcinomas, varying from well-differentiated, mucus-secreting papillary adenocarcinomas to poorly differentiated, colloid carcinomas with signet-ring cell differentiation. Rarely are SCCs and TCCs reported **(Option (C) is true)**.

As described above, urachal carcinomas develop along the course of the urachus and therefore should be predominantly extravesical in location **(Option (A) is true)**. Difficulty in diagnosis occurs when the tumor invades the bladder, in which case it can be impossible to determine whether the primary tumor arose from the bladder itself or from the urachus. Narumi et al. (1988) claim that nonurachal cancers of the dome of the bladder do not demonstrate extravesical growth and do not calcify. The presence of calcification is helpful in diagnosis, as it is present in 50 to 70% of urachal carcinomas **(Option (D) is true).** The separation of urachal and primary bladder adenocarcinoma may be arbitrary. Nonetheless, the Narumi criteria can be useful as guidelines for differential diagnosis.

Despite aggressive treatment, the prognosis in general has been poorer for urachal carcinomas than for bladder TCC. This reflects in part the later diagnosis of most urachal cancers and their extracystic growth **(Option (E) is false).** CT allows for earlier diagnosis and earlier institution of treatment. MRI may play a role in staging and treatment planning because of its ability to obtain direct axial, coronal, and sagittal images. Whether use of these imaging methods will improve the prognosis for urachal carcinoma has not been established.

Stanford M. Goldman, M.D.

SUGGESTED READINGS

URACHAL CARCINOMA

1. Brick SH, Friedman SC, Pollack HM, et al. Urachal carcinoma: CT findings. Radiology 1988; 169:377–381

2. Brick SH, Friedman SC, Pollack HM, Radecki PD. CT and MRI of urachal carcinoma. In: Goldman SM, Gatewood OMB (eds), CT and MRI of the genitourinary tract. New York: Churchill Livingstone; 1990:231–244

3. Han SY, Witten DM. Carcinoma of the urachus. AJR 1976; 127:351–353

4. Hill GS. Uropathology. New York: Churchill Livingstone; 1986:823–825

5. Korobkin M, Cambier L, Drake J. Computed tomography of urachal carcinoma. J Comput Assist Tomogr 1988; 12:981–987

6. Rosen L, Hoddick WK, Hricak H, Lue TF. Urachal carcinoma. Urol Radiol 1985; 7:174–177

7. Spataro RF, Davis RS, McLachlan MS, Linke CA, Barbaric ZL. Urachal abnormalities in the adult. Radiology 1983; 149:659–663

8. Wishnow KI. Endovesical ultrasonography of urachal carcinoma. Urol Radiol 1989; 11:53–54

OTHER MALIGNANT BLADDER TUMORS

9. Catalona WJ. Bladder cancer. In: Gillenwater JY, Grayhack JT, Howards SS, Duckett JW (eds), Adult and pediatric urology. Chicago: Yearbook Medical Publishers; 1987:1000–1043

10. Droller MJ. Transitional cell cancer: upper tracts and bladder. In: Walsh PC, Gittes RF, Perlmutter AD, Stamey TA (eds), Campbell's urology, 5th ed. Philadelphia: WB Saunders; 1986:1343–1440

11. Hahn D. Neoplasms of the urinary bladder. In: Pollack HM (ed), Clinical urography. Philadelphia: WB Saunders; 1990:1353–1380

12. Koss LG. Tumors of the urinary bladder. Washington, DC: Armed Forces Institute of Pathology; 1975

13. Narumi Y, Sato T, Hori S, et al. Squamous cell carcinoma of the uroepithelium: CT evaluation. Radiology 1989; 173:853–856

14. Narumi Y, Sato T, Kuriyama K, et al. Vesical dome tumors: significance of extravesical extension on CT. Radiology 1988; 169:383–385

15. Skinner DG, Lieskovsky G. Diagnosis and management of genitourinary cancer. Philadelphia: WB Saunders; 1988

CROHN'S DISEASE

16. Andrews MD, Papper S. The kidneys and the urinary tract. In: Berk JE (ed), Bockus gastroenterology, 4th ed. Philadelphia: WB Saunders; 1985:4613–4620

17. Bagby RJ, Clements JL Jr, Patrick JW, Rogers JV, Weens HS. Genitourinary complications of granulomatous bowel disease. AJR 1973; 117:297–306

18. Balfe DM, Bova JG. Genitourinary manifestations of gastrointestinal disease. In: Pollack HM (ed), Clinical urography. Philadelphia: WB Saunders; 1990:961–979

19. Boag GS, Nolan RL. Sonographic features of urinary bladder involvement in regional enteritis. J Ultrasound Med 1988; 7:125–128

20. Carson CC, Malek RS, Remine WH. Urologic aspects of vesicoenteric fistulas. J Urol 1978; 119:744–746

21. Fishman EK, Wolf EJ, Jones B, Bayless TM, Siegelman SS. CT evaluation of Crohn's disease: effect on patient management. AJR 1987; 148:537–540

22. Goldman SM, Fishman EK, Gatewood OM, Jones B, Siegelman SS. CT in the diagnosis of enterovesical fistulae. AJR 1985; 144:1229–1233
23. Klahr S, Buerker TJ, Morrison A. Urinary tract obstruction. In: Brenner BM, Rector FC Jr (eds), The kidney, 3rd ed. Philadelphia: WB Saunders; 1986:1443–1490
24. Koelbel G, Schmiedl U, Majer MC, et al. Diagnosis of fistulae and sinus tracts in patients with Crohn disease: value of MR imaging. AJR 1989; 152:999–1003
25. Sans JV, Tiegell JP, Redortz JP, Serrano MV, Gassol JMB. Review of 31 vesicointestinal fistulas: diagnosis and management. Eur Urol 1986; 12:21–27
26. Suits GS, Knoepp LF. A community experience with enterovesical fistulas. Am Surg 1985; 51:523–528
27. Williams RJ. Vesico-intestinal fistula and Crohn's disease. Br J Surg 1954; 42:179–187

SCHISTOSOMIASIS OF THE BLADDER

28. Dittrich M, Doehring E. Ultrasonographical aspects of urinary schistosomiasis: assessment of morphological lesions in the upper and lower urinary tract. Pediatr Radiol 1986; 16:225–230
29. Jorulf H, Lindstedt E. Urogenital schistosomiasis: CT evaluation. Radiology 1985; 157:745–749
30. Lautin EM, Becker RD, Fromowitz FB, Bezahler GH. Computed tomography of the lower urinary tract in schistosomiasis. J Comput Assist Tomogr 1983; 7:164–165

MALAKOPLAKIA

31. Hill GS. Uropathology. New York: Churchill Livingstone; 1986:401–404
32. Kenney PJ, Breatnach ES, Stanley RJ. Chronic inflammation. In: Pollack HM (ed), Clinical urography. Philadelphia: WB Saunders; 1990:822–843

EXSTROPHY OF THE BLADDER

33. Friedland GW, deVries PA, Nino-Murcia M, Cohen R, Rifkin MD. Congenital anomalies of the urinary tract. In: Pollack HM (ed), Clinical urography. Philadelphia: WB Saunders; 1990:559–787

Notes

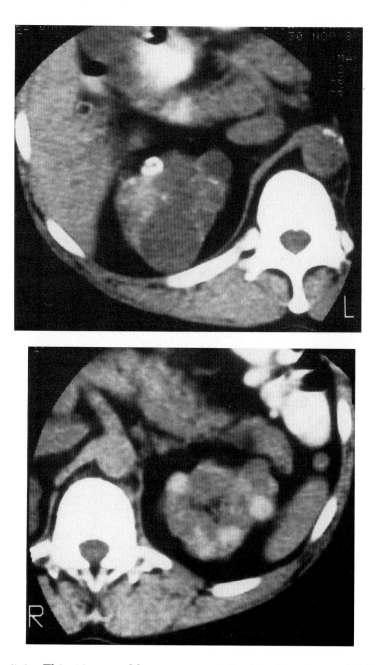

Figure 5-1. This 19-year-old man presented with chronic renal failure. You are shown two CT sections.

Case 5: Acquired Cystic Renal Disease

Question 18

Which *one* of the following is the MOST likely diagnosis?

(A) Autosomal dominant polycystic disease
(B) Medullary cystic disease
(C) Acquired cystic renal disease
(D) Autosomal recessive polycystic disease
(E) von Hippel-Lindau syndrome

The CT images (Figure 5-1A and B) show small right and left kidneys (see Figure 5-2). This can be ascertained by comparing the kidneys with the vertebral bodies. Virtually all of the parenchyma of both kidneys has been replaced by cysts of various densities. Both cortex and medulla are involved. Some of the cysts have attenuation values higher than that of water (arrowheads, Figure 5-2B) and represent areas of hemorrhage, pus, mucus, or a combination of these. In the right kidney (Figure 5-2A) there is coarse curvilinear calcification (arrow), which is the result of past intracystic hemorrhage. These findings are most consistent with acquired cystic kidney disease **(Option (C) is correct).**

Autosomal dominant polycystic disease (Option (A)) (Figure 5-3) (also called adult polycystic kidney disease) can be seen at any age but is classically diagnosed in middle-aged adults with hypertension or progressive renal insufficiency. History and family screening will usually establish the hereditary pattern. Initially the disease may develop asymmetrically, but when fully manifest, both kidneys are enlarged, often measuring between 16 and 22 cm in length. Several cysts of various sizes also develop in the liver. There is no correlation between the number of hepatic cysts and the severity of the renal disease. Cysts are also occasionally found in the pancreas and spleen. The fact that the kidneys are small in the test patient precludes autosomal dominant polycystic disease.

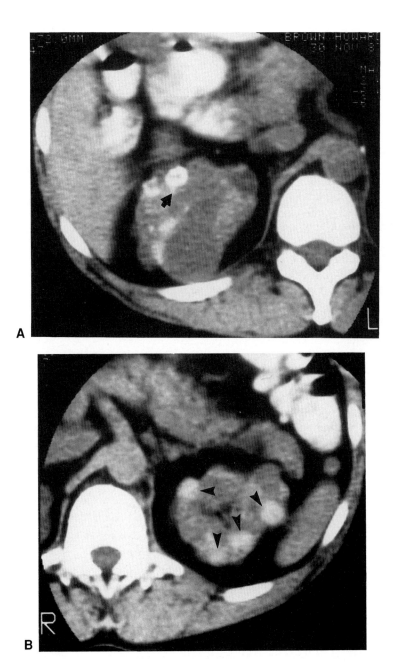

Figure 5-2 (Same as Figure 5-1). Acquired cystic kidney disease. The
kidneys are small when compared with the vertebral body. (A) In the right
kidney, there is coarse calcification (arrow) from previous hemorrhage.
(B) In the left kidney, several of the cysts are dense secondary to
hemorrhage (arrowheads).

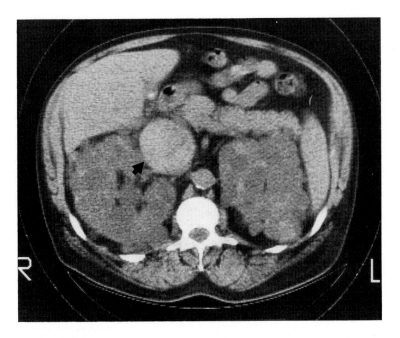

Figure 5-3. Adult polycystic kidney disease. CT scan shows that the kidneys are enlarged and are totally replaced by cysts. There are hemorrhagic cysts bilaterally. Note the especially large hemorrhagic cyst on the right (arrow).

Medullary cystic disease (Option (B)) (Figure 5-4) is also a hereditary disease; it is classically seen in teenagers and young adults. On CT, the kidneys of affected individuals are normal in size or, more likely, small. The cysts are confined to the medullary portion of the kidney. This disease is not consistent with the CT finding in the test case of both cortical and medullary cysts.

Autosomal recessive polycystic disease (Option (D)) is seen from the newborn period through the teen years. Most patients die from the renal disease in the neonatal period or in infancy. Patients with mild renal involvement succumb to cirrhosis-induced variceal bleeding in their twenties. The kidneys of patients with the mild form of the disease are small with changes that mimic those of medullary sponge kidney. In the newborn, the kidneys are enlarged. On ultrasonography (Figure 5-5) the kidneys are usually highly echogenic because the multiplicity of small cysts produces many interfaces. Because the cysts are more likely to be medullary, there may be a relatively hypoechoic rim as well (Figure 5-6). Iodinated contrast material should not be used in these patients because

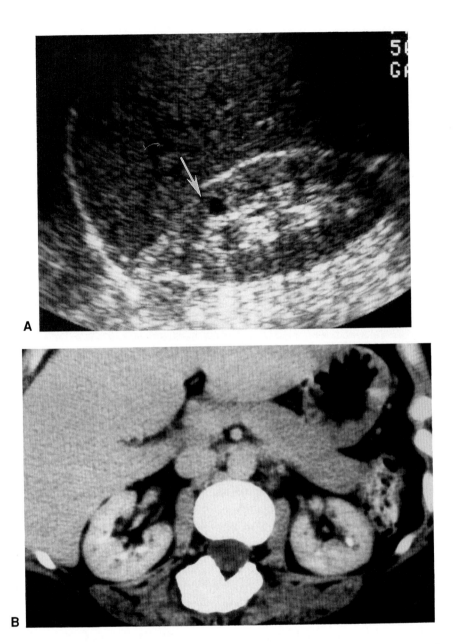

Figure 5-4. Medullary cystic kidney disease in a 25-year-old woman with a family history of renal failure due to medullary cystic kidney disease. (A) Sonogram demonstrates a single medullary cyst (arrow) in a normal-sized kidney. (B and C) Enhanced CT images demonstrate small, predominantly medullary cysts. Even the one larger cyst on the left (arrow) does not break through the cortex. (Case courtesy of Lee B. Talner, M.D., University of California, San Diego.)

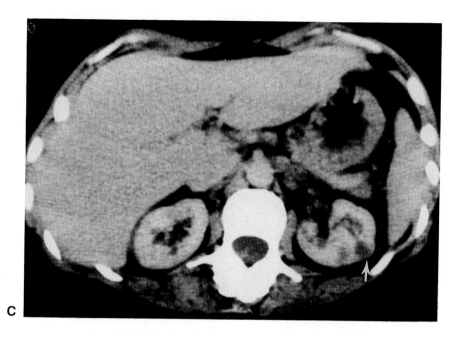

C

of the risk of renal toxicity. When a contrast agent is given for urography or CT, the nephrogram will persist for days. The CT findings shown in Figure 5-1 are not consistent with autosomal recessive polycystic disease.

von Hippel-Lindau syndrome (Option (E)) is yet another hereditary disease that affects the kidneys. Pathologically, the kidneys of patients with this syndrome contain cysts and multiple renal cell carcinomas. The kidneys are usually of normal size with normal parenchyma identified between the renal masses. von Hippel-Lindau syndrome is thus a less likely diagnosis in the test case.

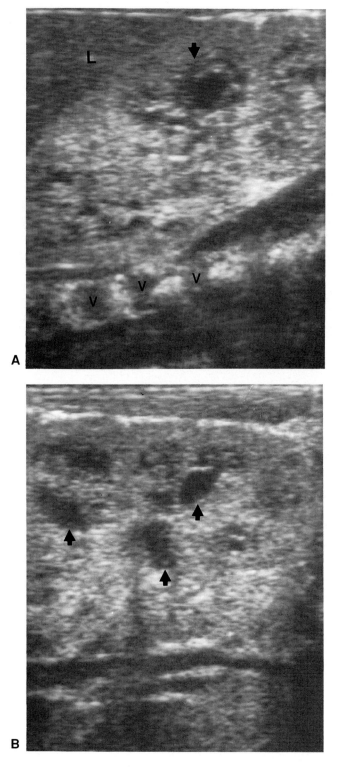

Figure 5-5. Autosomal recessive polycystic disease. Longitudinal ultra-sonograms of the right (A) and left (B) kidneys in a newborn show that the kidneys are enlarged (compare with vertebral-body [V] dimensions) and highly echogenic relative to the liver (L). Arrows point to a few larger cysts. (Case courtesy of Marilyn J. Siegel, M.D., Mallinckrodt Institute of Radiology, St. Louis, Mo.)

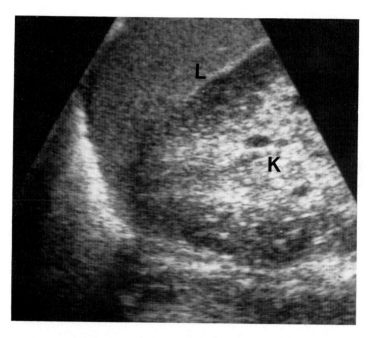

Figure 5-6. Autosomal recessive polycystic disease. Longitudinal ultra-sonogram of the right kidney in a newborn shows an enlarged, echogenic kidney with a hypoechoic rim. L = liver; K = kidney. (Case courtesy of Marilyn J. Siegel, M.D.)

Questions 19 through 22

For each numbered cystic disease listed below (Questions 19 through 22), select the *one* lettered pattern of inheritance (A, B, C, or D) that would be MOST closely associated with it if first diagnosed in the third decade of life. Each lettered pattern may be used once, more than once, or not at all.

19. Multicystic dysplastic kidney
20. Medullary sponge kidney
21. Medullary cystic disease
22. von Hippel-Lindau syndrome

   (A) Autosomal dominant
   (B) Autosomal recessive
   (C) Sex linked
   (D) No known hereditary pattern

There are a number of cystic diseases that have a hereditary pattern, whereas others have no clear hereditary pattern.

Multicystic dysplastic kidney is a unilateral process in which the entire kidney is affected, unless there is a duplication, in which case only one part of the duplication may be involved. There is a delayed union between the mesonephros and metanephros that leads to a nonfunctioning kidney. Although classically it was diagnosed in the newborn by the presence of a palpable mass, it can now be recognized by ultrasonography *in utero* as an enlarged kidney. Follow-up ultrasonography shows that many of these kidneys undergo atrophy. Multicystic dysplastic kidney may also be diagnosed initially in young adults with hypertension, a calcified cystic renal mass, or both (Figure 5-7). There are a few instances of familial multicystic dysplastic kidney. However, there is no known hereditary pattern in most patients with multicystic dysplastic kidney **(Option (D) is the correct answer to Question 19).** Some siblings of patients with multicystic dysplastic kidney may occasionally have ureteropelvic junction obstruction. More important, contralateral ureteropelvic junction obstruction, a treatable condition, may be identified in children with multicystic dysplastic kidney.

Medullary sponge kidneys are found in patients with developmentally dilated renal tubules (i.e., renal tubular ectasia). Within these tubules, there is slower urine flow, leading to an increased frequency of renal infection and intraluminal stone formation. There have been a few cases of familial medullary sponge kidney, but there is, in general, no known hereditary pattern **(Option (D) is the correct answer to Question 20).**

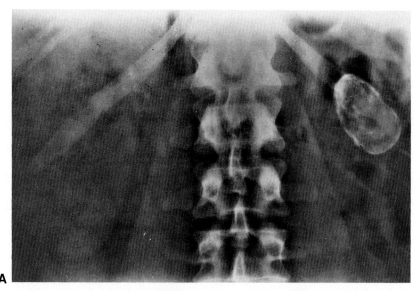

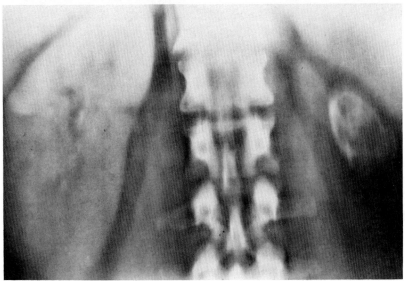

Figure 5-7. Left multicystic dysplastic kidney. (A) Radiograph shows small calcified kidney with compensatory right-sided hypertrophy. (B) Nephrographic phase of the intravenous urogram shows a right-sided nephrogram with no function on the left.

There is a well-recognized hereditary pattern in medullary cystic disease. In Europe, the disease was first recognized in teenagers and called "familial juvenile nephronophthisis." It has a recessive inheritance

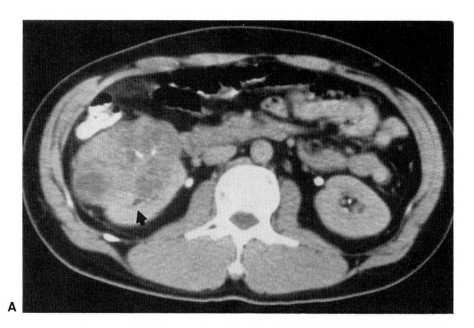

Figure 5-8. von Hippel-Lindau syndrome in a 49-year-old man. (A) CT scan shows a typical renal cell carcinoma of the right kidney (arrow). (B) CT scan at a higher level shows a pancreatic cystadenoma (cursor).

pattern. Besides the renal changes, the affected teenagers have red or blond hair; tapetoretinal degeneration, retinitis pigmentosa, and other optical anomalies; congenital hepatic fibrosis; skeletal dysplasia with cone-shaped epiphyses; and neurologic abnormalities. A young-adult form of the disease with a predominantly autosomal dominant hereditary pattern was described in the United States. In this group, the disease is confined to the kidney. Hence, in a patient in the third decade first diagnosed with medullary cystic disease, the autosomal dominant variant would be most likely **(Option (A) is the correct answer to Question 21).**

von Hippel-Lindau syndrome is inherited as an autosomal dominant gene with moderate penetrance and variable expressivity (Figure 5-8) **(Option (A) is the correct answer to Question 22).** There are more than 25 different abnormalities associated with von Hippel-Lindau syndrome. Four of these are considered basic to the syndrome: retinal angiomatosis, cerebellar hemangioblastomas, adrenal pheochromocytomas, and renal cell carcinomas. The additional association of small (0.5- to 3.0-cm) cysts, seen in as many as 75% of cases, is discussed above.

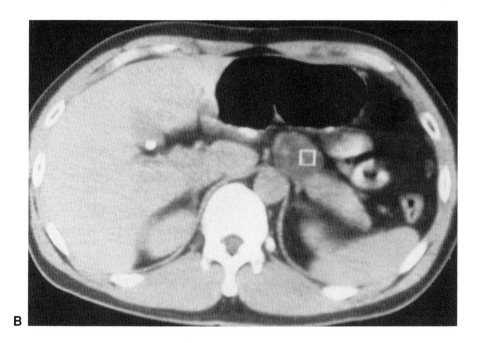

B

Renal cell carcinomas are found in about 40% of patients. They are bilateral in 75% of these and multifocal in 87%. Most recently, Choyke et al. reported finding epididymal cystadenomas, which were identified by sonographic screening, in 7 of 37 patients with von Hippel-Lindau syndrome.

RCC in 40%

Question 23

Concerning medullary cystic disease,

F (A) cortical cystic changes are noted in about 10% of cases
f (B) the angiographic pattern is indistinguishable from that of adult autosomal dominant polycystic disease
T (C) a thin cortical rim is identifiable on ultrasonography
T (D) it is a salt-wasting nephropathy

Medullary cystic disease predominantly affects the medulla or the corticomedullary junction. The cysts are small, varying from 0.1 to 1.0 cm in diameter. Tubular interstitial fibrosis and atrophy occur, and there is severe cortical parenchymal loss. Cortical cysts are rare, and, even when they are present, they are always covered by a rim of thinned cortical parenchyma **(Option (A) is false).**

Medullary cystic disease, or familial juvenile nephronophthisis, has a peak onset in teenagers (the autosomal recessive form seen in Europe) or in young adults (the predominantly autosomal dominant form described in the United States). In spite of the different hereditary pattern and age of onset, both forms are believed to be one and the same entity. The clinical presentation is that of a salt-wasting nephropathy **(Option (D) is true),** reflecting the tubular damage caused by the disease. Affected patients initially complain of polyuria, polydipsia, and enuresis. In children, anemia, growth retardation, and progressive renal failure are present. Bone pain secondary to renal osteodystrophy or a slipped femoral capital epiphysis may be the presenting complaint. Salt wasting, salt craving, and hypokalemia develop in both forms and are secondary to the loss of electrolytes at the tubular level. Hypertension may be present when the patient develops severe renal failure.

The pathologic differences between autosomal dominant polycystic disease and medullary cystic disease result in correspondingly different characteristic angiographic patterns **(Option (B) is false).** In patients with autosomal dominant polycystic disease, the kidneys are enlarged and the cysts affect both the medulla and the cortex. Some of the cortical cysts can be seen as thin-walled avascular masses breaking through the outer surface of the cortex. Angiographically, the intrarenal arteries are displaced and stretched by the cysts. In the nephrographic phase, multiple sharply defined cysts are identified throughout the kidney, with absence of cortical nephrogram where the cysts break the renal surface. On the other hand, angiograms in patients with medullary cystic disease demonstrate small or normal-sized kidneys. The cysts are much smaller and predominate in the medullary portion of the kidney. Most important, a thin rim of intact cortical tissue is noted over the cysts no matter how close they are to the cortical surface.

In general, ultrasonography (or, in older patients, computed tomography) is the method of choice in making this diagnosis. With high-resolution ultrasonography, the small fluid-filled medullary cysts can be seen in the normal-sized to small kidneys. Hyperechogenicity is present, reflecting the tubointerstitial fibrosis. The cysts do not break through the cortex, and a thin rim of residual cortex can be identified over the cysts **(Option (C) is true).**

Question 24

Concerning acquired cystic kidney disease,

F (A) it is seen only after hemodialysis
T (B) there is an increased risk of renal cell carcinoma
T (C) dystrophic calcification is often present
T (D) patients should be monitored by CT or ultrasonography
F (E) it is commonly seen in transplanted kidneys

Acquired cystic kidney disease was first described by Dunnill et al. in 1977. In their seminal paper, they reported the development of extensive cystic changes in 14 of 30 patients on chronic intermittent hemodialysis. These cystic changes have been shown to progress the longer the patient is on hemodialysis. Approximately 45 to 50% of patients on hemodialysis for 3 years ultimately develop the changes. The diagnosis should be suggested if at least 10 cysts are seen bilaterally or if there is evidence of cystic replacement of 40% of the remaining parenchyma. The cause of acquired cystic disease is not clear but has been variously thought to be due to (1) tubular occlusion by fibrosis or calcium oxalate crystals, (2) ischemia, (3) accumulation of an unknown uremic metabolite, and (4) deposition of unknown substances found in the hemodialysis fluid. This process is not confined to patients on hemodialysis but can also be seen in patients with long-standing uremia or in patients on peritoneal dialysis **(Option (A) is false)**. The cysts develop in the native kidneys, and it is believed that the disease can be arrested or may even regress with transplantation **(Option (E) is false)**.

One significant complication is hemorrhage with gross hematuria. The hemorrhage, which may be demonstrated on CT (Figure 5-9), MRI, and ultrasonography, is in various stages of resorption or development. This bleeding may be due to anticoagulation therapy or increased microvascular permeability and fragility, or both. Dystrophic calcification (Figure 5-10) and stone formation are seen quite frequently **(Option (C) is true)**.

The second major complication of hemodialysis is the development of renal tumors variously identified as adenomas, oncocytomas, or renal cell carcinomas (Figure 5-11). The incidence of renal neoplasms is reported to be seven times that in the normal population **(Option (B) is true)**. Although many consider these tumors to be of low grade, their propensity to metastasize has been documented. For this reason, some radiologists believe that once a tumor is detected, immediate surgical removal of the kidney is indicated. Others consider it safe to wait for the tumor to grow before treating it because of the supposition that the renal

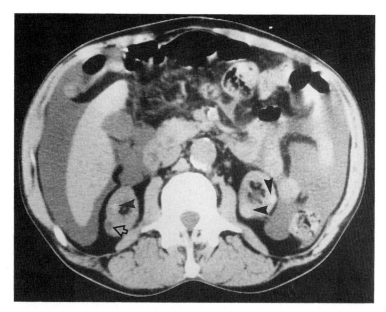

Figure 5-9. Acquired cystic kidney disease. CT scan of a patient on peritoneal dialysis shows that some cysts are hemorrhagic cysts (arrowheads), whereas others are simple, uncomplicated cysts (arrow). Note dialysis fluid in peritoneal cavity.

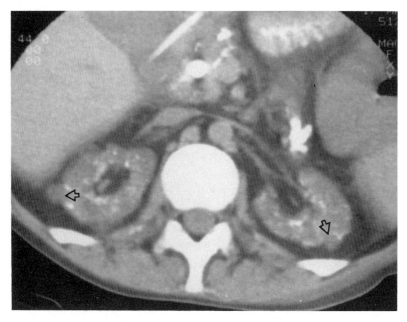

Figure 5-10. Acquired cystic kidney disease. CT scan shows extensive dystrophic calcification. Note the peripheral cysts with densities higher than that of water (arrows) (most likely due to hemorrhage).

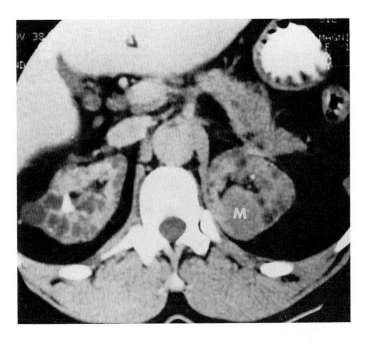

Figure 5-11. Adenocarcinoma of the kidney in a 47-year-old woman with acquired cystic kidney disease. Unenhanced CT demonstrates a solid mass (M) in the left kidney as well as the extensive bilateral cysts. (Case courtesy of Carl Sandler, M.D., University of Texas Medical School, Houston.)

tumors associated with acquired cystic kidney disease are either of low-grade malignancy or benign. It is important that all patients on dialysis be carefully monitored for tumor development. Various investigators have suggested interval ultrasonography, while others recommend CT at least on an annual or biannual basis **(Option (D) is true).** At present, MRI is too expensive a method for this purpose and is not sensitive enough. The place of contrast enhancement with gadolinium DTPA is as yet unknown. However, gadolinium DTPA probably will not identify the avascular or the hypovascular renal cell carcinomas. The problem of distinguishing hemorrhagic cysts from solid tumors in patients with acquired cystic disease has not been solved, but such cysts are usually observed unless growth is confirmed (Figure 5-12). Since neoplasms are often difficult to detect in these diffusely diseased kidneys, even with modern imaging modalities, careful follow-up studies to demonstrate change or growth of lesions are important.

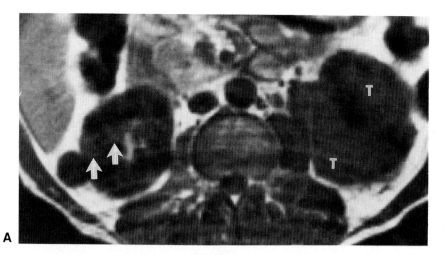

SE 500/17

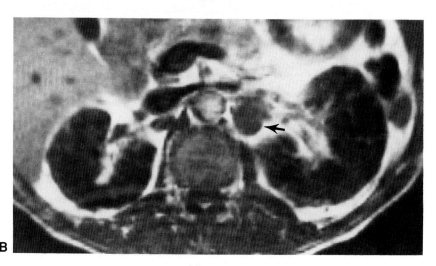

SE 500/17

Figure 5-12. Two renal cell carcinomas in a 46-year-old male with acquired cystic kidney disease. (A) T1-weighted image demonstrates two tumors (T) in the left kidney as well as extensive bilateral cysts. Hemorrhage (arrows) or infection is often indistinguishable from tumor. (B) T1-weighted image at the level of the hilum shows an enlarged lymph node filled with tumor (arrow). (Case courtesy of Errol Levine, M.D., Ph.D., University of Kansas Medical Center, Kansas City.)

Question 25

Concerning autosomal dominant polycystic disease,

T (A) approximately 50% of patients have associated hepatic cysts
T (B) hemorrhage into one or more cysts is common
F (C) the gene penetrance approaches 85%
F (D) it occurs as a spontaneous mutation in approximately 10% of patients
T (E) dystrophic calcification is common

Autosomal dominant polycystic disease is inherited with a gene penetrance of almost 100% **(Option (C) is false).** Although absence of a family history has been reported in 25% of cases, this may merely reflect one or more of the following: (1) family members may have been missed because they died prior to diagnosis, especially those who had the mild forms now being recognized by CT; (2) paternity may not have been known with certainty; or (3) family members may not have known about renal disease present in other branches or members of the family. There may be some rare spontaneous mutations, but 10% is an unrealistically high proportion **(Option (D) is false).** Clearly, when a case of autosomal dominant polycystic disease is found, the entire family should be studied by ultrasonography or CT. Careful follow-up evaluation and genetic counseling are mandatory to ensure early institution of treatment in affected patients before complications ensue and to aid family planning.

Some of the major complications of autosomal dominant polycystic disease are infection (believed by some investigators to be present in all patients, even when asymptomatic), hemorrhage, stone formation, cyst rupture, and obstruction. The hemorrhage may be severe enough to require nephrectomy. CT studies performed on almost all patients with advanced disease will demonstrate cyst hemorrhages in various states and of various ages **(Option (B) is true).** Because of the infection and hemorrhage, calcification is a frequent complication, being seen as stones or nephrocalcinosis (Figure 5-13) in more than half the cases reported by Greene and Barrett **(Option (E) is true).** Ultrasonography or CT will show hepatic cysts in up to 60% of patients **(Option (A) is true).** The hepatic cysts are usually asymptomatic and unassociated with hepatic functional abnormalities. There is no correlation between the number of cysts in the liver and the amount of kidney disease.

Stanford M. Goldman, M.D.

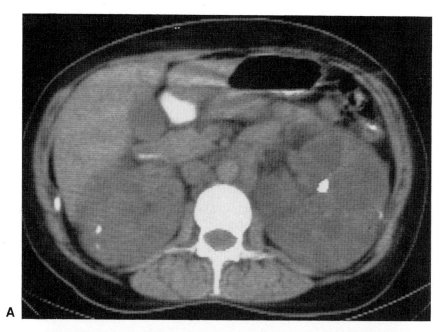

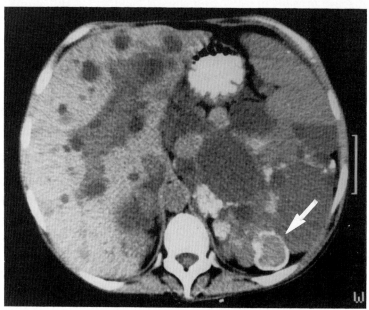

Figure 5-13. CT scans demonstrating different amounts of calcification in two different patients with autosomal dominant kidney disease. (A) Several areas of coarse calcification are noted. (B) Cyst with a heavily calcified wall (arrow) is noted. Multiple hepatic cysts are seen as well.

SUGGESTED READINGS

ACQUIRED CYSTIC RENAL DISEASE

1. Basile JJ, McCullough DL, Harrison LH, Dyer RB. End stage renal disease associated with acquired cystic disease and neoplasia. J Urol 1988; 140:938–943

2. Brendler CB, Albertsen PC, Goldman SM, Hill GS, Lowe FC, Millan JC. Acquired renal cystic disease in the end stage kidney: urological implications. J Urol 1984; 132:548–552

3. Cho C, Friedland GW, Swenson RS. Acquired renal cystic disease and renal neoplasms in hemodialysis patients. Urol Radiol 1984; 6:153–157

4. Dunnill MS, Millard PR, Oliver D. Acquired cystic disease of the kidneys: a hazard of long-term intermittent maintenance haemodialysis. J Clin Pathol 1977; 30:868–877

5. Ishikawa I. Uremic acquired cystic disease of kidney. Urology 1985; 26:101–108

6. Ishikawa I, Onouchi Z, Saito Y, et al. Sex differences in acquired cystic disease of the kidney on long-term dialysis. Nephron 1985; 39:336–340

7. Ishikawa I, Yuri T, Kitada H, Shinoda A. Regression of acquired cystic disease of the kidney after successful renal transplantation. Am J Nephrol 1983; 3:310–314

8. Jabour BA, Ralls PW, Tang WW, et al. Acquired cystic disease of the kidneys. Computed tomography and ultrasonography appraisal in patients on peritoneal and hemodialysis. Invest Radiol 1987; 22:728–732

9. Kutcher R, Amodio JB, Rosenblatt R. Uremic renal cystic disease: value of sonographic screening. Radiology 1983; 147:833–835

10. Levine E, Grantham JJ, Slusher SL, Greathouse JL, Krohn BP. CT of acquired cystic kidney disease and renal tumors in long-term dialysis patients. AJR 1984; 142:125–131

11. Levine E, Hartman DS, Smirniotopoulos JG. Renal cystic disease associated with renal neoplasms. In: Pollack HM (ed), Clinical urography. Philadelphia: WB Saunders; 1990:1126–1150

12. Takebayashi S. Sonographic evaluation of kidneys undergoing dialysis. Urol Radiol 1985; 7:69–74

AUTOSOMAL DOMINANT POLYCYSTIC DISEASE

13. Goldman SM, Hartman DS. Autosomal dominant polycystic kidney disease. In: Hartman DS (ed), Renal cystic disease. Philadelphia: WB Saunders; 1989:88–107

14. Goldman SM, Hartman DS. Autosomal dominant polycystic kidney disease. In: Pollack HM (ed), Clinical urography. Philadelphia: WB Saunders; 1990:1092–1112

15. Greene LF, Barrett DM. Renal cystic disease: radiologic appearance. In: Gardner KD Jr (ed), Cystic diseases of the kidney. New York: Wiley & Sons; 1976:91–113

16. Hatfield PM, Pfister RC. Adult polycystic disease of the kidneys (Potter type 3). JAMA 1972; 222:1527–1531

17. Hilpert PL, Friedman AC, Radecki PD, et al. MRI of hemorrhagic renal cysts in polycystic kidney disease. AJR 1986; 146:1167–1172
18. Lippert MC. Renal cystic disease. In: Gillenwater JY, Grayhack JT, Howards SS, Duckett JW (eds), Adult and pediatric urology. Chicago: Year Book Medical Publishers; 1987:620–647

MEDULLARY CYSTIC DISEASE

19. Resnick JS, Hartman DS. Medullary cystic disease of the kidney. In: Hartman DS (ed), Renal cystic disease. Philadelphia: WB Saunders; 1989:120–126
20. Resnick JS, Hartman DS. Medullary cystic disease of the kidney. In: Pollack HM (ed), Clinical urography. Philadelphia: WB Saunders; 1990:1178–1184

VON HIPPEL-LINDAU SYNDROME

21. Choyke PL, Filling-Katz MR, Shawker TH, et al. Von Hippel-Lindau disease: radiologic screening for visceral manifestations. Radiology 1990; 174:815–820
22. Levine E, Hartman DS, Smirniotopoulos JG. Renal cystic diseases associated with renal neoplasms. In: Hartman DS (ed), Renal cystic disease. Philadelphia: WB Saunders; 1989:38–72

MULTICYSTIC DYSPLASTIC KIDNEY

23. Hartman DS, Davis CJ. Multicystic dysplastic kidney. In: Hartman DS (ed), Renal cystic disease. Philadelphia: WB Saunders; 1989:127–145
24. Hartman DS, Davis CJ. Multicystic dysplastic kidney. In: Pollack HM (ed), Clinical urography. Philadelphia: WB Saunders; 1990:1151–1166

MEDULLARY SPONGE KIDNEY

25. Goldman SM, Hartman DS. Medullary sponge kidney. In: Hartman DS (ed), Renal cystic disease. Philadelphia: WB Saunders; 1989:108–120
26. Goldman SM, Hartman DS. Medullary sponge kidney. In: Pollack HM (ed), Clinical urography. Philadelphia: WB Saunders; 1990:1167–1177

RENAL CYSTIC DISEASE: GENERAL

27. Bernstein J. The classification of renal cysts. Nephron 1973; 11:91–100
28. Bernstein J, Gardner KD Jr. Renal cystic diseases and renal dysplasia. In: Walsh PC, Gittes RF, Perlmutter AD, Stamey TA (ed), Campbell's urology, 5th ed. Philadelphia: WB Saunders; 1986:1760–1803
29. Hayden CK Jr, Swischuk L. Renal cystic disease. Semin US CT MRI 1991; 12:361–373

Notes

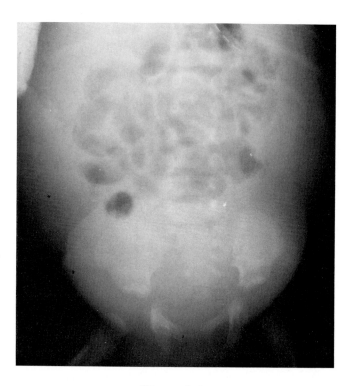

Figure 6-1
Figures 6-1 and 6-2. This newborn presented with a distended abdomen. You are shown an abdominal radiograph (Figure 6-1) and longitudinal sonograms of both kidneys (Figure 6-2A and B).

Case 6: Urine Ascites

Question 26

Which *one* of the following is the MOST likely diagnosis?

(A) Posterior urethral valves
(B) Multicystic dysplastic kidney
(C) Neurogenic bladder
(D) Megacystis-microcolon syndrome
(E) Prune belly syndrome

Evaluation of the abdominal radiograph (Figure 6-1) reveals the stomach and proximal and mid-small bowel to be located in the midabdomen. The small bowel loops are mildly dilated. The flank stripes are not visualized, and no loops of bowel can be identified near the bulging lateral walls of the abdomen. There is a paucity of bowel gas in the pelvis. This pattern is highly suggestive of a fluid-filled peritoneal cavity with bowel loops floating centrally. The longitudinal sonogram of the right kidney (Figure 6-2A) demonstrates a small amount of peritoneal fluid in the subhepatic space (arrows, Figure 6-3A). The parenchyma of the right kidney has increased echogenicity relative to the liver. Normally, in the newborn infant, the echogenicities of the kidney and liver are equal. The right renal pelvis is mildly dilated. The longitudinal sonogram of the left kidney (Figure 6-2B) demonstrates moderate hydronephrosis, increased renal parenchymal echogenicity, and a larger amount of free peritoneal fluid lateral to the kidney in the left infracolic space (Figure 6-3B).

A variety of causes must be considered in the differential diagnosis of ascites in a neonate. Erythroblastosis fetalis is commonly associated with ascites, but the radiograph will also show generalized edema. Hydronephrosis is not usually present. Other causes of intraperitoneal fluid in the newborn include congenital bowel anomalies (i.e., ileal atresia, ileal

---

Figures 6-1 through 6-4 were provided courtesy of Marilyn J. Siegel, M.D., Mallinckrodt Institute of Radiology, St. Louis, Mo.

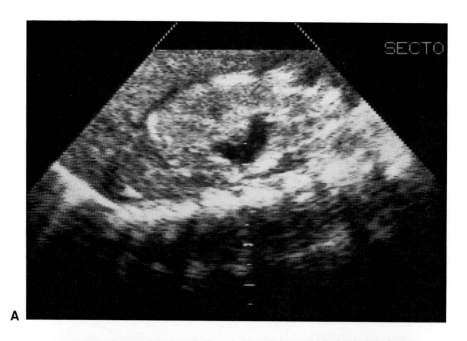

A

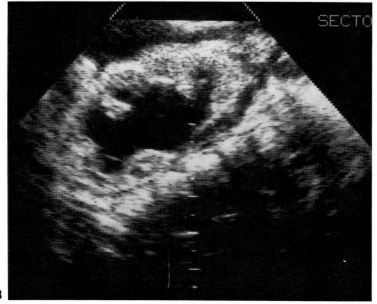

B

Figure 6-2

perforation, small bowel volvulus, etc.), hepatic failure, and cardiac failure. Birth trauma leading to rupture of the spleen, liver, or a bile duct is another important cause. However, none of these conditions causes hydronephrosis.

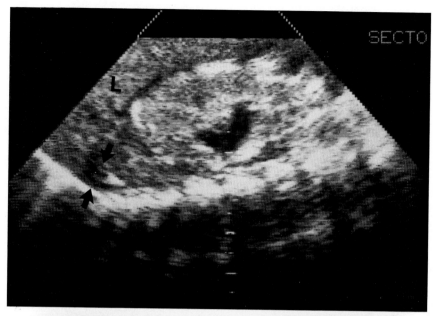

A

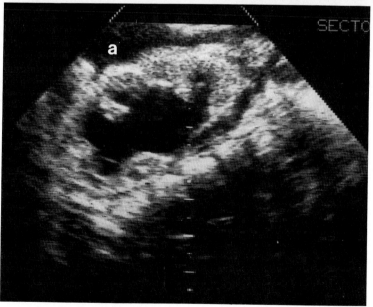

B

Figure 6-3 (Same as Figure 6-2). (A) The longitudinal sonogram of the right kidney demonstrates the kidney to be hyperechoic relative to the liver (L), mild dilatation of the renal pelvis, and ascitic fluid in the sub-hepatic space (arrows). (B) The corresponding image of the left kidney shows moderately marked hydronephrosis and a larger amount of ascitic fluid (a).

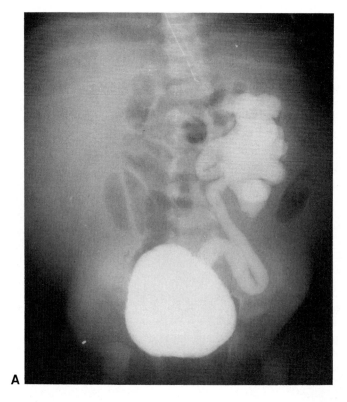

A

Figure 6-4. Same patient as in Figures 6-2 and 6-3. Full (A) and voiding (B) images of a cystourethrogram show left-sided reflux and characteristic findings of posterior urethral valves.

The most common cause of peritoneal fluid in the newborn is the intraperitoneal accumulation of urine as a result of bladder outlet obstruction with secondary rupture of either a calyceal fornix or the bladder itself. The most common cause of a bladder outlet obstruction in the newborn, and also of urine ascites, is posterior urethral valves **(Option (A) is correct).** This diagnosis was confirmed in the test patient at cystography (Figure 6-4A), which showed marked reflux into the left renal collecting system. The voiding cystourethrogram image (Figure 6-4B) demonstrates trabeculation of the bladder wall, a narrow bladder neck, a dilated prostatic urethra, and a normal anterior urethra. These findings are diagnostic of posterior urethral valves. The lack of significant right hydronephrosis in this patient is most likely the result of forniceal rupture *in utero*, which allowed the right collecting system to decompress and also led to the urine ascites. The increased echogenicity of both

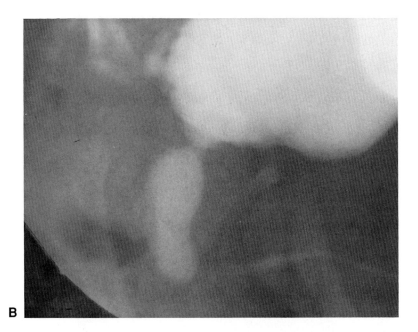

B

kidneys most likely represents the renal parenchymal dysplasia that is associated with *in utero* hydronephrosis.

Multicystic dysplastic kidney (Option (B)) (Figure 6-5) is a developmental anomaly characterized by a nonfunctioning cystic kidney secondary to an abnormality in the union between the mesonephros and metanephros. Sonography characteristically demonstrates multiple noncommunicating cysts of variable size and absence of normal renal parenchyma, in contrast to the typical findings of hydronephrosis in the test patient. The disease is unilateral for all practical purposes but may be associated with ureteropelvic junction (UPJ) obstruction on the opposite side. It should be noted that in Potter type IV cystic disease, bilateral dysplastic kidneys are present. This, however, is incompatible with life. Many of the patients with bilateral disease have bilaterally dilated ureters and have posterior urethral valves. For this reason, Potter type IV cystic disease may be considered a more severe form of the disorder seen in the test patient. Potter did not describe urine ascites as a routine finding in type IV cystic disease. Most have ascribed the dysplasia in these cases to be secondary to the effects of obstruction early in nephrogenesis. Henneberry and Stephens believe that the changes are unrelated to the outlet obstruction but are instead due to an abnormal positioning of the ureteral bud.

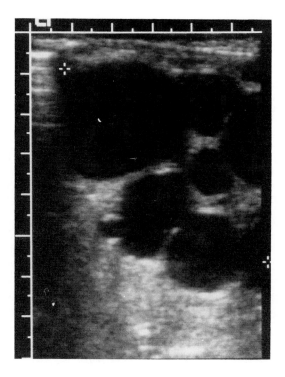

Figure 6-5. Longitudinal sonogram of multicystic dysplastic kidney in a newborn girl. There are multiple cysts of various sizes without a dominant central cyst. (Case courtesy of Sheila Sheth, M.D., Johns Hopkins University, Baltimore, Md.)

Neurogenic bladder in the newborn period (Option (C)) could theoretically cause a relative ureteric obstruction or pseudo-obstruction due to reflux. There is no evidence of a spinal anomaly or any history given to suggest neurogenic disease in the test case. Although a neurogenic bladder can cause urine ascites according to Tank et al., the occurrence of posterior urethral valves is a much more common etiology.

Megacystis-microcolon-intestinal hypoperistalsis syndrome, which is also known as megacystis-microcolon syndrome (Option (D)) (Figure 6-6), is more common in neonatal girls than in boys. The bladder is huge, with secondary nonobstructed refluxing ureters. The large bowel is small, with a dilated small bowel that is hypo- or aperistaltic. The large bowel is often malrotated, and the small bowel may be foreshortened and atretic. The cause of this syndrome is unknown. Nerve ganglia have been present in normal or even increased numbers in most patients, with only a few patients showing focal aganglionic areas. The urinary tract problem is

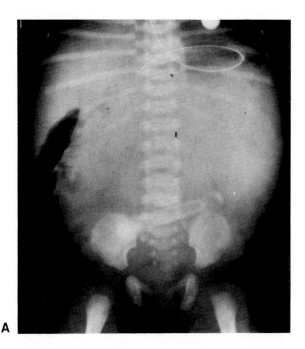

A

Figure 6-6. Two cases of megacystis-microcolon-intestinal hypoperistalsis syndrome. (A) Abdominal radiograph reveals a somewhat distended abdomen. The bowel hugs the lateral flank stripes. There is no evidence of floating loops indicative of ascites. There is a suggestion of an enlarged bladder extending out of the pelvis. (B) A lateral radiograph of the same patient obtained after both barium enema and contrast cystography examinations demonstrates a microcolon and a huge bladder (B). (C) A longitudinal sonogram of the kidney in the second patient demonstrates marked hydronephrosis. (D) A longitudinal sonogram of the mid-abdomen demonstrates multiple, dilated, fluid-filled loops of small bowel. (Panels A and B courtesy of Kook Sang Oh, M.D., Allegheny General Hospital, Pittsburgh, Penn.; panels C and D courtesy of Marilyn J. Siegel, M.D., Mallinckrodt Institute of Radiology, St. Louis, Mo.)

manageable by use of a suprapubic tube, but the use of intestinal alimentations, parasympathomimetics, synthetic gastrointestinal stimulants, etc., has been for the most part unsuccessful. Prognosis is poor. In the test patient, the absence of a markedly enlarged bladder and the relatively mild small bowel dilatation suggest that this is not the correct diagnosis. Additionally, dilated, refluxing ureters were not seen sonographically and the patient is a boy.

Prune belly, or Eagle-Barrett syndrome (Option (E)) (Figure 6-7), is a complex of abnormalities that is seen almost exclusively in boys but has

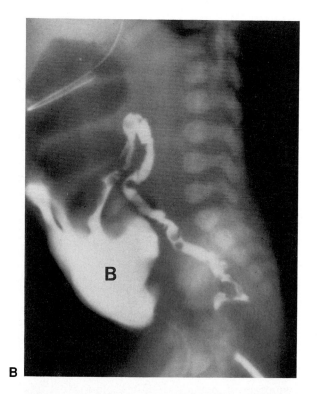

B

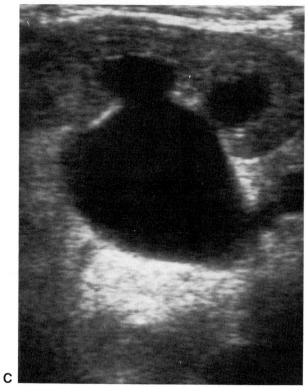

C

108

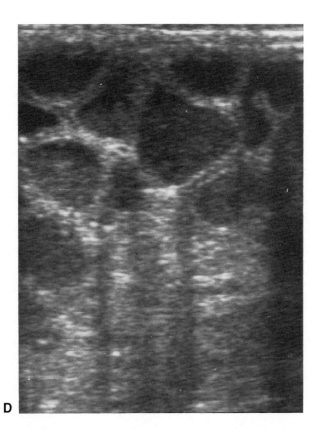

D

been found occasionally in girls (fewer than 30 cases). Its manifestations include absence of the abdominal wall muscles (either diffusely or in a scattered fashion); a large hypotonic bladder; dilated, tortuous ureters; and bilateral cryptorchidism. Ascites at birth is rarely present in these patients. The radiographs in the test case show ascites. The test patient did not have the cryptorchidism or absent abdominal wall musculature indicative of prune belly syndrome (PBS), which should have been readily apparent on physical examination.

Urine ascites is most commonly seen in boys (7:1 male/female ratio). In addition to posterior urethral valves, other obstructive causes include ureteroceles, urethral atresia, and bilateral ureteral stenosis. Two unusual causes reported in the literature include a perforation of the urachus during umbilical catheterization (Vordermark et al. and Mata et al.) and a presacral neuroblastoma causing bladder outlet obstruction (Weller and Miller). In most cases of urine ascites, evidence of a forniceal rupture or, less commonly, a bladder rupture is present. An actual

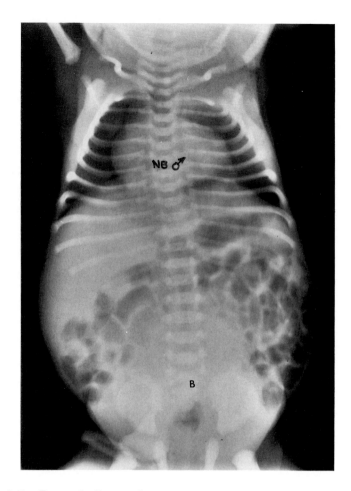

Figure 6-7. Prune belly syndrome in a newborn boy. The radiograph reveals a distended bladder (B) with the bowel hugging the lateral flank stripes.

communication with the peritoneum has been identified between the kidney or the perinephric space at surgery or autopsy or by imaging techniques. In the few cases in which a tear is not seen, a renal transudate across the peritoneum has been postulated as the cause of ascites. These ruptures may have a beneficial effect by limiting the renal parenchymal damage from the back-pressure of obstruction. The bladder or forniceal rupture decompresses the system.

Decompressive procedures such as placement of a suprapubic tube or a Foley catheter, nephrostomy, or immediate surgical intervention to resect the urethral valves have led to survival rates in the range of 70%, as reported by Tank et al. This improves to almost 85%, according to Scott, if the child survives longer than 72 hours. Similarly, Rittenberg et al. reported that all three of their patients with posterior urethral valves and ascites did well with serum creatinines below 1 mg/dL. Other clinical problems that must be addressed in these neonates are associated electrolyte imbalances or pulmonary hypoplasia. The latter is a consequence of the oligohydramnios, associated with the *in utero* obstruction of the bladder outlet, and of the increased pressure of the uterus on the fetal chest. At birth, pulmonary hypoplasia is often associated with pneumothorax or mediastinal emphysema occurring during mechanical ventilation.

Question 27

Concerning posterior urethral valves,

(A) they are associated with "spinning-top" urethra
(B) the most common type extends just distal to the verumontanum as a circumferential diaphragm
(C) hypertrophy of the external sphincter is common
(D) retrograde urethrography is the most accurate method of diagnosis
(E) they are usually associated with renal dysplasia

Posterior urethral valves were first classified into three types by Young in 1919. The most common type is classified as a type I valve (Figure 6-8). It consists of thickened normal tissue derived from the plicae colliculi. These valves extend inferiorly from the lower edge of the verumontanum at the level of the membranous urethra and course sagittally. Type II valves supposedly result from mucosal folds running anteriorly and superiorly towards the bladder neck from the verumontanum. At present, there is doubt whether a true type II valve exists. The type III valve is described as an iris-type diaphragm attached around the circumference of the urethra, distal to the verumontanum and transverse in orientation. The ratio of type I to type III valves is 4:1 **(Option (B) is false).**

The diagnosis of posterior urethral valves is made by ultrasonography or on voiding cystourethrography, which shows a dilated prostatic urethra during voiding. The type I valves are seen as bulging crescentic radiolucent defects (the "spinnaker sail" sign). In type III valves, the membranes may prolapse into the bulbous urethra, giving a "windsock" deformity. Use of retrograde urethrography is not appropriate when a

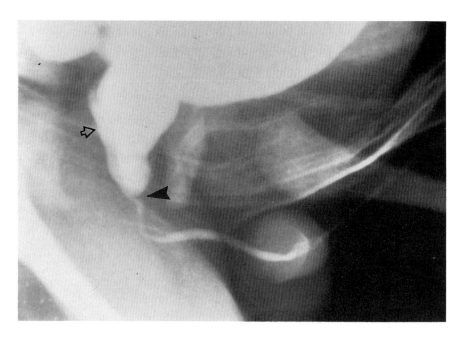

Figure 6-8. Voiding cystourethrogram showing type I posterior urethral valves (arrowhead). Note the distended prostatic urethra, normal anterior urethra, and reflux into Cowper's gland (arrow).

posterior urethral valve is suspected. With this technique, there will be a tendency to actually compress the valves against the urethra, disguising the presence of an obstruction **(Option (D) is false).**

Vesicoureteral reflux accompanies posterior urethral valves in 30 to 70% of cases. Renal dysplasia is present in 15 to 20% of fetuses with obstructing urethral valves and either is secondary to the obstruction or represents an associated primary bud anomaly. In an excellent review on the subject, Hill reviews both the clinical and experimental data that show that ureteral obstruction during nephrogenesis will lead to cystic dysplastic changes, whereas obstruction occurring after nephrogenesis leads only to hydronephrosis. In addition, the aberrant origin of the ureter occasionally found in these cases would lead to renal dysplasia, as described in the Mackie-Stephens ureteral bud theory of ureteral development. One should be aware of the association of renal dysplasia, even though it is not a common finding **(Option (E) is false).**

The external sphincter in male subjects is found in the urogenital diaphragm and plays the major role in urinary continence. The external sphincter is distal to the site where valves are found, and so hypertrophy does not occur **(Option (C) is false).**

From the 1950s to the 1970s the term "acorn deformity" or "spinning-top deformity" was in common usage. It was used for female patients with meatal stenosis. The meatal "stenosis" reputedly caused the urethra to dilate, and the relative proximal narrowing represented the bladder neck, which was hypertrophied. Urologists would then dilate the meatal stenosis and not infrequently operate on the bladder neck, with resultant incontinence because the urinary sphincter was inadvertently dilated or torn. Since then, many have questioned the existence of meatal stenosis in female patients. It is now believed by most pediatric radiologists that the "spinning-top deformity" is normal and is merely an expression of volume and flow rate. However, Saxton et al. believe it to be a sign of bladder instability. The term "spinning-top deformity" is also sometimes mistakenly used for the dilatation of the urethra behind a posterior urethral valve **(Option (A) is false).**

Question 28

Concerning prune belly syndrome,

T (A) ureteral reflux is common
T (B) maternal oligohydramnios is usually present
T (C) bilateral cryptorchidism is present
F (D) renal dysplasia is not a significant feature
F (E) on voiding cystourethrography, urethral valves are usually present

The multiple urinary tract abnormalities in patients with PBS cause the other two findings of the triad, i.e., absence of abdominal wall musculature and cryptorchidism **(Option (C) is true).** At this time, the etiology of PBS is still controversial. Snow and Duckett describe four possible explanations. Of these, the theory of urethral outlet obstruction *in utero* as the primary cause is ideal for remembering the numerous elements that make up the syndrome. The outlet obstruction leads to bladder and ureteral distention. This causes destruction of the abdominal wall musculature and prevents the testes from reaching the scrotal sac. In those cases where urethral valves are not present, recanalization is thought to have occurred. Stephens has suggested that the yolk sac being retained within the embryo causes the abdominal wall redundance and the bladder and urachal anomalies. However, this theory fails to explain the ureteral and testicular anomalies. Similarly, a lateral mesenchymal plate defect really only explains the abdominal wall defect. Many believe that the urinary tract and abdominal wall abnormalities result from a single insult occurring at a vulnerable stage of development and affecting both systems simultaneously. As reviewed by Woodard and Trulock, other explanations for the failure of descent of the testes without invoking a mechanical obstruction by the distention include (1) absence of the gubernaculum testis (according to this theory, the latter could be viewed as a "guidewire" leading the testis to its appropriate location) and (2) intrinsic abnormality of the testis itself.

Although a normal pregnancy is possible with PBS, maternal oligohydramnios is more common **(Option (B) is true).** This leads to both pulmonary and skeletal abnormalities. The resultant pulmonary hypoplasia is partly due to the direct compression of the fetus by the uterus because of the inadequate volume of intrauterine fluid and possibly secondary to the compression of the lungs by the distended abdomen. Mechanical ventilation is associated with an increased frequency of pneumothorax and pneumomediastinum in infants with pulmonary hypoplasia. It is important to note that children with PBS also have respiratory problems secondary to absent abdominal musculature, which is needed for a powerful expiration (i.e., cough). The oligohydramnios also leads to limb deformities as a result of uterine compression of the fetus. The important deformities include club feet, absence of lower limbs, congenital hip dislocation, dysplastic hips, and elbow and knee dimples. The latter are the sites of compression of the child's extremities, which are in an exaggerated fetal position *in utero* caused by the oligohydramnios.

The ureters are characteristically tortuous and dilated, with the lower ends more severely affected. They are hypotonic, with poor peristalsis and emptying. Ureteral kinks and functional obstruction result. The ureterovesical junction is markedly abnormal, and vesicoureteral reflux is present in ureters in most but not all PBS patients (Figure 6-9) **(Option (A) is true).**

The kidneys in children with PBS may not be affected. More typically, hydronephrosis and renal dysplasia are present **(Option (D) is false).** The latter may determine the ultimate prognosis and is most severe in patients with urethral stenosis, megalourethra, or imperforate anus. The dysplasia may affect either one kidney or both kidneys. In its most severe form, it presents as a nonfunctioning multicystic dysplastic kidney. Several theories have been advanced for the dysplasia, as reviewed by Snow and Duckett. These include (1) early outlet obstruction causing secondary renal changes; (2) intrinsic abnormality in the metanephros, including possibly incomplete development of the primitive streak; (3)

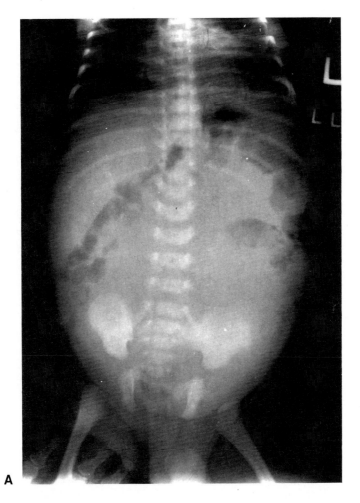

A

Figure 6-9. Prune belly syndrome in a 16-day-old boy. (A) Radiograph shows the bowel hugging the lateral abdominal wall in a patient with absent abdominal musculature. (B) Cystogram reveals bilateral reflux with dilated, tortuous ureters.

ectopic ureteric bud development, according to the Mackie-Stephens theory of ureteral development; and (4) ischemia to the kidney and ascending ureter, leading to ureteric atresia and renal hypoplasia because of failure to acquire appropriate stepwise blood supply with renal ascent from the pelvis *in utero*.

Megalourethra is more common in PBS than in any other condition. It may be scaphoid or fusiform; the latter type is more serious. Megalourethra is an anterior urethral dilation due to absence of the corpus

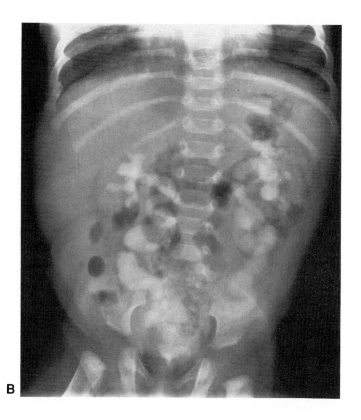

B

spongiosa. Currarino reports that on voiding cystourethrography, the bladder neck is high, with the proximal posterior urethra dilated and elongated. The membranous and anterior urethras have normal widths, with a sharp transition mimicking a true obstruction. As such, the voiding cystourethrogram is often misinterpreted by the inexperienced as showing posterior urethral valves. Part of this configuration may reflect failure of the external sphincter to relax. Posterior urethral valves, urethral stenosis, urethral atresia, and hypoplasia have been seen in autopsy series; these infants are stillborn or will not survive for long after birth. Posterior urethral valves in the total picture of clinically diagnosed PBS are rare **(Option (E) is false).**

Question 29

Concerning multicystic dysplastic kidney,

(A) it is predominantly an abnormality of the metanephros
(B) children with higher ureteral obstructions have a better prognosis than do those with lower ureteral obstructions
(C) contralateral ureteropelvic junction obstruction is present in about 40% of live-born infants
(D) it is difficult to distinguish from severe ureteropelvic junction obstruction by ultrasonography alone
(E) the risk of malignant degeneration necessitates nephrectomy

There are two theories concerning the development of multicystic dysplastic kidney. One theory postulates an unknown intrinsic parenchymal cause. Most investigators believe that the primary problem lies in an abnormality in the mesonephros, the primordial tissue from which the collecting system develops **(Option (A) is false).** The ampullae of the mesonephros perform two functions. One is the successive dichotomous branching into the calyces, collecting ducts, and tubules, and the other is the induction of nephrons from the metanephric blastema. It is failure of one or both of these functions that leads to multicystic dysplastic kidney formation.

Pathologically, multicystic dysplastic kidney can be thought of as occurring in two forms. In one, the ureteric "malfunction" occurs below or, more likely, at the UPJ. In this situation, the ureter is atretic or stenosed at this site. The kidney above the site of obstruction becomes "cystic," but there is one dominant or larger "cyst," which can be looked upon as a dilated renal pelvis. The rest of the kidney will be dysplastic, with cysts of various sizes. In the other form, the atresia or stenosis in the collecting system (i.e., mesonephros) can be looked upon as having occurred in the renal pelvis or extended intrarenally from the UPJ. As a result, no dominant cyst may be present. By definition, there is always ureteral atresia, ureteral agenesis, or UPJ occlusion. According to de Klerk et al., patients with higher ureteral stenoses have better prognoses than do those with lower ones because the lower ones are associated with more-severe contralateral anomalies **(Option (B) is true).**

Multicystic dysplastic kidney is the most common unilateral abdominal mass in the newborn. It is most important to evaluate the opposite kidney and ureters to exclude any abnormalities that may be present. In autopsy series, contralateral abnormalities are present in 30 to 100% of cases. However, this incidence is clearly less in live births. Thus, Taxy reported that in live patients the incidence of additional anomalies is only 14%. These include ectopia, horseshoe kidney, UPJ obstruction, and vesicoureteral reflux. For example, a contralateral UPJ obstruction was present in 3 of 38 cases reported by Greene et al. In clinical practice, contralateral UPJ obstruction occurs in approximately 10% (and no more than 20%) of cases **(Option (C) is false).**

In a child presenting with an abdominal mass, ultrasonography is currently the imaging method of choice (Figure 6-5). On ultrasonography, multicystic dysplastic kidney is relatively easy to diagnose when the kidney is completely replaced by cysts of various sizes with no dominant cyst seen. On the other hand, when the kidney contains a single dominant cyst, it is often impossible to differentiate a multicystic dysplastic kidney from a severe UPJ obstruction **(Option (D) is true).** Even pathologists have difficulty making this distinction.

In the past, removal of a multicystic dysplastic kidney was believed to be mandatory because of a perceived risk of malignant degeneration. Although there are a few reported cases of adenocarcinomas in multicystic dysplastic kidney in patients in the 15- to 33-year age range, malignant degeneration is very rare; therefore, nephrectomy is no longer indicated **(Option (E) is false).** Lippert, Glassberg and Filmer, and others advocate periodic follow-up imaging of the kidneys. In most cases, the multicystic dysplastic kidney will spontaneously regress or remain as an asymptomatic mass. If pain, hypertension, infection, or increase in size of the dysplastic kidney is noted, surgery can be performed.

Stanford M. Goldman, M.D.

SUGGESTED READINGS

URINE ASCITES

1. Adzick NS, Harrison MR, Flake AW, deLorimier AA. Urinary extravasation in the fetus with obstructive uropathy. J Pediatr Surg 1985; 20:608–615
2. Cass AS, Khan AU, Smith S, Godec C. Neonatal perirenal urinary extravasation with posterior urethral valves. Urology 1981; 18:258–261
3. Griscom NT, Colodny AH, Rosenberg HK, Fliegel CP, Hardy BE. Diagnostic aspects of neonatal ascites: report of 27 cases. AJR 1977; 128:961–970
4. Mata JA, Livne PM, Gibbons MD. Urinary ascites: complication of umbilical artery catheterization. Urology 1987; 30:375–377
5. Mitchell ME, Garrett RA. Perirenal urinary extravasation associated with urethral valves in infants. J Urol 1980; 124:688–691

6. Rittenberg MH, Hulbert WC, Snyder HM III, Duckett JW. Protective factors in posterior urethral valves. J Urol 1988; 140:993–996

7. Scott TW. Urinary ascites secondary to posterior urethral valves. J Urol 1976; 116:87–91

8. Tank ES, Carey TC, Seifert AL. Management of neonatal urinary ascites. Urology 1980; 16:270–273

9. Vordermark JS II, Buck AS, Dresner ML. Urinary ascites resulting from umbilical artery catheterization. J Urol 1980; 124:751

10. Weller MH, Miller K. Unusual aspects of urine ascites. Radiology 1973; 109:665–669

POSTERIOR URETHRAL VALVES

11. Colodny A. Urethral lesions in infants and children. In: Gillenwater JY, Grayhack JT, Howards SS, Duckett JW (eds), Adult and pediatric urology. Chicago: Yearbook Medical Publishers; 1987:1782–1808

12. Cremin BJ, Aaronson IA. Ultrasonic diagnosis of posterior urethral valve in neonates. Br J Radiol 1983; 56:435–438

13. Duckett JW, Snow BW. Disorders of the urethra and penis. In: Walsh PC, Gittes RG, Perlmutter AD, Stamey TA (eds), Campbell's urology, 5th ed. Philadelphia: WB Saunders; 1986:2000–2030

14. Elder JS, Duckett JW. Perinatal urology. In: Gillenwater JY, Grayhack JT, Howards SS, Duckett JW (eds), Adult and pediatric urology. Chicago: Yearbook Medical Publishers; 1987:1512–1603

15. Henneberry MO, Stephens FD. Renal hypoplasia and dysplasia in infants with posterior urethral valves. J Urol 1980; 123:912–915

16. Osathanondh V, Potter EL. Pathogenesis of polycystic kidneys. Type 4 due to urethral obstruction. Arch Pathol 1964; 77:502–509

17. Saxton HM, Borzyskowski M, Mundy AR, Vivian GC. Spinning top urethra: not a normal variant. Radiology 1988; 168:147–150

18. Talner LB. Specific causes of obstruction. In: Pollack HM (ed), Clinical urography. Philadelphia: WB Saunders; 1990:1629–1751

19. Tank ES, Carey TC, Seifert AL. Management of neonatal urinary ascites. Urology 1980; 16:270–273

MULTICYSTIC DYSPLASTIC KIDNEY

20. Barrett DM, Wineland RE. Renal cell carcinoma in multicystic dysplastic kidney. Urology 1980; 15:152–154

21. Bernstein J, Gardner CD Jr. Renal cystic disease and renal dysplasia. In: Walsh PC, Gittes RF, Perlmutter AD, Stamey TA (eds), Campbell's urology, 5th ed. Philadelphia: WB Saunders; 1986:1760–1803

22. Birken G, King D, Vane D, Lloyd T. Renal cell carcinoma arising in a multicystic dysplastic kidney. J Pediatr Surg 1985; 20:619–621

23. de Klerk DP, Marshall FF, Jeffs RD. Multicystic dysplastic kidney. J Urol 1977; 118:306–308

24. Glassberg K, Filmer RB. Renal dysplasia, renal hypoplasia and cystic disease of the kidney. In: Kelatis PO, King LR (eds), Clinical pediatric urology, vol 2. Philadelphia: WB Saunders; 1985:922–971

25. Greene LF, Feinzaig W, Dahlin DC. Multicystic dysplasia of the kidney with special reference to the contralateral kidney. J Urol 1971; 105:482–487

26. Hartman DS, Davis CJ. Multicystic dysplastic kidneys. In: Hartman DS (ed), Renal cystic disease. Philadelphia: WB Saunders; 1989:127–145

27. Hartman DS, Davis CJ. Multicystic dysplastic kidney. In: Pollack HM (ed), Clinical urography. Philadelphia: WB Saunders; 1990:1151–1166

28. Hartman GE, Smolik LM, Shochat SJ. The dilemma of the multicystic dysplastic kidney. Am J Dis Child 1986; 140:925–928

29. Hill GS. Uropathology. New York: Churchill Livingstone; 1989:81–133

30. Kleiner B, Filly RA, Mack L, Callen PW. Multicystic dysplastic kidney: observations of contralateral disease in the fetal population. Radiology 1986; 161:27–29

31. Kyaw MM. Roentgenologic triad of congenital multicystic kidney. AJR 1973; 119:710–719

32. Kyaw MM. The radiological diagnosis of congenital multicystic kidney "Radiological Triad." Clin Radiol 1974; 25:45–62

33. Lippert MC. Renal cystic disease. In: Gillenwater JY, Grayhack JT, Howards SS, Duckett JW (eds), Adult and pediatric urology. Chicago: Yearbook Medical Publishers; 1987:620–647

34. Raffensperger J, Abousleiman A. Abdominal masses in children under one year of age. Surgery 1968; 63:514–521

35. Shirai M, Kitagawa T, Nakata H, Urano Y. Renal cell carcinoma originating from dysplastic kidney. Acta Pathol Jpn 1986; 36:1263–1269

36. Taxy JB. Renal dysplasia: a review. Pathol Annu 1985; 20:139–159

MEGACYSTIS-MICROCOLON SYNDROME

37. Amoury RA, Fellows RA, Goodwin CD, Hall RT, Holder TM, Ashcraft KW. Megacystis-microcolon-intestinal hypoperistalsis syndrome: a cause of intestinal obstruction in the newborn. J Pediatr Surg 1977; 12:1063–1065

38. Berdon WE, Baker DH, Blanc WA, Gay B, Santulli TV, Donovan C. Megacystis-microcolon-intestinal hypoperistalsis syndrome: a new cause of intestinal obstruction in the newborn. Report of radiologic findings in five newborn girls. AJR 1976; 126:957–964

39. Friedland GW, deVries PA, Nino-Murcia M, Cohen R, Rifkin MD. Congenital anomalies of the urinary tract. In: Pollack HM (ed), Clinical urography. Philadelphia: WB Saunders; 1990:559–787

40. Hoehn W, Thomas GG, Mearadji M. Urologic evaluation of megacystis-microcolon-intestinal hypoperistalsis syndrome. Urology 1981; 17:465–466

41. Krook PM. Megacystis-microcolon-intestinal hypoperistalsis syndrome in a male infant. Radiology 1980; 136:649–650

42. Willard DA, Gabriele OF. Megacystis-microcolon-intestinal hypoperistalsis syndrome in a male infant. JCU 1986; 14:481–485

PRUNE BELLY SYNDROME

43. Aaronson IA, Cremin BJ. Prune belly syndrome in young females. Urol Radiol 1979–1980; 1:151–155

44. Currarino G. The genitourinary tract. In: Silverman FN (ed), Caffey's pediatric X-ray diagnosis, 8th ed. Chicago: Yearbook Medical Publishers; 1985:1696–1698
45. Moerman P, Fryns JP, Goddeeris P, Lauweryns JM. Pathogenesis of prune-belly syndrome: a functional urethral obstruction caused by prostatic hypoplasia. Pediatrics 1984; 73:470–475
46. Monie IW, Monie BJ. Prune belly syndrome and fetal ascites. Teratology 1979; 19:111–117
47. Snow BW, Duckett JW. Prune belly syndrome. In: Gillenwater JY, Grayhack JT, Howards SS, Duckett JW (eds), Adult and pediatric urology. Chicago: Yearbook Medical Publishers; 1987:1709–1725
48. Woodard JR, Trulock TS. Prune belly syndrome. In: Walsh PC, Gittes RF, Perlmutter AD, Stamey TA (eds), Campbell's urology, 5th ed. Philadelphia: WB Saunders; 1986:2159–2178

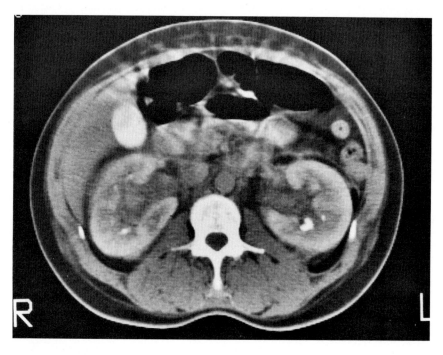

Figure 7-1. This 60-year-old man presented with oliguria. You are shown a CT scan obtained 24 hours after administration of contrast material for an excretory urogram.

Case 7: Renal Sinus Hemorrhage

Question 30

Which *one* of the following is the MOST likely diagnosis?

   (A) Bilateral ureteral obstruction
   (B) Lymphoma
   (C) Renal sinus hemorrhage
   (D) Uric acid nephropathy
   (E) Shock

The CT scan obtained 24 hours after injection of contrast agent (Figure 7-1) reveals mixed-attenuation collections filling the renal sinuses and essentially obliterating the fat density normally present in the sinuses. No para-aortic adenopathy or other masses are present. There are prominent bilateral nephrograms, as well as persistence of excreted contrast medium within mildly ectatic calyces. The opacification of the gallbladder is a result of vicarious excretion of the contrast material. The CT findings are most consistent with renal sinus hemorrhage **(Option (C) is correct).**

Bilateral ureteral obstruction (Option (A)) could certainly cause the patient's oliguria. However, collecting-system dilatation is not a prominent feature of the test image, and no ureteral dilatation is present. At 24 hours after contrast agent administration, most of the retained contrast agent should be in the collecting system and ureters (rather than in the renal parenchyma) in a patient with ureteral obstruction. Moreover, ureteral obstruction would not explain the high-attenuation collections in the renal sinuses.

Lymphoma (Option (B)) could explain the soft tissue density in the renal sinuses. The lack of periaortic adenopathy or renal masses makes this diagnosis less likely. Renal lymphoma may occur as a result of hematogenous spread or may be secondary to direct extension from adjacent lymph nodes. The most common appearance of renal lymphoma is one of discrete parenchymal masses. Renal sinus involvement may also

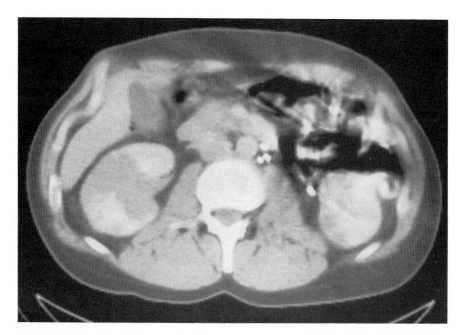

Figure 7-2. Renal lymphoma. Contrast-enhanced CT scan. On the right there is an irregular low-attenuation cortical mass, which extends into the renal sinus. Several masses involving the left renal parenchyma were seen on other sections.

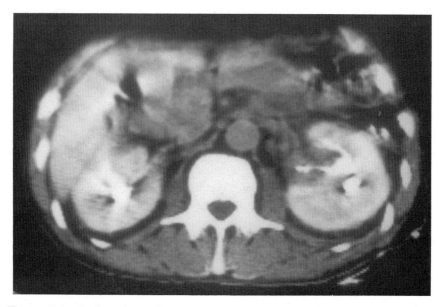

Figure 7-3. Isolated renal sinus lymphoma. There is a mixed-attenuation soft tissue mass occupying the left renal sinus and compressing the renal pelvis. (Reprinted with permission from Ruchman et al. [15].)

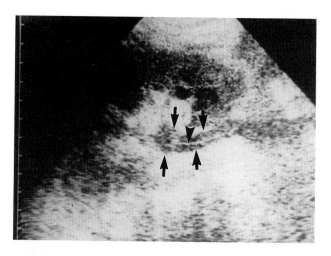

Figure 7-4. Renal sinus lymphoma. The compressed renal pelvis and proximal ureter are seen on this longitudinal sonogram as a linear echogenic structure (arrowhead) surrounded by the hypoechoic lymphoma (arrows). (Courtesy of H.-C. Yeh, M.D., The Mount Sinai Hospital, New York, N.Y.)

occur as direct extension from the parenchyma. Figure 7-2 shows the CT findings in such a patient. Note the low-attenuation cortical mass in the right kidney associated with renal sinus extension. Figure 7-3 is a CT scan of another patient, who presented with flank pain and fever. The compressed renal pelvis was a result of isolated renal sinus lymphoma. There was no evidence of disease elsewhere in this patient. Because deposits of lymphoma often appear anechoic or hypoechoic, the sonographic pattern of lymphoma may lead to an incorrect diagnosis of hydronephrosis. Careful sonographic examination will demonstrate a central linear echo representing the collapsed compressed collecting system (Figure 7-4).

Uric acid nephropathy (Option (D)) and shock (Option (E)) could both result in dense nephrograms and oliguria. Neither condition, however, would produce soft tissue density in the renal sinuses.

The renal sinus is the space that surrounds the pelvicalyceal system. It is composed of fibrofatty tissue that communicates directly with the perirenal fat. The renal lymphatics and extraparenchymal vessels traverse the renal sinus. It is the pathway for egress of urine in spontaneous renal extravasation associated with acutely obstructing renal calculi and in pyelosinus extravasation during retrograde pyelography.

Bleeding into the renal sinus is most often associated with anticoagulant therapy. The test patient was taking warfarin following a myocardial

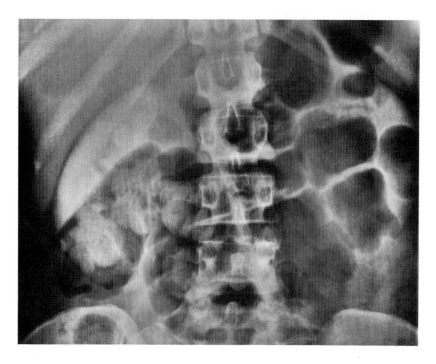

Figure 7-5. Same patient as in Figure 7-1. Conventional abdominal radiograph taken 24 hours after the intravenous urogram demonstrates persistent dense nephrograms. No dilatation of the renal pelves or ureters is seen.

infarction and had a prothrombin time of 52 seconds with a laboratory control of 12 seconds. Other causes of renal sinus hemorrhage include occult neoplasm and leaking aneurysm, although one would not expect these conditions to be bilateral. In addition, bleeding associated with renal neoplasms is usually subcapsular or perirenal. Vasculitis and blood dyscrasias are other possible causes of bilateral renal sinus hemorrhage. The presence of fresh blood could have been better demonstrated by its high attenuation on an unenhanced CT scan; however, the test patient had received contrast material 24 hours prior to his hospital admission, and so CT confirmation of the presence of fresh blood was not possible.

Renal sinus hemorrhage will resorb in 2 to 4 weeks once the patient's coagulation defect is corrected. The excretory urographic finding of bilateral dense nephrograms in the test patient (Figure 7-5) is not surprising, because the accumulated blood caused acute compression of the pelvicalyceal system. This bilateral pelvicalyceal compression (and resultant pelvicalyceal obstruction) was also responsible for the patient's oliguria.

Question 31

Concerning bilateral ureteral obstruction,

F (A) ureteral dilatation on sonography establishes the diagnosis
T (B) it is usually due to tumor
F (C) antegrade placement of stents is preferable to retrograde placement
F (D) early dialysis is recommended

Ureteral obstruction usually leads to ureteral dilatation. This is not always the case, however. Diseases such as retroperitoneal fibrosis and metastatic carcinoma can encase the ureters and lead to obstruction with little or no dilatation. In addition, periureteral inflammation with or without fibrosis may inhibit normal ureteral peristalsis, leading to a degree of functional obstruction. Chronic incomplete obstruction of the ureters due to carcinomatosis has also been described. Curry et al. believe that a superimposed acute event in such patients, e.g., infection or ureteral impaction with debris, could lead to acute obstruction and renal failure before significant dilatation occurred. It is also important to remember that ureteral dilatation is not synonymous with obstruction. Primary megaureter, reflux, and ureteral atony are other causes of dilatation without obstruction. Thus, the presence of dilated ureters on imaging studies is not diagnostic of obstruction **(Option (A) is false).**

Ureteral obstruction may be due to primary intrinsic lesions, such as stenoses, valves, atresia, ureteroceles, primary urothelial tumors, or, most commonly, obstructing calculi. Secondary or extrinsic causes include urethral valves, bladder diverticula, benign prostatic hypertrophy, neurogenic bladder, bladder tumors, periureteral fibrosis or inflammation, periureteral neoplasms, and endometriosis. In clinical practice, many of these conditions are uncommon. One must also differentiate between secondary dilatation of the ureters from bladder outlet obstruction, as in benign prostatic hypertrophy, and bilateral obstruction due to direct ureteral involvement. The most common cause of bilateral ureteral obstruction in adults is direct extension from prostatic, colorectal, or gynecologic tumors (Figure 7-6A) **(Option (B) is true).** Norman et al. reported a series of 50 patients with renal failure due to bilateral ureteral obstruction. Thirty-eight of these patients (76%) had underlying malignant disease as the cause of the obstruction. The most common cause in women was carcinoma of the cervix (11 cases). Carcinoma of the prostate (8 cases) was the most common cause in men. Colonic, bladder, and ovarian carcinomas were the cause of the obstruction in 15 of the patients (5 cases of each). The most common treatment for malignant ureteral

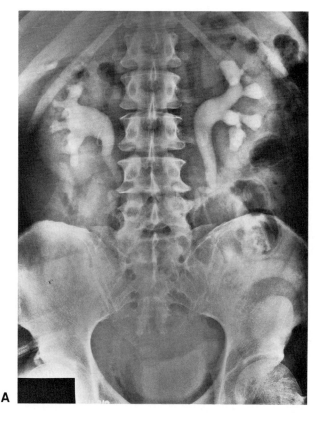

A

Figure 7-6. Bilateral ureteral obstruction due to recurrent infiltrating colonic carcinoma. (A) Urogram. In this patient the ureters are obstructed at the level of the lumbosacral junction. Note the increased density in the pelvis as a result of the mass. There is a colostomy projecting over the left iliac bone. (B) In another patient with the same diagnosis, bilateral ureteral stents have been placed to bypass the obstruction.

obstruction (34 patients) was placement of a stent or nephrostomy (Figure 7-6B). The nonpelvic malignant tumor that most commonly metastasizes to the retroperitoneum and causes ureteral obstruction is breast carcinoma.

Benign causes of bilateral obstruction are less common. Although bilateral renal pelvicalyceal calculi occur frequently, it is rare for both ureters to be obstructed at the same time (Figure 7-7).

Antegrade placement of ureteral stents requires puncture of the renal parenchyma. Although the risk associated with percutaneous nephrostomy is low, it is still the preferred clinical practice to place stents by the retrograde approach when feasible **(Option (C) is false).** Some patients

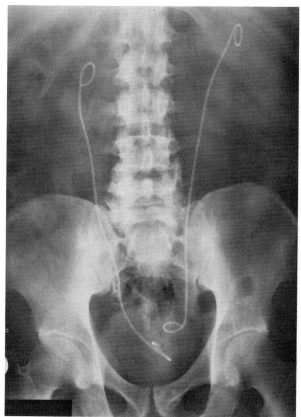

B

present with sepsis and require percutaneous drainage of the obstructed collecting system. If these patients require ureteral stents, then antegrade placement via the nephrostomy tract is indicated once the infection has been controlled.

Ureteral obstruction *per se* is not an indication for dialysis **(Option (D) is false).** Obstructed ureters are treated by ureteral catheter drainage, percutaneous nephrostomy, placement of ureteral stents, or surgical diversion as necessary. Relief of obstruction, if effective, will prevent development of renal failure and obviate dialysis.

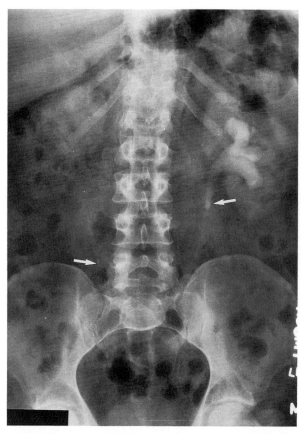

Figure 7-7. Bilateral ureteral obstruction due to ureteral calculi. Radio-paque stones (arrows) are seen in both ureters. The degree of obstruction is greater on the right, accounting for the poorer opacification of the right collecting system.

Question 32

Concerning renal sinus hemorrhage,

T (A) it is often related to anticoagulation

F (B) the suburothelial tissue is not involved

F (C) surgical decompression is indicated

F (D) it is often associated with perinephric hemorrhage

Renal sinus hemorrhage, as well as suburothelial hemorrhage, has been found most commonly in patients receiving anticoagulants **(Option (A) is true).** Warfarin is responsible for most of the reported cases of renal sinus hemorrhage. Fishman et al. reported four such patients.

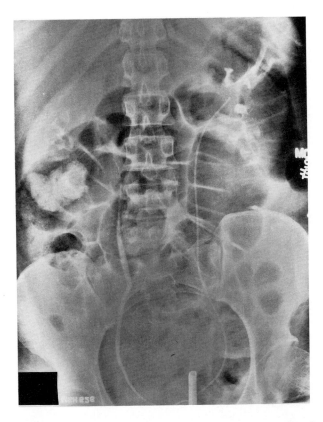

Figure 7-8. Renal sinus hemorrhage in a patient who is receiving warfarin and has an excessively prolonged prothrombin time. This patient has had ureteral catheters placed for bilateral drainage. There is essentially no calyceal dilatation; this is due in part to extrinsic pressure on the collecting system by the blood in the renal sinus.

Three of my patients with renal sinus hemorrhage were receiving warfarin and had prothrombin times approximately fourfold longer than the control value. Heparin is a less common cause, probably because of its short duration of action coupled with the practice of administering it in the hospital and frequently monitoring the patient's partial thromboplastin time. Other reported causes have included acquired circulating anticoagulants and thrombocytopenia. Reports have described both suburothelial location of the blood **(Option (B) is false)** and accumulation in the renal sinus. Since many of these patients have hematuria, it is quite likely that the blood dissects into the collecting system from the suburothelial collections. Correcting the underlying bleeding diathesis is the primary treatment. Severely compressed collecting systems may require temporary ureteral catheterization via the cystoscopic route

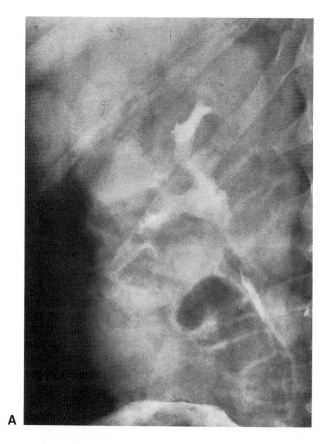

A

Figure 7-9. Suburothelial hemorrhage with resolution. The patient had a prothrombin time four times the control value. (A) The initial urogram demonstrates an irregular renal pelvis with several lucent areas due to submucosal hemorrhage. (B) A repeat excretory urogram several months later reveals a smooth collecting system with no residual defects. This effectively excludes a coexisting mucosal lesion. There is some residual barium in the colon.

(Figure 7-8). Surgical decompression is not indicated, however **(Option (C) is false).** Extension of blood into the perinephric space has been described but is not common **(Option (D) is false).** The differential diagnosis of renal sinus hemorrhage includes renal artery aneurysm and lymphoma as described above. A blood-filled peripelvic cyst can also produce a high-attenuation density in the renal sinus. Another common cause of local increased density in the renal sinus on CT is mass due to transitional cell carcinoma of the renal pelvis.

The radiologic findings and the abnormal bleeding parameters should lead to the correct diagnosis. Not all cases of renal sinus or suburothelial

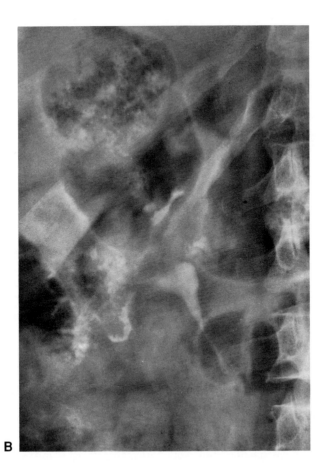

B

hemorrhage are as extensive as that illustrated in Figure 7-1. Patients with suburothelial blood may have only local defects in the contours of the renal pelvis or ureter, which may be difficult to differentiate from other lesions, including transitional cell carcinoma. In addition, a coexisting lesion such as a transitional cell carcinoma may be associated with the suburothelial bleeding. This possibility can be excluded by follow-up urographic or imaging studies to confirm the return to a normal appearance (Figure 7-9), which typically occurs in 3 to 4 weeks.

Question 33

Causes of dense nephrograms include:

T (A) acute tubular necrosis
T (B) uric acid nephropathy
T (C) renal vein thrombosis
T (D) multiple myeloma
F (E) amyloidosis

The nephrogram has been described as having an angiographic component and a tubular component. The angiographic nephrogram is a result of the distribution of 80% of renal blood flow to the cortex. Thus, a CT examination of the kidney with bolus administration of contrast medium shows early opacification of the cortex, largely as a result of the angiographic phase of the nephrogram. The urographic or tubular nephrogram results from the glomerular filtration of the contrast material and its concentration in tubular urine, the magnitude of the latter effect depending on the patient's state of hydration and consequently on the tubular reabsorption of water from the filtrate. Davidson classified dense nephrograms as being either increasingly dense or immediate, dense, and persistent. The increasingly dense nephrogram is due to an increase in tubular transit time and a reduced clearance of contrast material. Water continues to be absorbed from the filtrate, and so glomerular filtration does not cease entirely. In addition, some contrast material may accumulate in the interstitial spaces. The most common cause of the increasingly dense nephrogram is acute ureteral obstruction by a calculus. The resultant increased pressure in the collecting system leads to increased hydrostatic pressure in the tubules. Diminished perfusion pressure associated with hypotension or renal artery stenosis has also been described as a cause of increasingly dense nephrograms. Acute tubular necrosis may be associated with an increasingly dense nephrogram or an immediate, dense, persistent nephrogram **(Option (A) is true).**

An increasingly dense nephrogram is seen with intratubular obstruction by uric acid crystals **(Option (B) is true),** casts of myeloma proteins **(Option (D) is true),** and Tamm-Horsfall proteins.

Renal vein thrombosis (Figure 7-10) may lead to a dense nephrogram **(Option (C) is true).** This may be due to tubular obstruction by edema or hemorrhage or to an associated decrease in arterial perfusion. Leakage of contrast material into the interstitial spaces has also been suggested as a contributing mechanism in renal vein thrombosis.

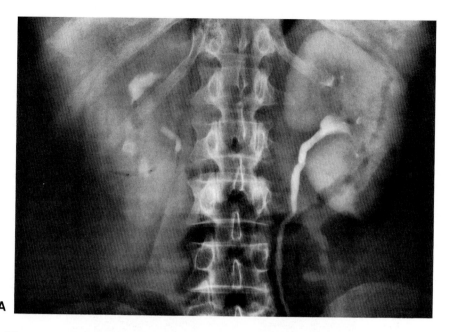

A

Figure 7-10. Renal vein thrombosis. (A) Left retrograde pyelogram performed 2 hours after the excretory urogram. There is a persistent dense nephrogram on the left. No obstructive lesion was present. (B) Venogram. Injection into the renal vein reveals the thrombus (arrows). There is also a catheter in the renal artery (A), as well as in the ureter (U). V = venous catheter.

Amyloidosis is characterized by enlarged smooth kidneys early in the disease. Subsequent ischemia and fibrosis lead eventually to small kidneys. The nephrogram is normal early in the disease and diminishes in intensity as the disease progresses. Dense nephrograms are not a feature of renal amyloidosis **(Option (E) is false).**

Harold A. Mitty, M.D.

obst
hypotension (art.)
renal vein thrombosis (vein)
ATN
uric acid nephropathy
mult. myeloma

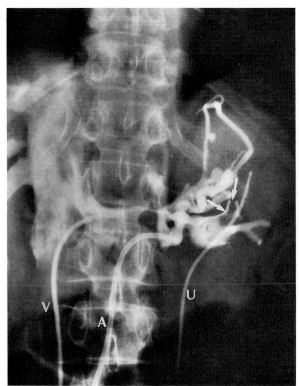

B

SUGGESTED READINGS

RENAL SINUS HEMORRHAGE

1. Brannen GE, Wettlaufer JN, Stables DP, Weill R III. Intramural bleeding into a renal allograft pelvis during heparin anticoagulation. Br J Radiol 1979; 52:838–840
2. Eisenberg RL, Clark RE. Filling defects in the renal pelvis and ureter owing to bleeding secondary to acquired circulating anticoagulants. J Urol 1976; 116:662–663
3. Fishman MC, Pollack HM, Arger PH, Banner MP. Radiographic manifestations of spontaneous renal sinus hemorrhage. AJR 1984; 142:1161–1164
4. Kossol JM, Patel SK. Suburothelial hemorrhage: the value of preinfusion computed tomography. J Comput Assist Tomogr 1986; 10:157–158
5. Miller V, Witten DM, Shin MS. Computed tomographic findings in suburothelial hemorrhage. Urol Radiol 1982; 4:11–14

BILATERAL URETERAL OBSTRUCTION

6. Curry NS, Gobien RP, Schabel SI. Minimal-dilatation obstructive nephropathy. Radiology 1982; 143:531–534

7. Maillet PJ, Pelle-Francoz D, Laville M, Gay F, Pinet A. Nondilated obstructive acute renal failure: diagnostic procedures and therapeutic management. Radiology 1986; 160:659–662

8. Mitty HA, Train JS, Dan SJ. Placement of ureteral stents by antegrade and retrograde techniques. Radiol Clin North Am 1986; 24:587–600

9. Naidich JB, Rackson ME, Moosey RT, Stein HL. Nondilated obstructive uropathy: percutaneous nephrostomy performed to reverse renal failure. Radiology 1986; 160:653–657

10. Norman RW, Mack FG, Awad SA, Belitsky P, Schwarz RD, Lannon SG. Acute renal failure secondary to bilateral ureteric obstruction: review of 50 cases. Can Med Assoc J 1982; 12:601–604

11. Richie JP, Withers G, Ehrlich RM. Ureteral obstruction secondary to metastatic tumors. Surg Gynecol Obstet 1979; 148:355–357

12. Schlegel PN, Epstein JI, Fishman EK, Brendler CB. Rapidly progressive bilateral ureteral obstruction. J Urol 1990; 144:957–960

LYMPHOMA

13. Hartman DS, David CJ Jr, Goldman SM, Friedman AC, Fritzsche P. Renal lymphoma: radiologic-pathologic correlation of 21 cases. Radiology 1982; 144:759–766

14. Heiken JP, McClennan BL, Gold RP. Renal lymphoma. Semin Ultrasound CT MR 1986; 7:58–66

15. Ruchman RB, Yeh HC, Mitty HA, et al. Ultrasonographic and computed tomographic features of renal sinus lymphoma. JCU 1988; 16:35–40

NEPHROGRAM

16. Davidson AJ. Radiology of the kidney. Philadelphia: WB Saunders; 1985:569–595

17. Friedenberg RM. Excretory urography in the adult. In: Pollack HM (ed), Clinical urography. Philadelphia: WB Saunders; 1990:101–207

18. Love L, Lind JA Jr, Olson MC. Persistent CT nephrogram: significance in the diagnosis of contrast nephropathy. Radiology 1989; 172:125–129

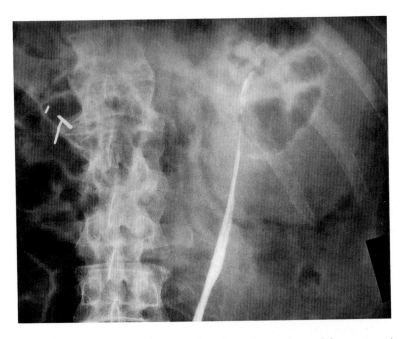

Figure 8-1. This 56-year-old man developed anuria and hypertension 1 day after extracorporeal shock wave lithotripsy (ESWL) for a calculus in a solitary kidney. You are shown a left retrograde pyelogram with the catheter tip just below the ureteropelvic junction.

Case 8: Extracorporeal Shock Wave Lithotripsy

Question 34

Which *one* of the following is the MOST likely diagnosis?

(A) Arterial occlusion
(B) Subcapsular hematoma
(C) Failure to use a ureteral stent
(D) Renal vein thrombosis
(E) Steinstrasse

The left retrograde pyeloureterogram (Figure 8-1) demonstrates a com-pressed, poorly filled renal pelvis. The kidney is enlarged, but its contour is smooth and sharply defined. These findings are most compatible with a subcapsular hematoma **(Option (B) is correct).** An unenhanced CT scan of the test patient (Figure 8-2) confirmed the diagnosis of left subcap-sular hematoma. Note the higher attenuation of the fresh blood. The compression of the renal parenchyma by the hematoma caused inade-quate perfusion of this solitary kidney, which led to anuria. The asso-ciated renal ischemia also explains the development of hypertension.

Subcapsular or perirenal bleeding is a recognized complication of extra-corporeal shock wave lithotripsy (ESWL). The reported frequency of this complication varies depending on the modalities used to evaluate the kidney following treatment. Clinically, patients with subcapsular bleed-ing with or without a perinephric component following ESWL have per-sistent flank pain, and many patients require narcotics. A fall in hemo-globin values is common, and blood transfusions may be necessary in as many as one-third of patients with clinical evidence of this complication.

Renal arterial occlusion (Option (A)) certainly could cause anuria and hyperreninemic hypertension in a patient with a solitary kidney, but neither arterial thrombosis nor dissection causing occlusion is a recog-

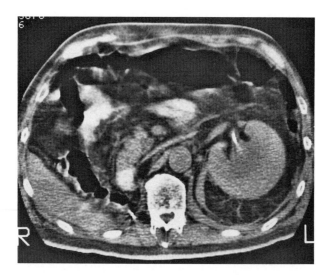

Figure 8-2. Same patient as in Figure 8-1. Unenhanced CT scan shows a left subcapsular hematoma. Note that the fresh blood has higher attenuation than does the more central compressed renal parenchyma. The perirenal fascia is thickened medially, and there is some prominence of perirenal fascial strands. The increased density in the renal pelvis is the upper end of a ureteral stent placed after ESWL to aid drainage.

nized complication of ESWL. Arterial occlusion would not be expected to result in an enlarged kidney.

Ureteral stents are frequently used during ESWL to facilitate drainage and stone fragment passage. The lack of hydronephrosis confirms that the patient is not suffering from an obstructive process, and thus failure to use a ureteral stent (Option (C)) is not the cause of the problem.

Renal vein thrombosis (Option (D)) of a solitary kidney would explain the anuria, hypertension, and enlarged kidney in the test patient. It is conceivable that severe parenchymal edema and hemorrhage might explain the compressed renal pelvis. Thus, these radiographic findings are compatible with severe renal vein thrombosis. However, renal vein thrombosis is not a reported complication of ESWL.

Steinstrasse (literally "stone street") (Option (E)) is a term that describes the filling of a length of ureter with stone fragments following ESWL (Figure 8-3). Steinstrasse may be associated with pain and obstruction. This complication of ESWL can be treated by appropriate ureteral stents or percutaneous nephrostomy. Placement of stents before ESWL decreases the incidence of symptomatic steinstrasse. There is no evidence of steinstrasse in the test patient's retrograde pyelogram.

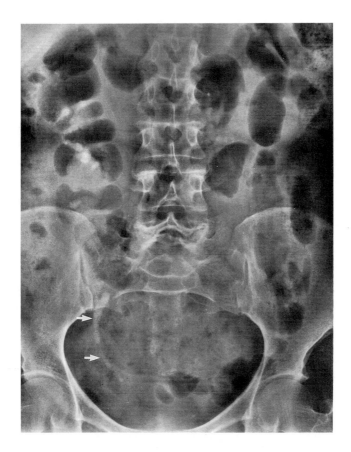

Figure 8-3. Steinstrasse. There are many small stone fragments in the distal right ureter (arrows). Fragments also remain in the collecting system.

Question 35

Concerning subcapsular hematomas after ESWL,

(A) Page kidney occasionally results
(B) they are more common with calyceal calculi
(C) preexisting hypertension is a risk factor
(D) surgical evacuation is the treatment of choice
(E) bleeding is from the capsular arteries

ESWL is associated with alterations in renal morphology. MRI indicates that more than 60% of patients have perirenal fluid, subcapsular hematomas, or loss of corticomedullary differentiation. The shock waves produced by ESWL affect the kidney like other forms of blunt renal trauma. The effects vary from simple edema to intrarenal, subcapsular, and perinephric hemorrhage. Several large series of patients treated with the HM3 Dornier lithotriptor have been evaluated by renal ultrasonography 24 hours after treatment. Knapp et al. evaluated 3,620 patients and reported a 0.66% frequency of subcapsular hematoma. These patients had normal coagulation profiles. The frequency of hematoma showed no correlation with the number of shocks administered or the size or weight of the patient. In addition, the size and location of the stone did not correlate with the formation of a hematoma **(Option (B) is false).** The frequency of subcapsular hematoma reported by Knapp et al. was 2.5% in patients with preexisting hypertension **(Option (C) is true)** and rose to 3.8% in patients whose hypertension had been poorly controlled. The site of bleeding is the renal parenchymal vessels **(Option (E) is false).** Thus, the bleeding is generally between the renal parenchyma and the true capsule. Rupture into the perinephric space is common. One-third of patients with hematoma in the series of Knapp et al. required blood transfusion, but surgical evacuation of the hematoma is rarely required **(Option (D) is false).** It is recommended that patients with subcapsular or perirenal hematoma be observed by sonography or CT to be sure that the collection has resolved. In addition, the blood pressure should be closely monitored. The combination of an organized hematoma and extrinsic pressure on the renal parenchyma can lead to ischemia with resultant increased renin formation: the so-called Page kidney **(Option (A) is true).** Clinical experience has shown that prelithotripsy urinary tract infections, as well as bilateral ESWL, increase the risk of developing a subcapsular hematoma.

CT is more sensitive than ultrasonography in demonstrating the renal and perirenal changes following ESWL. Rubin et al. reported the post-ESWL CT findings in 50 patients, including 3 with bilateral treatment. Eight (15%) had subcapsular hematomas, none of which were symptomatic. Two (4%) had small intrarenal hematomas. The overall size of the treated kidney also increased in 9% of patients. Thirty-seven of the treated renal fossae (70%) showed evidence of edema in the form of fascial thickening or "soft tissue stranding." Despite the high frequency of posttreatment findings on CT scans, ESWL is generally well tolerated, with significant permanent renal damage being quite rare.

Question 36

Concerning ureteral stents in ESWL,

T (A) insertion prior to the procedure is recommended for calculi larger than 2 cm
F (B) they provide a lumen for passage of the calculus fragments
T (C) they allow vesicoureteral reflux
F (D) they cause steinstrasse

It became apparent early in the course of clinical evaluation of ESWL that intervention to treat complications related to the passage of stone fragments was necessary in about 30% of patients. A popular method of providing urine drainage while stone fragments are being passed is to insert a ureteral stent. These stents are generally inserted just prior to the ESWL for stones 2 cm or larger **(Option (A) is true).** Stents not only provide a lumen for the passage of urine down the ureter, but they also allow the stone fragment to pass between the outer stent wall and the ureter **(Option (B) is false).** Ureteral stents of the double-J or double-pigtail variety allow free reflux of urine into the renal pelvis **(Option (C) is true).** This may aid the passage of stone fragments by increasing the amount of antegrade urine flow. Since the stent relieves or prevents obstruction, patients with stents inserted are generally free of renal colic while they pass the post-ESWL stone fragments. Two additional benefits of ureteral stents often cited by those administering the treatment are related to localization of the calculus: (1) the stent provides a target adjacent to stones that are poorly visualized during treatments done under fluoroscopic guidance, and (2) the stent prevents migration of the calculus just prior to therapy. Stents may cause local bladder irritation. In addition, some patients may experience flank pain associated with reflux during the elevated bladder pressure that accompanies micturition. Preminger et al. questioned the accepted routine use of stents in patients undergoing ESWL for calculi 3 cm or smaller. They cited a higher prevalence of bladder irritation, hematuria, and urinary frequency in the patients with ureteral stents. The stone-free rate was the same in patients treated with and without stents. However, Preminger et al. continued to support the use of stents in patients with larger stone burdens or solitary kidneys.

Steinstrasse is not a result of the placement of a ureteral stent **(Option (D) is false).** It may occur with or without a stent in the ureter (Figure 8-4). It appears that stone fragments are less likely to impact in patients with ureteral stents.

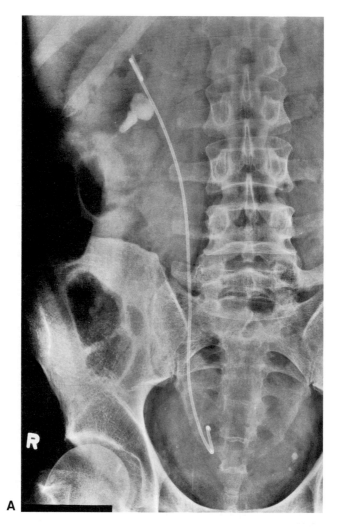

Figure 8-4. Use of ureteral stent in conjunction with ESWL. (A) Pre-ESWL. There is a large calculus occupying the renal pelvis and extending into the lower pole. A double-pigtail stent was inserted just prior to ESWL. (B) Post-ESWL. Some fragments remain in the lower pole. There is a steinstrasse in the distal right ureter just lateral to the sacrum (arrows).

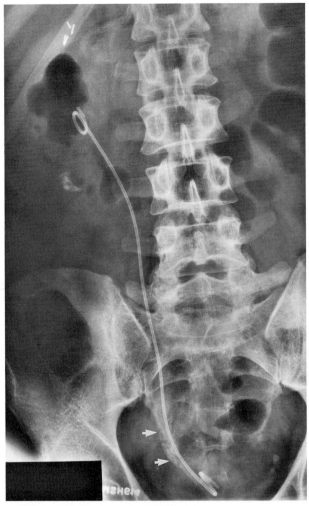

B

Question 37

Concerning ESWL,

T (A) new stones will form in up to 8% of patients by 1 year after treatment
F (B) associated hematuria is primarily due to ureteral passage of stone fragments
F (C) persistent hypertension is a complication in 15% of patients
F (D) it has virtually eliminated percutaneous nephrostolithotomy for staghorn calculi

Extracorporeal shock wave lithotriptors consist of four basic parts: (1) a stone localization system, (2) a shock wave source, (3) a shock wave focusing device, and (4) a coupling medium. The original HM3 Dornier lithotriptor produces the shock waves by means of a spark-gap electrode immersed in a water bath. The shock waves are focused by a semiellipsoidal reflector. The patient is placed in the water bath (coupling medium) in a supine position so that the flank is submerged. In this way, the shock wave travels through water and is focused on the fluoroscopically localized stone.

There are now a variety of commercially available machines with different localization systems. Technomed, Northgate, EDAP, and Wolf lithotriptors use ultrasound as a means of localization. Different methods of generating a shock wave are also available. The Siemens Lithostar has an electromagnetic source, whereas the EDAP and Wolf machines use a piezoelectric energy source. The coupling mediums now available include water cushions, water basins, and gel disks.

Most upper urinary tract stones requiring treatment are treated by ESWL or a combination of ESWL and percutaneous techniques. Fewer than 5% of patients come to open surgery in centers where these methods are available.

The early success rate reported for ESWL therapy of renal calculi is quite good, with 90% of patients being stone-free within 3 months after treatment for 1-cm calculi. However, ESWL is less successful in achieving a stone-free state when it is the only means of treating patients with larger calculi, such as staghorn stones. Only 50% of these patients are stone-free 3 months after treatment. Post-ESWL monitoring shows that new stones form in up to 8% of patients followed for 1 year **(Option (A) is true)**. Residual stone fragments increase in size in about 25% of patients monitored for 2 years after ESWL.

Transient decreases in renal function in the treated kidney have been reported. Function returns to normal by 3 weeks after ESWL. Mild abdominal distension due to colonic ileus occurs frequently and usually resolves within 48 hours after treatment.

Transient hematuria occurs in most patients who undergo ESWL. This is due to the direct effect of the shock waves on the renal parenchyma and epithelium **(Option (B) is false)**. Some patients may experience hematuria due to passage of stone fragments, but the parenchymal source of bleeding is more common.

There has been great concern about the long-term effects of ESWL on the renal parenchyma. Thus far, the major long-term adverse effect is suspected to be the development of hypertension. The frequency of hypertension has been reported to be as high as 8% **(Option (C) is false)** 2 years following treatment. These reports have been open to question for a variety of reasons, including the variations in the incidence of

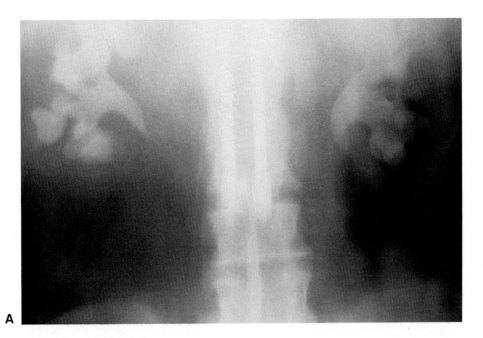

A

Figure 8-5. ESWL of left staghorn calculus in a 39-year-old paraplegic man. (A) Tomogram reveals bilateral staghorn calculi. (B) Radiograph obtained following two sessions of ESWL on the left. Fine gravel is present in the collecting system. A percutaneous nephrostomy tube is in place. (C) Radiograph obtained following a third session of ESWL on the left and a single session on the right. The left system is essentially stone-free. The pelvic portion of the right staghorn calculus has been treated.

new-onset hypertension reported in the general population. In any event, there is agreement that a prospective randomized study is needed to determine whether the incidence of new hypertension is greater in patients undergoing ESWL than it is in the general population.

Since ESWL therapy alone for staghorn calculi is difficult (Figure 8-5), many centers use percutaneous nephrostolithotomy as a means of debulking large calculi **(Option (D) is false).** This is followed by ESWL of the fragments. Most of these patients also have ureteral stents inserted to aid the passage of fragments.

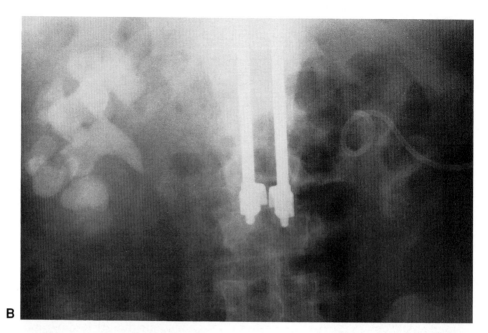

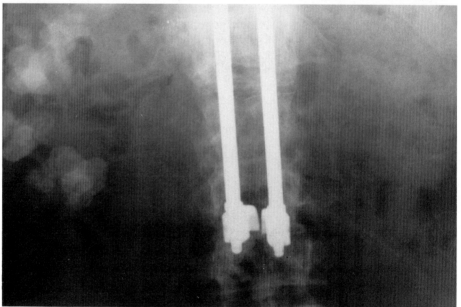

Questions 38 through 41

For each of the calculi listed below (Questions 38 through 41), select the *one* lettered therapeutic approach (A, B, C, D, or E) that is MOST effective. Each lettered therapy may be used once, more than once, or not at all.

C 38. A 4-cm uric acid calculus in the renal pelvis
E 39. A 4-cm struvite calculus in the renal pelvis
D 40. A 2-mm calcium phosphate ureteral calculus
A 41. A 4-cm calcium oxalate calculus in the renal pelvis

    (A) Stent, then ESWL
    (B) Ureteroscopy
    (C) Sodium bicarbonate
    (D) No intervention
    (E) Antibiotics, stent, then ESWL

Uric acid calculi may be treated effectively by alkalinizing the urine. Sodium bicarbonate solution may also be infused directly into the kidney so that the stone is bathed in the alkaline solution **(Option (C) is the correct answer to Question 38).** When this approach is used, a catheter for infusion is placed with its end hole directed on the stone. A percutaneous nephrostomy is left in place to allow drainage of the infused solution (Figure 8-6). Since uric acid stones are nonopaque, they do not lend themselves to fluoroscopy-guided ESWL. A uric acid calculus is a physically hard calculus, which does not fragment easily.

A 4-cm struvite calculus can be fragmented effectively with ESWL. Since struvite calculi are associated with infection (*Proteus mirabilis* in 72% of cases), appropriate antibiotic treatment is indicated before, during, and after ESWL until the patient is stone-free. Urease-producing bacteria are found in the stone interstices and will lead to new stone growth if all fragments are not passed **(Option (E) is the correct answer to Question 39).** In most centers, a double-J stent also would be inserted before ESWL of a kidney containing a stone of this size.

The number of modalities and devices available to aid in the treatment of renal calculi continues to increase. However, not all calculi require intervention. A 2-mm calcium phosphate calculus will most probably pass spontaneously **(Option (D) is the correct answer to Question 40).** Intervention in the form of a ureteral catheter may be necessary if the patient experiences incapacitating pain or spontaneous extravasation into the renal sinus from a ruptured fornix. Infection superimposed on a blocked ureter requires prompt drainage via percutaneous nephrostomy, as well as antibiotic treatment. Ureteroscopic retrieval, ultrasonic litho-

struvite = Proteus infxn

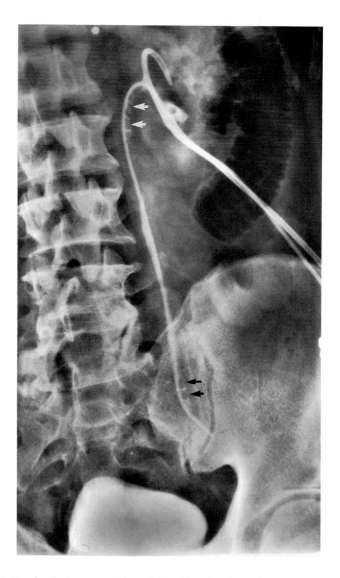

Figure 8-6. Catheters positioned for dissolution of uric acid calculi. The catheter used for infusion of sodium bicarbonate solution is in the ureter at the level of an obstructing calculus. Other lucent calculi are seen (arrows) following injection of contrast material. The proximal nephrostomy tube serves as a route for drainage of both the infused solution and urine.

tripsy, and laser lithotripsy are alternative treatments for impacted ureteral calculi.

Calcium oxalate calculi are usually treated by ESWL if they are too large to pass spontaneously. A 4-cm stone of this composition would be treated by ESWL. A ureteral stent would be used in most centers **(Option (A) is the correct answer to Question 41).**

Harold A. Mitty, M.D.

SUGGESTED READINGS

SUBCAPSULAR HEMATOMA

1. Kaude JV, Williams CM, Millner MR, Scott KN, Finlayson B. Renal morphology and function immediately after extracorporeal shock-wave lithotripsy. AJR 1985; 143:305–313
2. Knapp PM, Kulb TB, Lingeman JE, et al. Extracorporeal shock wave lithotripsy-induced perirenal hematomas. J Urol 1988; 139:700–703
3. Lingeman JE, McAteer JA, Kempson SA, Evan AP. Bioeffects of extracorporeal shock-wave lithotripsy. Strategy for research and treatment. Urol Clin North Am 1988; 15:507–514
4. Rubin JI, Arger PH, Pollack HM, et al. Kidney changes after extracorporeal shock wave lithotripsy: CT evaluation. Radiology 1987; 162:21–24

URETERAL STENTS

5. Bregg K, Riehle RA Jr. Morbidity associated with indwelling ureteral stents after shock wave lithotripsy. J Urol 1989; 141:510–512
6. Fine H, Gordon RL, Lebensart PD. Extracorporeal shock wave lithotripsy and stents: fluoroscopic observations and a hypothesis on the mechanisms of stent function. Urol Radiol 1989; 11:37–41
7. Libby JM, Meacham RB, Griffith DP. The role of silicone ureteral stents in extracorporeal shock wave lithotripsy of large renal calculi. J Urol 1988; 139:15–17
8. Pollard SG, Mcfarlane R. Symptoms arising from double-J ureteral stents. J Urol 1988; 139:37–38
9. Preminger GM, Kettelhut MC, Elkins SL, Seger J, Fetner CD. Ureteral stenting during extracorporeal shock wave lithotripsy: help or hindrance? J Urol 1989; 142:32–36
10. Shore N, Somers W, Riehle RA Jr. Evolution of pre-treatment stenting and local anesthesia for extracorporeal shock wave lithotripsy at a single university center. J Urol 1990; 143:257–260

EXTRACORPOREAL SHOCK WAVE LITHOTRIPSY

11. Chaussy CG, Fuchs GJ. Current state and future developments of noninvasive treatment of human urinary stones with extracorporeal shock wave lithotripsy. J Urol 1989; 141:782–789
12. Cochran ST. Extracorporeal shock wave lithotripsy: clinical results. Urol Radiol 1988; 10:46–47
13. Grantham JR, Millner MR, Kaude JV, Finlayson B, Hunter PT II, Newman RC. Renal stone disease treated with extracorporeal shock wave lithotripsy: short-term observations in 100 patients. Radiology 1986; 158:203–206
14. Lingeman JE, Woods JR, Toth PD. Blood pressure changes following extracorporeal shock wave lithotripsy and other forms of treatment for nephrolithiasis. JAMA 1990; 263:1789–1794
15. Newman DM, Scott JW, Lingeman JE. Two-year follow-up of patients treated with extracorporeal shock wave lithotripsy. J Endourol 1988; 3:163–171
16. Pfister RC, Papanicolaou N, Yoder IC. Urinary extracorporeal shock wave lithotripsy: equipment, techniques, and overview. Urol Radiol 1988; 10:39–45

RENAL CALCULUS

17. Fuchs GJ, Chaussy CG, Stenzl A. Current management concepts in the treatment of ureteral stones. J Endourol 1988; 2:119–121
18. Lerner SP, Gleeson MJ, Griffith DP. Infection stones. J Urol 1989; 141:753–758
19. Rodman JS. Prophylaxis of uric acid stones with alternate day doses of alkaline potassium salts. J Urol 1991; 145:97–99
20. Smith LH. The medical aspects of urolithiasis: an overview. J Urol 1989; 141:707–710
21. Winfield HN, Clayman RV, Chaussy CG, Weyman PJ, Fuchs GJ, Lupu AN. Monotherapy of staghorn renal calculi: a comparative study between percutaneous nephrolithotomy and extracorporeal shock wave lithotripsy. J Urol 1988; 139:895–899

Notes

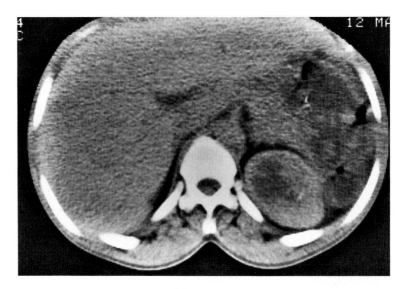

Figure 9-1

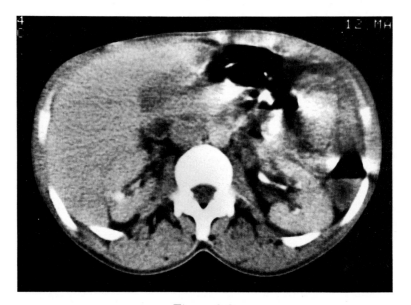

Figure 9-2
Figures 9-1 and 9-2. This 40-year-old man with diabetes mellitus presented with left flank pain and fever. You are shown two contrast-enhanced CT scans.

Case 9: Renal Abscess

Question 42

Which *one* of the following is the MOST likely diagnosis?

(A) Necrotic renal cell carcinoma
(B) Focal acute pyelonephritis
(C) Abscess
(D) Segmental infarction
(E) Focal xanthogranulomatous pyelonephritis

The enhanced CT scan (Figure 9-1) demonstrates an irregular low-attenuation area in the medial aspect of the upper pole of the kidney. (This area can be considered to be unenhanced water density consistent with fluid, necrotic tissue, or pus.) The renal contour appears smooth, and the perirenal fat is not involved. Figure 9-2 is from the same study at the level of the renal hilum. There is normal renal opacification, with a nondilated collecting system. The CT findings in a diabetic patient with flank pain and fever are most consistent with a renal abscess **(Option (C) is correct).**

The diagnosis of necrotic renal cell carcinoma (Option (A)) cannot be excluded solely on the basis of the CT findings, even though there is no discrete renal mass on the test images. Renal cell carcinomas may have the appearance of necrotic cystic masses on CT (Figure 9-3). The wall of a cystic-appearing renal cell carcinoma may represent non-necrotic residual tumor, adjacent normal parenchyma, or both. Similarly, an abscess may produce an enhancing wall as a result of peripheral granulation tissue, compressed adjacent parenchyma, or both. Figure 9-1 shows an irregular interface rather than a discrete wall. It is unlikely that the lesion is composed totally of necrotic tumor. In addition, the age and clinical history of the test patient are less consistent with the diagnosis of renal cell carcinoma than with renal abscess.

Renal cell carcinoma is most common among patients 50 to 70 years old, with a median age at onset of 57 years. The classic presenting signs

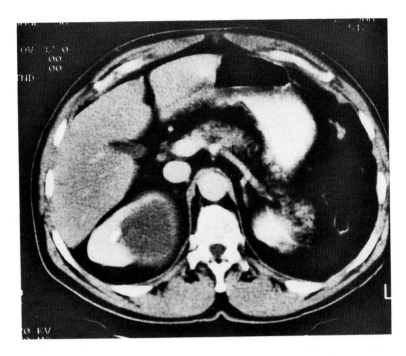

Figure 9-3. Necrotic renal cell carcinoma. This contrast-enhanced CT scan demonstrates a low-attenuation mass density in the medial aspect of the upper pole of the right kidney. The medial wall proved to be a combination of tumor and parenchyma.

of flank pain, hematuria, and a palpable mass are encountered in only 10% of cases. More often, only one of these signs is present. In fact, the widespread use of CT and sonography has led to the detection of 25% of cases in patients with no genitourinary tract symptoms.

The clinical features of focal acute pyelonephritis (Option (B)) are often the same as those of a renal abscess. Untreated pyelonephritis may progress to abscess formation. However, with acute focal pyelonephritis the excretory urogram appears normal in 75% of cases. Twenty percent of patients will have some smooth renal enlargement on the urogram. This may be difficult to appreciate since a prior study is rarely available during the acute phase. Patients who have significant parenchymal involvement by the inflammatory process may have diminished opacification. This finding is present in 15% of cases. A striated nephrogram has been described as a rare finding in acute pyelonephritis. This is most likely to be detected when tomography is part of the urographic study. The appearance is due to the presence of inflammatory cells, edema, and

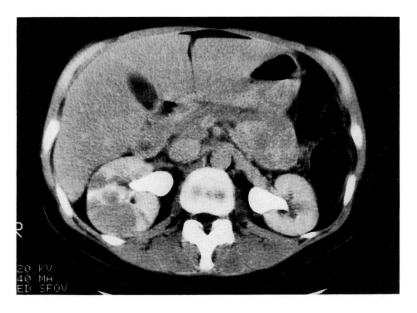

Figure 9-4. Focal acute pyelonephritis. On this postcontrast CT scan, the right kidney is swollen and contains focal areas of decreased attenuation (without liquefaction). There is no obstruction.

vasospasm alternating with areas of functioning parenchyma. Another rare finding is edema of the normally smooth renal pelvis, which gives the renal pelvis a nodular or tree-bark appearance. Dilatation of the collecting system and ureter, which is a form of nonobstructing hydronephrosis, occurs infrequently. This finding is due to atony of the collecting system in response to the acute process. The most common CT pattern of acute pyelonephritis is that of zones of diminished attenuation on a contrast-enhanced scan (Figure 9-4). A more severe form of this process described on CT scans has been called focal bacterial nephritis. The area of involvement is typically rounded and still enhances but is 20 to 40 HU less than the adjacent normal parenchyma. In addition, lower-density zones due to liquefaction may be present. These zones may resolve with treatment or may coalesce to form a frank abscess. Abscesses are well-marginated low-attenuation masses. The liquified purulent material does not enhance (Figure 9-1). CT is the best method of establishing the extent of inflammatory processes, but CT findings are not specific for inflammation. Other conditions that may mimic renal inflammatory conditions include lymphoma, infarction, necrotic tumor, metastatic tumor, and renal vein thrombosis. For this reason, the CT

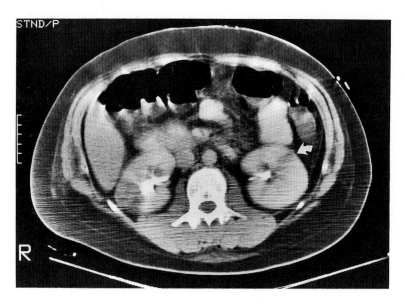

Figure 9-5. Segmental renal infarction. This patient had a history of heart disease. This contrast-enhanced CT scan was performed because the patient was experiencing flank pain. Note the area of decreased enhancement at the posterolateral aspect of the right kidney. A smaller area of decreased enhancement is seen anteriorly on the left (arrow).

findings must be correlated with the clinical and laboratory findings to arrive at the correct diagnosis. Sonography detects acute pyelonephritis and focal bacterial nephritis as areas of decreased echogenicity. This is due to the presence of edema fluid within the normal tissue. This process also results in loss of the normal corticomedullary junction on the sonogram. Sonography of a renal abscess demonstrates fluid accumulation within a mass. Internal echoes that move with change of position represent debris within the cavity. It is important to remember that hemorrhagic or infected cysts and necrotic renal tumors may have a similar sonographic appearance.

Segmental infarction (Option (D)) is most commonly due to embolism in patients with heart disease. Thrombotic causes include sickle cell disease and vasculitis of various types. Trauma with occlusion of the main renal artery or one of its branches is a common cause encountered in institutions with active trauma services. A cortical rim sign is seen in about 50% of cases of segmental or global renal infarction. This represents maintained peripheral cortical perfusion because of collateral flow to the renal parenchyma via the renal capsular, peripelvic, and periureteric branches in the presence of renal artery occlusion. The cortical rim sign may be seen on nephrotomography, but it is best demonstrated on CT due to the higher contrast resolution of this modality. On contrast-enhanced CT, segmental infarction typically appears as a wedge-shaped zone of decreased attenuation without significant associated mass effect or parenchymal fluid accumulation (Figure 9-5). This appearance may be difficult to differentiate from areas of acute pyelonephritis. Clinical correlation is mandatory. Subcapsular fluid collections were seen in 21% of patients with infarctions described by Wong et al. They believed that this was most likely the residuum of a hemorrhagic component of the infarct. They also noted that 6% of their patients had thickened renal fascia associated with the infarction. Ultrasonography may show no abnormality in acute renal infarctions unless a Doppler examination is performed as well (Figure 9-6). The typical wedge-shaped peripheral defect in the renal cortex is due to absent perfusion via the obstructed vessel. This defect may be well shown by renal cortical scintigraphy with either Tc-99m glucoheptonate or Tc-99m dimercaptosuccinic acid.

Focal xanthogranulomatous pyelonephritis (Option (E)) is usually recognized by the presence of one or more dilated calyces, most often associated with an obstructing stone. The kidney is usually enlarged in the area of the disease, although the reniform shape is often maintained.

Urinary tract infection is common, but the complication of renal abscess occurs most often in patients with predisposing factors such as calculi, immunosuppression, and diabetes mellitus. The excretory urogram usually shows a mass. The sonographic pattern is variable and depends on the degree of liquefaction of the contents of the abscess. The wall of an abscess is not as sharply defined as that of a simple cyst. It may be difficult to distinguish between necrotic tumor and abscess even on CT examination. Soulen et al. have shown that both history and follow-up CT studies are important when evaluating some of these patients. Focal or diffuse swelling was present in 12 of their 17 patients. This swelling persisted in 6 of 7 patients rescanned within 2 weeks and in all 4 patients rescanned at 2 to 4 weeks. In doubtful cases, percutaneous aspiration to confirm the presence of pus may be vital for diagnosis and management. In any event, percutaneous drainage has revolutionized the treatment of patients with renal abscesses.

Figure 9-7 shows the drainage catheter placed in the abscess cavity in the test patient. Following 5 days of percutaneous drainage and 2 weeks of antibiotic therapy, no further intervention was necessary.

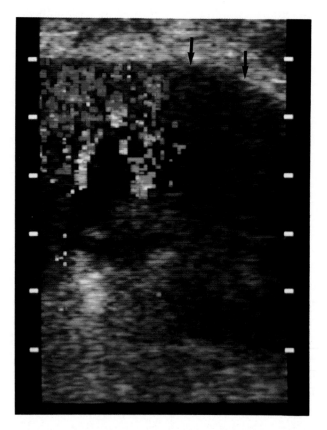

Figure 9-6. Longitudinal color-flow Doppler sonogram of segmental renal infarction in a transplanted kidney. The color-flow pattern of the perfused portion of the kidney is seen on the left side of the image. An area with absent flow (arrows) is seen on the right.

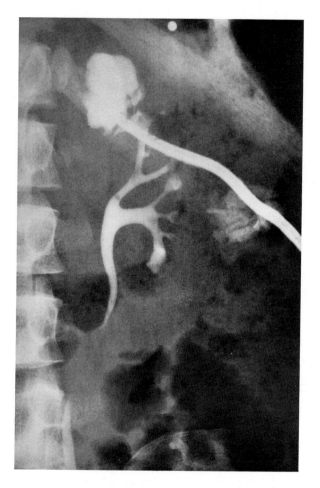

Figure 9-7. Same patient as in Figures 9-1 and 9-2. Abscess drainage. This urogram of the test patient shows a sump catheter in the abscess at the upper pole. The cavity has been opacificed by injection of contrast material through the catheter.

Question 43

Concerning renal abscess,

T (A) percutaneous drainage is effective in about 60% of cases
F (B) when it is associated with struvite calculi, *Klebsiella pneumoniae* is the most common organism
F (C) it is a hematogenous infection in most patients
F (D) perinephric involvement is present in fewer than 10% of cases

Although percutaneous drainage of renal abscesses has become the treatment of choice, only a few large series of patients have been reported. Sacks et al. described a series of 18 patients with renal and related retroperitoneal abscesses. The indications for percutaneous drainage included failure to respond to parenteral antibiotic treatment and persistent fever and leukocytosis. Half of their patients had extension to the perirenal space, pararenal space, or the psoas muscle. The decision to perform percutaneous drainage is based on finding a safe route of access for catheter placement as demonstrated by CT. The pleural space or peritoneal cavity should not be traversed. Organs at risk include the liver on the right and the spleen on the left. Sacks described one case of erosion of the drainage catheter into the adjacent duodenum. One patient had urosepsis and another had transient fever associated with the catheter manipulations. The extent of success of the percutaneous route depends to a large degree on the associated underlying problem. For example, abscesses associated with calculi will not respond favorably if the calculi are not adequately treated. Often, the associated renal damage necessitates nephrectomy or partial nephrectomy once the abscess is controlled. Similarly, an immunosuppressed patient is more prone to recurrence of the abscess. Sacks et al. reported successful management with only percutaneous drainage and antibiotic therapy in 11 of 18 patients (61%) with renal abscesses **(Option (A) is true).**

The organism responsible for most renal abscesses is *Escherichia coli* or *Proteus mirabilis*. *Klebsiella pneumoniae* has also been reported as a less common cause in some series. When there are associated struvite calculi, *Proteus mirabilis* is the most common cause of the abscess **(Option (B) is false).**

Most renal infection occurs in women 20 to 40 years old. The infection begins in the lower urinary tract and ascends to the kidney. Patients with the additional complication of diabetes mellitus, corticosteroid therapy, or immunosuppression are likely to have more-severe renal infections that can progress to abscess formation. The abscesses that form

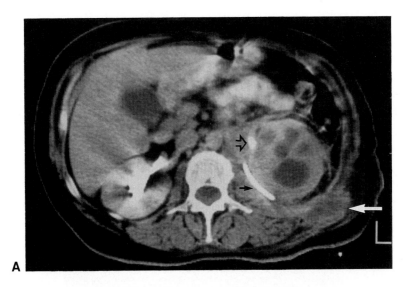

Figure 9-8. Pyonephrosis with perinephric abscess. Initial drainage of pus was performed, and an 8 French drainage tube was inserted. An antegrade study was not performed because of concern about distending an infected system and causing sepsis. (A) CT scan. The left kidney has multiple lucent areas in the parenchyma, which represent dilated calyces as well as abscesses. The drainage tube (black arrow) is in the expanded perirenal space. A calculus is seen in the medial aspect of the kidney (open arrow). The posterior pararenal space and subcutaneous tissue also show a mixed-attenuation collection (white arrow). (B) Abdominal radiograph after placement of tube in the kidney. The more medial tube is in the perinephric space and corresponds to the tube on the CT scan. The upper tube is in the pyonephrotic collecting system. Two renal calculi are also seen. This kidney was eventually removed. There were diffuse xantho-granulomatous changes, as well as cortical abscesses and the pyo-nephrosis.

begin as ascending urinary tract infections **(Option (C) is false).** The hematogenous route of infection is more likely in patients with a history of intravenous drug abuse. Staphylococcal infections are often of hema-togenous origin and are more likely to cause cavitation than infections with other organisms.

Renal abscesses have perinephric extension in 50% of cases when they present clinically **(Option (D) is false).** Drainage of both the intrarenal and perinephric components is often necessary (Figure 9-8). Conservative medical management is an option in selected patients who respond to antibiotics. Soulen et al. reported that 8 of 13 patients with renal ab-scesses responded to antibiotics alone. Serial CT or sonographic examina-

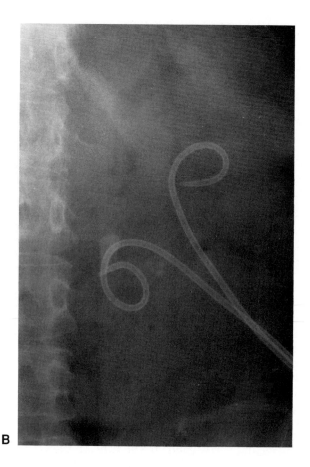

B

tions are necessary to confirm resolution of the condition (Figure 9-9). Swelling and areas of changing enhancement may persist for months. New scars may eventually appear on CT examination in as many as 50% of patients who have acute infections with or without abscess formation. This reflects the greater sensitivity of CT as compared to excretory urography as a means of demonstrating changes in the cortical contour.

Percutaneous drainage can be performed under CT, sonographic, or fluoroscopic guidance. The type of catheter used for drainage depends on the size of the cavity and the preference of the operator. For example, 8 French pigtail catheters can be adequate for small liquid collections, whereas larger collections may require 12 to 16 French sump catheters (Figure 9-7). Excessive injection of contrast material during the initial drainage should be avoided because it may cause bacteremia and septic shock. Catheters can be left in place with simple drainage into a collection

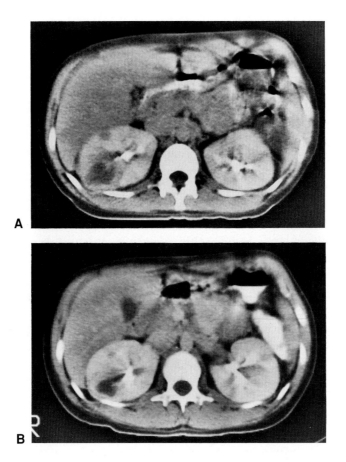

Figure 9-9. Serial CT scans of a renal abscess treated by antibiotics. (A) The first pretreatment CT scan demonstrates an area of low attenuation and liquefaction in the posterolateral aspect of the swollen right kidney. A similar, smaller area is seen anteriorly. (B) Two weeks later, after administration of antibiotics, the swelling has diminished. The area of liquefaction is smaller and sharply circumscribed. The anterior lesion is also considerably smaller.

bag. Irrigation is usually not necessary. When resolution of the collection has been confirmed by appropriate imaging studies, the drainage tube may be removed. The usual period of drainage is 1 to 4 weeks, depending on the size of the collection. Antibiotic therapy is continued during drainage.

Question 44

Concerning xanthogranulomatous pyelonephritis,

T (A) it usually occurs in the presence of calculi and obstruction
T (B) a common predisposing organism is *Proteus mirabilis*
T (C) perinephric extension is common
F (D) the tumefactive variety is the most common form

Xanthogranulomatous pyelonephritis is characterized by destruction of renal parenchyma and by the presence of lipid-laden macrophages. Chronic infection, which is usually associated with collecting system calculi and obstruction, leads to this chronic granulomatous process. The cells of chronic infection include lymphocytes, fibroblasts, histiocytes, and giant cells. Histiocytes, or macrophages, engulf debris and organisms related to the process. The characteristic histiocyte in xanthogranulomatous pyelonephritis is the xanthoma cell, which is a lipid-laden macrophage. These cells accumulate in the destroyed parenchyma as yellowish deposits. This xanthogranulomatous process may also extend into the perinephric and posterior pararenal spaces. Patients most commonly present with pain and signs of urinary tract infection, including dysuria, nocturia, and leukocytosis. A palpable mass is present in approximately 50% of cases. The most common predisposing organisms are *Proteus mirabilis* and *Escherichia coli* (**Option (B) is true**).

The excretory urogram usually demonstrates one or more renal calculi and poor renal function. Sonography and CT will confirm the presence of calculi and obstruction (**Option (A) is true**) in most cases. Pararenal and perirenal space involvement has been reported to be common (**Option (C) is true**). Of 18 patients reported by Goldman et al. in 1984, 11 had perirenal involvement and 13 had pararenal extension. CT most often reveals replacement of the normal parenchyma by low-density areas corresponding to the dilated obstructed calyces (Figure 9-10). Enhancing rims may be present; they correspond to compressed normal parenchyma, inflammatory granulation tissue, or both. Since perinephric and pararenal space involvement is common, particular attention to the extent of disease is important. Focal or tumefactive xanthogranulomatous pyelonephritis is a less common form; it may occur when only a portion of the kidney is involved (**Option (D) is false**). This may be due to local intrarenal obstruction by a calculus or involvement of one moiety of a duplication.

Therapy is usually surgical. The resected kidneys contain calculi and dilated calyces. Sheets of lipid-laden macrophages result in characteristic

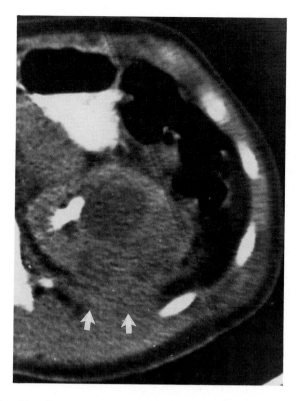

Figure 9-10. Focal xanthogranulomatous pyelonephritis. There is an area of decreased attenuation representing a focal dilated calyx proximal to the medially situated calculus. The posterior aspect of the renal capsule and Gerota's fascia are adherent as a result of extension of disease into the posterior pararenal space (arrows). (Reprinted with permission from Goldman et al. [11].)

yellowish deposits in the parenchyma adjacent to the calyces. Extension of this granulomatous material into the perinephric space, as well as involvement of the psoas muscle and soft tissues of the flank, is common.

Harold A. Mitty, M.D.

ABSCESS

1. Bernardino ME, Baumgartner BR. Abscess drainage in the genitourinary tract. Radiol Clin North Am 1986; 24:539–549
2. Gordon DH, Macchia RJ, Glanz S, Koser MW, Laungani GB. Percutaneous management of retroperitoneal abscesses. Urology 1987; 30:299–306
3. Sacks D, Banner MP, Meranze SG, Burke DR, Robinson M, McLean GK. Renal and related retroperitoneal abscesses: percutaneous drainage. Radiology 1988; 167:447–451
4. Soulen MC, Fishman EK, Goldman SM, Gatewood OM. Bacterial renal infection: role of CT. Radiology 1989; 171:703–707

FOCAL ACUTE PYELONEPHRITIS

5. Gold RP, McClennan BL. Acute infections of the renal parenchyma. In: Pollack HM (ed), Clinical urography. Philadelphia: WB Saunders; 1990:799–821
6. Goldman SM. Acute and chronic urinary infection: present concepts and controversies. Urol Radiol 1988; 10:17–24
7. Rosenfield AT, Glickman MG, Taylor KJ, Crade M, Hodson J. Acute focal bacterial nephritis (acute lobar nephronia). Radiology 1979; 132:553–561
8. Soulen MC, Fishman EK, Goldman SM. Sequelae of acute renal infections: CT evaluation. Radiology 1989; 173:423–426

INFARCTION

9. Freeman LM, Zuckier LS, Lutzker LG, Rosenthall L. Anatomic lesions of the kidney. In: Blaufox MD (ed), Evaluation of renal function and disease with radionuclides: the upper urinary tract, 2nd ed. Basel: Karger; 1989:350–372
10. Wong WS, Moss AA, Federle MP, Cochran ST, London SS. Renal infarction: CT diagnosis and correlation between CT findings and etiologies. Radiology 1984; 150:201–205

XANTHOGRANULOMATOUS PYELONEPHRITIS

11. Goldman SM, Hartman DS, Fishman EK, Finizio JP, Gatewood OM, Siegelman SS. CT of xanthogranulomatous pyelonephritis; radiologic-pathologic correlation. AJR 1984; 142:963–969
12. Hartman DS, Davis CJ Jr, Goldman SM, Isbister SS, Sanders RS. Xanthogranulomatous pyelonephritis sonographic–pathologic correlation of 16 cases. J Ultrasound Med 1984; 3:481–488
13. Subramanyam BR, Megibow AJ, Raghavendra BN, Bosniak MA. Diffuse xanthogranulomatous pyelonephritis: analysis by computed tomography and sonography. Urol Radiol 1982; 4:5–9

Notes

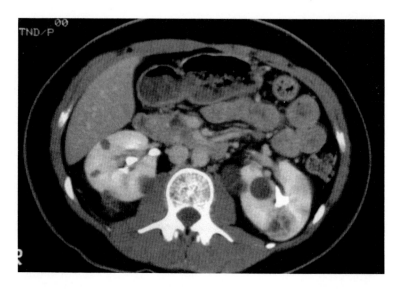

Figure 10-1. This 35-year-old woman has hematuria. You are shown a contrast-enhanced abdominal CT scan.

Case 10: von Hippel-Lindau Disease

Question 45

Which *one* of the following is the MOST likely diagnosis?

(A) Autosomal dominant polycystic kidney disease
(B) Acquired cystic kidney disease
(C) von Hippel-Lindau disease
(D) Tuberous sclerosis
(E) Multilocular cystic nephroma

The contrast-enhanced abdominal CT examination (Figure 10-1) reveals both solid and cystic renal masses in both kidneys. Since simple cortical renal cysts are common, it is possible that they are unrelated to the solid masses. However, the young age of the patient and the multiplicity of the renal cysts argue against this. The differential diagnosis of both solid renal neoplasms and renal cysts includes tuberous sclerosis, von Hippel-Lindau disease, and acquired cystic kidney disease.

The solid neoplasms of tuberous sclerosis are angiomyolipomas, which are usually recognized by the low density of the fatty component. There is no evidence for a fatty component in the solid lesions seen in Figure 10-1. Acquired cystic kidney disease occurs in patients with chronic renal failure. The normal renal size and normal renal function evidenced by parenchymal opacification and contrast excretion in the test image exclude chronic renal failure. The low-density area in the liver indicates focal fatty infiltration and is unrelated. Thus, von Hippel-Lindau disease is the most likely diagnosis **(Option (C) is correct).**

Patients with autosomal dominant polycystic kidney disease (Option (A)) may present with hematuria but do not have solid renal neoplasms. The kidneys are riddled with parenchymal cysts of various sizes and are usually markedly enlarged.

Acquired cystic kidney disease (Option (B)) is seen in patients with renal failure. The cysts may be present in patients who have never been on dialysis, but they continue to increase in size and number after dialysis has been instituted. Presumably, they are caused by an endogenous

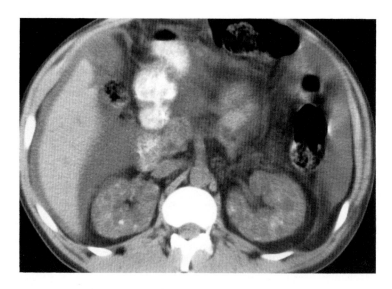

Figure 10-2. Acquired cystic kidney disease. An unenhanced abdominal CT scan demonstrates multiple small cysts and dystrophic calcification. The patient is on chronic ambulatory peritoneal dialysis, and fluid is seen in the peritoneal cavity.

substance that is not removed by either hemodialysis or peritoneal dialysis. There is also an increased incidence of solid neoplasms, which are found in as many as 7% of patients with acquired cystic disease. However, only about half of these neoplasms are histologically malignant. Even those with malignant features on histologic examination do not seem as biologically aggressive as sporadic renal adenocarcinomas. The kidneys are small, which reflects the chronic renal failure. Multiple small cysts are detected by either CT or sonography. Dystrophic calcification is common (Figure 10-2). Intravenous contrast material is often not used because of the renal failure, and this makes detection of the occasional solid neoplasm difficult.

Tuberous sclerosis (Option (D)) is a multisystem disease that includes both cutaneous and neurologic manifestations. It is inherited as an autosomal dominant trait with variable expressivity. The syndrome includes epilepsy, mental retardation, retinal phakomas, adenoma sebaceum, and various hamartomas. Approximately 80% of patients with the tuberous sclerosis syndrome have renal angiomyolipomas, and renal cysts are common.

A multilocular cystic nephroma (Option (E)) is a congenital renal lesion, which is not genetically transmitted. Male and female patients are affected equally; however, boys are usually younger than 2 years of age when affected and present with an abdominal mass. Almost 90% of female patients are over 4 years of age when the lesion is detected, often as an incidental finding. Unlike the findings in the test patient, the cystic mass of a multilocular cystic nephroma is usually solitary and unilateral.

Question 46

Patients with autosomal dominant polycystic kidney disease have an increased incidence of:

T (A) hypertension
T (B) renal infection
F (C) renal adenocarcinoma
T (D) berry aneurysms
F (E) hepatic fibrosis

Autosomal dominant polycystic kidney disease (ADPKD) is the most common inherited form of renal disease and is the underlying disease in 5 to 12% of patients on chronic dialysis. Although ADPKD is transmitted as an autosomal dominant trait, the variable expressivity and occasional spontaneous mutations of the responsible gene mean that as many as 50% of patients have no family history of ADPKD.

Since the disease is genetically transmitted, it is important to make the diagnosis before patients reach childbearing age. Since renal cysts occur in only 0.2% of children, their identification in an individual with a family history of ADPKD is strongly suggestive. Sonography has largely replaced excretory urography for this purpose.

Patients most often present during the fourth or fifth decade, complaining of abdominal or flank pain. The enlarged kidneys are often palpable. Innumerable cysts of various sizes are seen throughout the renal parenchyma (Figure 10-3). Hypertension occurs in over half the patients with ADPKD **(Option (A) is true)** and is most often due to increased renin production by the kidneys.

There is an increased incidence of renal infection in patients with ADPKD **(Option (B) is true).** Experimental evidence suggests not only that polycystic kidneys may be infected more easily but also that the infection may play a role in the development of these cysts. Pelvicalyceal obstruction from extrinsic compression by large cysts or from blood clots

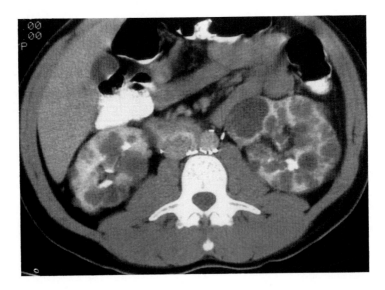

Figure 10-3. Autosomal dominant polycystic kidney disease. A contrast-enhanced abdominal CT scan reveals innumerable cysts throughout both kidneys.

or stones within the collecting system also predisposes to infection. In some patients, the cysts themselves may become infected.

Hemorrhage into a renal cyst is common in patients with ADPKD. Hemorrhagic cysts shown by CT may occur in as many as 70% of patients (Figure 10-4). This high prevalence of hemorrhagic cysts is presumably due to the erosion of cysts upon one another, the presence of systemic hypertension, and impaired hemostasis in patients with renal failure. Despite the frequency of hemorrhage into renal cysts, perinephric hemorrhage remains rare.

Although there is an increased incidence of renal adenocarcinoma in patients with von Hippel-Lindau disease and acquired cystic kidney disease, there is no association of renal carcinoma with ADPKD **(Option (C) is false).**

Almost half of patients with ADPKD have aneurysms of intracerebral arteries (berry aneurysms) near the circle of Willis **(Option (D) is true).** Stroke resulting from rupture of one of these aneurysms causes significant morbidity and mortality.

Extrarenal cysts are common in patients with ADPKD. Approximately 50% of patients have associated hepatic cysts (Figure 10-5), but cysts may also occur in other organs, such as the spleen and pancreas. Despite occasionally numerous liver cysts, hepatic function remains normal.

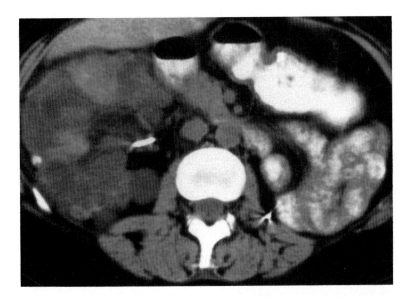

Figure 10-4. Autosomal dominant polycystic kidney disease. There has been a left nephrectomy. The right kidney is enlarged with numerous cysts. The high-density material on this unenhanced scan indicates hemorrhage.

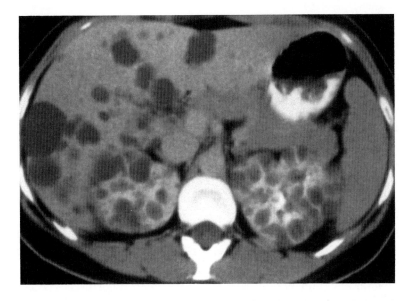

Figure 10-5. Autosomal dominant polycystic kidney disease. A contrast-enhanced abdominal CT scan demonstrates numerous renal cysts consistent with ADPKD. The well-defined water-density hepatic lesions represent liver cysts, which are seen in approximately 50% of patients with ADPKD.

Hepatic fibrosis is seen in patients with autosomal recessive polycystic kidney disease (ARPKD). In the perinatal form of ARPKD there is massive renal enlargement and severe renal failure. The diminished urine output *in utero* leads to marked oligohydramnios and secondary pulmonary hypoplasia. In the childhood form of ARPKD, renal involvement is less severe and consists of medullary tubular ectasia and modest nephromegaly. The clinical manifestations are dominated by hepatic fibrosis, which may progress to portal hypertension or hepatic failure. Hepatic fibrosis is not seen in patients with ADPKD **(Option (E) is false)**.

Question 47

Findings associated with von Hippel-Lindau disease include:

T (A) retinal angiomas
F (B) adenoma sebaceum
T (C) pancreatic cysts
T (D) pheochromocytoma
F (E) hemihypertrophy

von Hippel-Lindau disease is a multisystem disorder transmitted by autosomal dominant inheritance. In 1904, von Hippel reported two patients with retinal hemangiomas ("von Hippel tumor"). A subsequent autopsy on one of these patients revealed tumors of the nervous system, bones, and kidneys, as well as pancreatic and renal cysts. Later, Lindau discovered the cerebellar hemangioblastomas ("Lindau tumor") and cysts. In a 1926 monograph, he summarized the findings in 24 previously reported cases and 16 additional cases of his own. von Hippel-Lindau disease includes benign angiomas of the eyes and central nervous system, as well as cysts and neoplasms of the kidneys, pancreas, adrenal glands, and epididymis.

Retinal angiomas were one of the earliest recognized manifestations of the disease **(Option (A) is true)**. They may be multiple and are often associated with adjacent cysts.

Although nevi and café-au-lait spots have been reported in von Hippel-Lindau disease, other cutaneous manifestations have not. Adenoma sebaceum occurs in patients with tuberous sclerosis, not in those with von Hippel-Lindau disease **(Option (B) is false)**.

A variety of pancreatic cysts and neoplasms have been reported to occur in patients with von Hippel-Lindau disease **(Option (C) is true)**. The

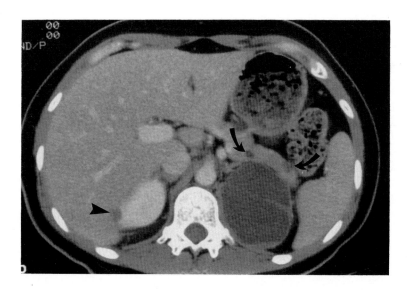

Figure 10-6. von Hippel-Lindau disease. A contrast-enhanced abdominal CT scan demonstrates two small pancreatic cysts (arrows). A large cyst is present in the upper pole of the left kidney, and a small cyst (arrowhead) can be seen in the lateral aspect of the right kidney.

earliest pancreatic manifestations are small cysts, which may calcify (Figure 10-6). As more cysts develop and enlarge, there may be sufficient replacement of pancreatic parenchyma to cause pancreatic insufficiency.

Solid pancreatic neoplasms, including hemangiomas, islet cell tumors, and serous cystadenomas, are also seen but are less frequent than pancreatic cysts. A single case of an associated pancreatic adenocarcinoma has been reported. A recent review of 43 patients with von Hippel-Lindau disease found islet cell tumors in 6 of the 36 patients (17%) who had cross-sectional imaging studies. None of these six patients presented for evaluation of endocrine dysfunction. However, three of the six islet cell tumors were malignant.

Pheochromocytomas occur in 10 to 20% of patients with von Hippel-Lindau disease **(Option (D) is true).** The incidence of pheochromocytomas is even higher among patients who also have pancreatic islet cell tumors, suggesting an extension of the multiple endocrine neoplasia syndromes.

Although cysts and anomalies of diploic vessels have been found in the bones of patients with von Hippel-Lindau disease, there is no association with hemihypertrophy **(Option (E) is false).** Hemihypertrophy is associated with Wilms' tumor and may be either ipsilateral or contralateral to the affected kidney.

Question 48

Findings associated with tuberous sclerosis include:

F (A) cerebellar hemangioblastoma
T (B) retinal phakomas
F (C) hypertension
F (D) renal adenocarcinomas
T (E) periungual fibromas

Tuberous sclerosis is a developmental anomaly characterized by tumor-like malformations called hamartomas. The lesions occur in ectodermal tissue, such as the brain, retinas, or skin, and in mesenchymal tissue, especially the kidneys, heart, lungs, and bone. Although the cerebral lesions of tuberous sclerosis were first described by von Recklinghausen in 1862, Bourneville first recognized the clinical triad of epilepsy, mental retardation, and adenoma sebaceum. Thus, tuberous sclerosis is also referred to as Bourneville's disease.

Tuberous sclerosis is transmitted as an autosomal dominant trait with incomplete penetrance. However, patients with tuberous sclerosis have diminished effective fertility, and so transmission beyond two generations is uncommon.

Giant cell Astrocytomas

The cerebral lesions are hamartomas, which are tumor-like malformations in which there is abnormal mixing of the tissue components that occur normally in the organ. Malignant transformation of abnormal glial cells occurs in 10 to 15% of patients; the characteristic tumor is the subependymal giant cell astrocytoma. Cerebellar hemangioblastomas, however, do not occur in tuberous sclerosis **(Option (A) is false)**, but rather are a characteristic feature of von Hippel-Lindau disease.

The clinical manifestations of tuberous sclerosis are dominated by the lesions in the central nervous system. Epilepsy is present in the vast majority of patients, and mental retardation is common. Pathognomonic retinal phakomas may be recognized on fundoscopic examination as large, yellow-to-white nodules arranged in clusters **(Option (B) is true).**

Pulmonary lesions may cause dyspnea or chest pain, and rupture of a subpleural cyst may result in pneumothorax. Renal lesions are usually asymptomatic, but hemorrhage from an angiomyolipoma may cause pain

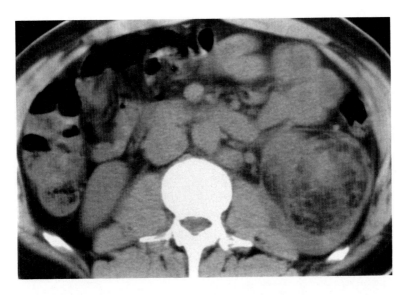

Figure 10-7. Angiomyolipoma. Subcapsular hemorrhage resulted in acute left-flank pain. This unenhanced abdominal CT scan reveals the characteristic fat of an angiomyolipoma.

(Figure 10-7). Hypertension, common in patients with ADPKD, is not seen in those with tuberous sclerosis **(Option (C) is false).**

The renal involvement includes angiomyolipomas and cysts. From 70 to 95% of patients with tuberous sclerosis have angiomyolipomas, which are usually multiple and bilateral. Renal cysts are present in approximately 20% of patients. The cysts of tuberous sclerosis have a hyperplastic eosinophilic epithelial lining that projects into the lumen of the cyst. Severe involvement by cysts occasionally leads to renal failure.

Angiomyolipomas are hamartomas composed of vascular, muscular, and fatty tissues. The morphologic appearance on imaging studies depends on the relative amount of each of these tissues in the lesion. There is seldom enough fat to identify an angiomyolipoma by its decreased density on excretory urography. Sonography may reveal an echogenic mass, which is often characteristic (Figure 10-8). However, CT is the most definitive imaging technique, since the density of the fatty component can be measured. Narrow collimation is recommended to minimize partial-volume artifact.

Although there are scattered reports of renal adenocarcinoma in patients with tuberous sclerosis, there have not been enough cases to document a statistical association **(Option (D) is false).**

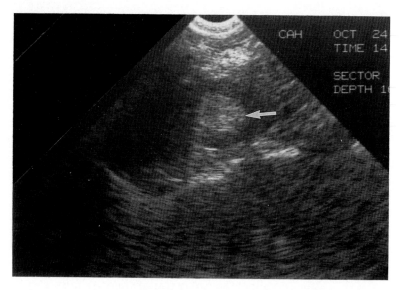

Figure 10-8. Angiomyolipoma. This longitudinal renal sonogram reveals a highly echogenic mass (arrow) typical of an angiomyolipoma.

Cutaneous manifestations of tuberous sclerosis are common. The characteristic adenoma sebaceum is actually a facial angiofibroma. It is not an adenoma, and the sebaceous glands are only secondarily drawn into the angiofibroma. Subungual or periungual angiofibromas are also common **(Option (E) is true).** Other skin lesions, such as areas of skin thickening (shagreen patches) and regions of hypopigmentation, are also common in patients with tuberous sclerosis.

Question 49

Concerning multilocular cystic nephroma,

F (A) it is often malignant
T (B) it occasionally herniates into the renal pelvis
F (C) most patients have hypertension
T (D) in adults, it is more common in women than in men
F (E) it is most accurately diagnosed by arteriography

A multilocular cystic nephroma (MLCN) is a well-defined renal mass consisting of multiple, noncommunicating cysts separated by thick,

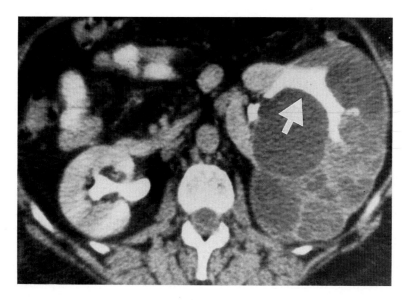

Figure 10-9. Multilocular cystic nephroma. A large cystic mass with multiple septations is shown on this enhanced abdominal CT scan. Protrusion into the renal pelvis (arrow) is a typical finding with multilocular cystic nephroma.

fibrous septa. It is a benign cystic neoplasm, which does not metastasize and is not locally invasive **(Option (A) is false).** Many synonyms have been used to describe this entity, including Perlman's tumor, benign cystic nephroma, multicystic nephroma, multilocular cyst, cystic nephroblastoma, cystic Wilms' tumor, segmental multicystic kidney, cystic adenoma, cystic hamartoma, lymphangioma, and segmental polycystic kidney.

The cystic mass is usually solitary and unilateral. A well-defined, thick capsule separates it from the adjacent renal parenchyma. Calcification is not uncommon. The mass arises within the renal parenchyma and often protrudes into the renal pelvis (Figure 10-9); this gives it a characteristic appearance on CT or excretory urography **(Option (B) is true).** This sign is not specific, as it is also seen in some patients with renal adenocarcinoma or Wilms' tumor.

MLCN may be discovered in childhood, when an abdominal mass is palpated. Occasionally, hematuria or a urinary tract infection is the initial manifestation. Lesions in adults are usually an incidental finding during an imaging examination for an unrelated complaint. However, some patients complain of abdominal pain, which may be due to the

MLCN. Hypertension, although occurring occasionally, is uncommon **(Option (C) is false)**.

Overall, the prevalence of MLCN is equal in both sexes. However, there are differences when the age of the patients is considered. In male patients, the vast majority of the lesions are detected in the first few years of life, whereas female patients more often present either between the ages of 4 and 20 years or after 40 years of age. In a series of 58 patients with MLCN reported from the Armed Forces Institute of Pathology, 88% of the male patients were under 2 years of age, whereas over 50% of female patients were between the ages of 40 and 60 years **(Option (D) is true)**.

Since the renal masses are large, they are usually seen on excretory urography. They are hypovascular, are usually well defined, and may show protrusion into the renal pelvis. When the cysts are large, sonography is very useful. The finding of multiple cystic locules separated by echogenic stroma is characteristic. However, if the cysts are small, they may not be recognized, and the echogenic mass cannot then be distinguished from a renal carcinoma.

The CT appearance is often characteristic. A large, well-defined cystic mass is sharply demarcated from the normal renal parenchyma (Figure 10-10). The lesion is hypovascular, but the thick septations will enhance with intravenous contrast material injection. If the cysts are small, the mass may have a pitted appearance.

Arteriography clearly defines the hypovascular nature of the mass. Abnormal vessels can be seen supplying the thick, fibrous capsule and numerous septations (Figure 10-11). However, this angiographic appearance is not sufficiently characteristic to diagnose MLCN or to exclude a hypovascular cancer, and arteriography is seldom used in the evaluation of these patients **(Option (E) is false)**.

The treatment of MLCN is nephrectomy. In some patients, surgical excision is indicated to alleviate symptoms of pain, hematuria, or urinary tract infection. In most patients, surgical removal is indicated because a renal cancer cannot be excluded on the basis of the imaging studies. If typical features of MLCN are present, a simple tumorectomy may be considered rather than the more radical formal nephrectomy, which would be performed if a renal adenocarcinoma were expected.

N. Reed Dunnick, M.D.

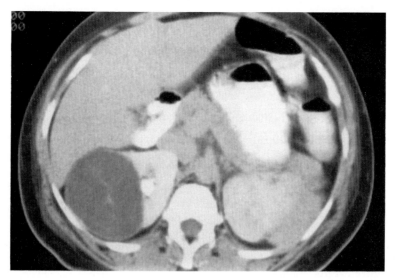

Figure 10-10. Multilocular cystic nephroma. A contrast-enhanced abdominal CT scan reveals a well-defined right renal mass. Several internal septations are seen in a cystic lesion.

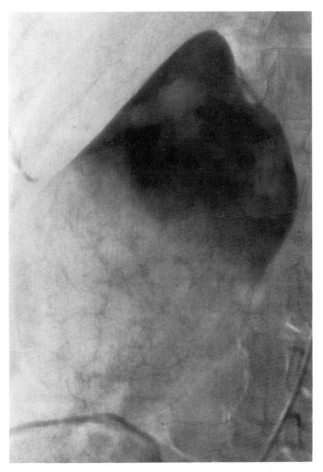

Figure 10-11. Multilocular cystic nephroma. This subtraction arteriogram demonstrates a hypovascular right renal mass. The fine vascularity is supplying the septations and cyst wall.

183

SUGGESTED READINGS

VON HIPPEL-LINDAU DISEASE

1. Binkovitz LA, Johnson CD, Stephens DH. Islet cell tumors in von Hippel-Lindau disease: increased prevalence and relationship to the multiple endocrine neoplasias. AJR 1990; 155:501–505
2. Choyke PL, Filling-Katz MR, Shawker TH, et al. Von Hippel-Lindau disease: radiologic screening for visceral manifestations. Radiology 1990; 174:815–820
3. Dunnick NR, McCallum RW, Sandler CM. A textbook of uroradiology. Baltimore: Williams & Wilkins; 1991:107–108
4. Levine E, Collins DL, Horton WA, Schimke RN. CT screening of the abdomen in von Hippel-Lindau disease. AJR 1982; 139:505–510
5. Melmon KL, Rosen SW. Lindau's disease: review of the literature and study of a large kindred. Am J Med 1964; 36:595–617

AUTOSOMAL DOMINANT POLYCYSTIC KIDNEY DISEASE

6. Levine E, Cook LT, Grantham JJ. Liver cysts in autosomal-dominant polycystic kidney disease: clinical and computed tomographic study. AJR 1985; 145:229–233
7. Levine E, Grantham JJ. Perinephric hemorrhage in autosomal dominant polycystic kidney disease: CT and MR findings. J Comput Assist Tomogr 1987; 11:108–111
8. McHugh K, Stringer DA, Hebert D, Babiak CA. Simple renal cysts in children: diagnosis and follow-up with US. Radiology 1991; 178:383–385
9. Parfrey PS, Bear JC, Morgan J, et al. The diagnosis and prognosis of autosomal dominant polycystic kidney disease. N Engl J Med 1990; 323:1085–1090
10. Walker FC Jr, Loney LC, Root ER, Melson GL, McAlister WH, Cole BR. Diagnostic evaluation of adult polycystic kidney disease in childhood. AJR 1984; 142:1273–1277

ACQUIRED CYSTIC KIDNEY DISEASE

11. Basile JJ, McCullough DL, Harrison LH, Dyer RB. End stage renal disease associated with acquired cystic disease and neoplasia. J Urol 1988; 140:938–943
12. Cho C, Friedland GW, Swenson RS. Acquired renal cystic disease and renal neoplasms in hemodialysis patients. Urol Radiol 1984; 6:153–157
13. Levine E, Grantham JJ, Slusher SL, Greathouse JL, Krohn BP. CT of acquired cystic kidney disease and renal tumors in long-term dialysis patients. AJR 1984; 142:125–131
14. Mindell HJ. Imaging studies for screening native kidneys in long-term dialysis patients. AJR 1989; 153:761–769
15. Taylor AJ, Cohen EP, Erickson SJ, Olson DL, Foley WD. Renal imaging in long-term dialysis patients: a comparison of CT and sonography. AJR 1989; 153:765–767

TUBEROUS SCLEROSIS

16. Bissada NK, White HJ, Sun CN, Smith PL, Barbour GL, Redman JF. Tuberous sclerosis complex and renal angiomyolipoma. Collective review. Urology 1975; 6:105–113
17. Bosniak MA, Megibow AJ, Hulnick DH, Horii S, Raghavendra BN. CT diagnosis of renal angiomyolipoma: the importance of detecting small amounts of fat. AJR 1988; 151:497–501
18. Mitnick JS, Bosniak MA, Hilton S, Raghavendra BN, Subramanyam BR, Genieser NB. Cystic renal disease in tuberous sclerosis. Radiology 1983; 147:85–87
19. Stillwell TJ, Gomez MR, Kelalis PP. Renal lesions in tuberous sclerosis. J Urol 1987; 138:477–481

MULTILOCULAR CYSTIC NEPHROMA

20. Banner MP, Pollack HM, Chatten J, Witzleben C. Multilocular renal cysts: radiologic-pathologic correlation. AJR 1981; 136:239–247
21. Madewell JE, Goldman SM, Davis CJ Jr, Hartman DS, Feigin DS, Lichtenstein JE. Multilocular cystic nephroma: a radiographic-pathologic correlation of 58 patients. Radiology 1983; 146:309–321
22. Parienty RA, Pradel J, Imbert MC, Picard JD, Savart P. Computed tomography of multilocular cystic nephroma. Radiology 1981; 140:135–139

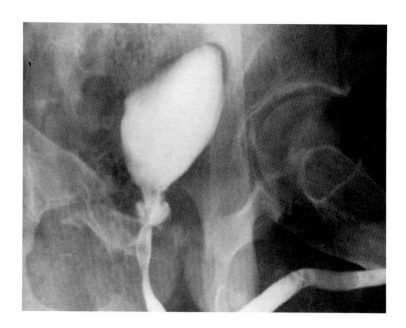

Figure 11-1

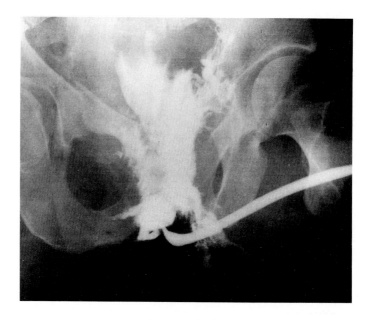

Figure 11-2
Figures 11-1 through 11-4. Four patients underwent urethrography after sustaining blunt pelvic trauma. You are shown a retrograde urethrogram from each patient.

Case 11: Urethral Injury

Questions 50 through 53

For each patient's retrograde urethrogram (Questions 50 through 53), select the *one* lettered condition (A, B, C, D, or E) that BEST corresponds to that image. Each condition may be used once, more than once, or not at all.

E 50. Figure 11-1
B 51. Figure 11-2
D 52. Figure 11-3
A 53. Figure 11-4

       (A) Complete Type II urethral injury
       (B) Partial Type III urethral injury
       (C) Complete Type III urethral rupture
       (D) Straddle injury
       (E) Extraperitoneal bladder rupture

Figure 11-1 demonstrates leakage of contrast material into the pelvic extraperitoneal space surrounding the bladder neck (arrow, Figure 11-5). An acute fracture of the right superior pubic ramus is present. The urethra distal to the verumontanum is clearly visualized and appears normal. Because posterior urethral injuries associated with pelvic fracture occur at the level of the membranous urethra, the injury demonstrated in this patient represents an extraperitoneal bladder rupture rather than an injury of the posterior urethra **(Option (E) is the correct answer to Question 50).** Extraperitoneal bladder rupture generally occurs in association with a pelvic fracture. The classically described mechanism for such injuries is laceration of the base of the bladder by a spicule of bone in association with the fracture itself. Recent data, which demonstrate that the area of contrast material leakage is associated with the area of the fracture in only 35% of the cases, suggest that a variety of other mechanisms may also result in extraperitoneal rupture (see Case 15). With simple extraperitoneal bladder rupture the leakage is limited to the pelvic extraperitoneal space, whereas with complex extraperitoneal

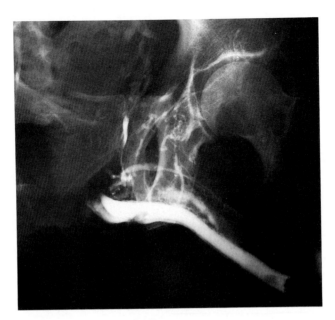

Figure 11-3

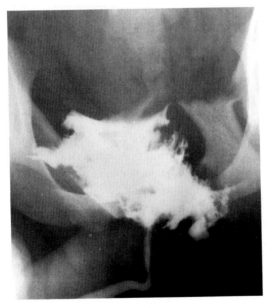

Figure 11-4

bladder rupture the leakage extends beyond the perivesicle space into the anterior abdominal wall, the scrotum, the thigh, or the perineum.

Figure 11-2 demonstrates an acute pelvic fracture and leakage of contrast material into both the pelvic extraperitoneal space and the

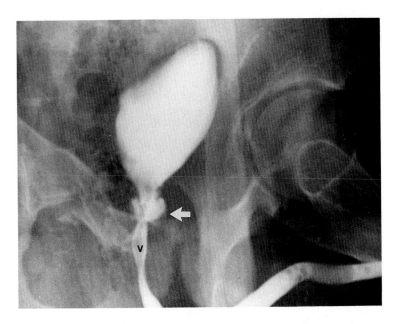

Figure 11-5 (Same as Figure 11-1). Extraperitoneal bladder rupture. There is leakage of contrast material from the bladder neck (arrow) above the level of the verumontanum (V). This indicates that the injury represents an extraperitoneal bladder rupture rather than a urethral injury. The visualized portions of the urethra are normal. Lucencies at the penoscrotal junction represent air bubbles introduced during the study.

perineum from an injury of the posterior urethra. Some filling of the bladder (B in Figure 11-6) is present, however, indicating that the urethra is not completely transected; the injury therefore represents an incomplete or partial Type III urethral injury **(Option (B) is the correct answer to Question 51).**

Figure 11-3 demonstrates a defect in the bulbous urethra, venous intravasation, and leakage of contrast material into the corpus spongiosum, as well as a pelvic fracture (Figure 11-7). All of these findings, except the fracture (see below), are typical of a straddle injury **(Option (D) is the correct answer to Question 52).**

Figure 11-4 also shows a pelvic fracture and demonstrates leakage of contrast material into the pelvic extraperitoneal space above an intact urogenital diaphragm from an injury of the membranoprostatic urethra. There is no filling of the bladder, indicating that the urethra is completely transected. The injury is therefore a complete Type II posterior urethral injury **(Option (A) is the correct answer to Question 53).** The clas-

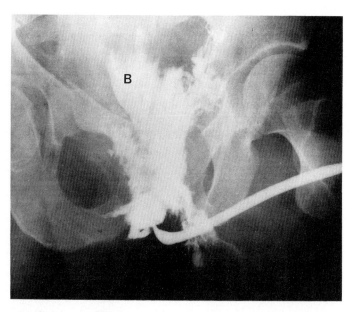

Figure 11-6 (Same as Figure 11-2). Partial Type III urethral injury. Extensive contrast material leakage from the membranous urethra is present; however, the leakage extends both above and below the expected position of the urogenital diaphragm. The injury is therefore considered Type III urethral rupture. However, as there is some filling of the urinary bladder (B), the damage is an incomplete or partial injury rather than a complete urethral disruption.

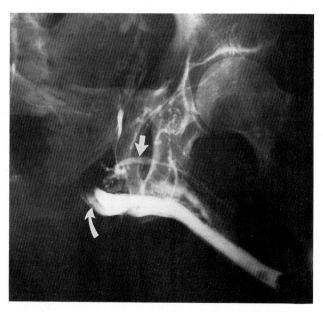

Figure 11-7 (Same as Figure 11-3). Straddle injury. There is partial disruption of the proximal bulbous urethra, with contrast leakage that extends into the corpus spongiosum (curved arrow) and is associated with venous intravasation (straight arrow). These findings indicate a straddle injury of the anterior urethra. There is no filling of the posterior urethra, most probably because of spasm of the external urethral sphincter.

sification and the differential diagnosis of the various types of urethral injuries are discussed in greater detail below.

Question 54

Concerning posterior urethral injuries from blunt pelvic trauma,

T (A) a pelvic fracture is generally present
F (B) they are caused by laceration of the prostatic urethra by a bone spicule
T (C) they are generally classified by their relationship to the urogenital diaphragm
F (D) on urethrography, the urogenital diaphragm prevents contrast material leakage from extending into the perineum in the majority of cases
T (E) the puboprostatic ligaments are generally ruptured

The male urethra is divided into anterior and posterior portions at the level of the urogenital diaphragm. The anterior urethra is subdivided into the penile or pendulous urethra and the bulbous urethra, and the posterior urethra is subdivided into the membranous urethra and the prostatic urethra. The verumontanum marks the boundary between the prostatic urethra and the membranous urethra, which is wholly contained within the urogenital diaphragm. Injuries to the male urethra following blunt pelvic trauma are classified into two groups: (1) those associated with pelvic fracture, generally referred to as posterior urethral injuries, which occur at the level of the membranous urethra **(Option (A) is true),** and (2) those associated with straddle injury involving the anterior urethra generally at the level of the bulbous urethra, in which a pelvic fracture is commonly, but not always, absent. Because of its short length and its mobility, the female urethra is very rarely injured as a result of blunt pelvic trauma.

On physical examination the classical triad of blood at the urethral meatus, inability to urinate, and a palpable urinary bladder may be found. In addition, a high-riding prostate may be palpated on digital rectal examination. The prostate is dislocated from its normal position because its attachments to the urogenital diaphragm are severed (see discussion below). Of these clinical indicators, the finding of blood at the meatus is the most reliable; McAninch found blood at the meatus in all patients with urethral injuries. Although these clinical findings are valuable indicators of possible urethral injury, none are specific and their absence does not preclude injury. Thus the diagnosis of a suspected urethral injury must be established by retrograde urethrography. It is

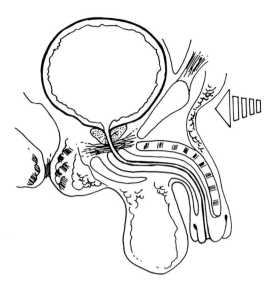

Figure 11-8. Mechanism of urethral injury associated with pelvic fracture. A shearing force disrupts the ligamentous attachment of the prostate to the urogenital diaphragm, resulting in tearing of the membranoprostatic urethra.

especially important that such a study be performed prior to any attempt at passage of a Foley catheter. Urethral instrumentation in a male patient with a potential urethral injury is contraindicated because it carries the risk of converting a partial urethral injury into a complete tear (causing additional hemorrhage) and contaminating a previously sterile hematoma. Therefore, retrograde urethrography must be performed prior to any attempt at urethral catheterization in every male patient with an anterior pelvic arch fracture, whether or not blood at the urethral meatus is present.

The vast majority of injuries of the posterior urethra occur as a result of pelvic fracture, especially one involving the anterior pelvic arch. The urethral injury generally occurs as a consequence of a shearing force (Figure 11-8) that disrupts the urethra during the pelvic fracture rather than as a consequence of an active laceration of the soft tissues by a bone spicule **(Option (B) is false).** The puboprostatic ligaments are generally ruptured **(Option (E) is true)** as the prostate is severed from its connection to the urogenital diaphragm. With a complete urethral transection, the bladder and attached prostate rise out of the true pelvis, giving rise to the so-called "pie-in-the-sky" bladder and to the high-riding prostate found on physical examination. A hematoma results in the retropubic and perivesicle spaces. Although the precise incidence of posterior urethral injury varies somewhat among the reported series, Palmer et al. found the frequency to be 5.5% among male patients in a series encompassing 200 patients with pelvic fractures. Only two case reports of posterior urethral injuries in male patients without pelvic fracture have been described.

Both the diagnostic classification of and the therapeutic approach to injuries of the posterior urethra following blunt trauma have undergone tremendous revision in recent years. The current classification presented below replaces the one found in an earlier syllabus of the Self-Evaluation Program, the first *Genitourinary Tract Disease Syllabus* (volume 3). The classically described injury of the posterior urethra following pelvic fracture is rupture of the membranoprostatic urethra above an intact urogenital diaphragm. Extension of the injury into the proximal bulbous urethra and rupture of the urogenital diaphragm itself had been considered rare. A urethrogram performed in such a patient would show leakage of contrast material into the pelvic extraperitoneal space limited inferiorly by the intact urogenital diaphragm. This description of a "classic" posterior urethral injury was based on the surgical findings in patients who were operated on shortly after the injury for immediate repair of the urethral damage. In recent years, however, the use of delayed surgical repair, which has been found to result in decreased patient morbidity (see discussion below), has increased the need for accurate diagnosis by urethrography. Increased experience with urethrography, however, demonstrated that the classically described injury was rarely seen. In 1977, Colapinto and McCallum proposed a new classification of posterior urethral injuries that was based on the relationship of urethrographic patterns of contrast material leakage to the urogenital diaphragm **(Option (C) is true)** rather than on surgical findings. In this system urethral injuries were classified into Types I, II, and III injuries as follows.

In Type I injuries the posterior urethra is stretched because the puboprostatic ligaments are ruptured, resulting in displacement of the bladder out of the pelvis. Although the urethra is stretched, it remains intact and there is no leakage of contrast material on urethrography. A Foley catheter may be carefully inserted, and no further therapy is typically required (Figure 11-9).

In Type II injuries the membranoprostatic urethra is ruptured above an intact urogenital diaphragm. This is the classically described injury, which results in leakage of contrast material into the pelvic extraperi-

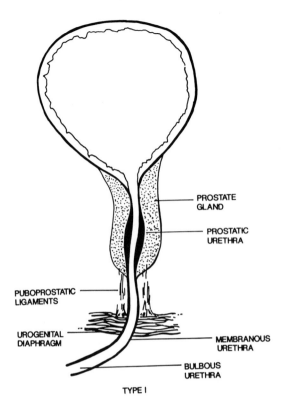

PROSTATE
GLAND

PROSTATIC
URETHRA

PUBOPROSTATIC
LIGAMENTS

UROGENITAL
DIAPHRAGM

MEMBRANOUS
URETHRA

BULBOUS
URETHRA

TYPE I

Figure 11-9. Type I urethral injury. The posterior urethra is stretched and elongated but remains intact. There is no leakage of contrast material on urethrography.

toneal space limited inferiorly by an intact urogenital diaphragm on urethrography (Figure 11-10).

In Type III injuries the membranous urethra is disrupted; however, the injury extends into the proximal bulbous urethra, or the urogenital diaphragm itself is ruptured, or both. On urethrography, there is leakage of contrast material into the perineum below the level of the urogenital diaphragm (Figure 11-11).

In their original series, Colapinto and McCallum reported that 13 of 15 patients had Type III injuries; there were no Type II injuries in the series **(Option (D) is false).** Sandler et al. subsequently confirmed the validity of this classification and reported that a spectrum of Type III leakage could be present. In some patients with Type III injuries, the leakage was predominantly into the pelvis; in some patients there were approximately equal amounts of pelvic and perineal leakage; and in still

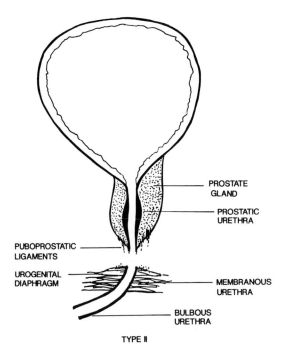

TYPE II

Figure 11-10. Type II urethral injury. The urethra is disrupted along the urogenital diaphragm, resulting in leakage of contrast material into the pelvic extraperitoneal space on urethrography. Because the urogenital diaphragm remains intact, contrast leakage is prevented from extending into the perineum.

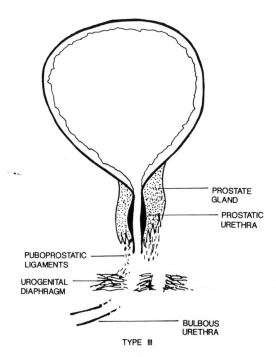

TYPE III

Figure 11-11. Type III urethral injury. The urethral injury extends into the proximal bulbous urethra or there is disruption of the urogenital diaphragm itself, allowing contrast material leakage to extend into the perineum on urethrography.

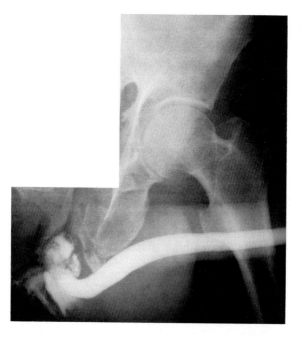

Figure 11-12. Type III urethral injury with predominantly perineal leakage of contrast material demonstrated by urethrography.

others the leakage was predominantly perineal (Figure 11-12). These researchers speculated that the pattern of leakage depended on the degree of disruption of the urogenital diaphragm and the degree of extension of injury into the bulbous urethra. With greater disruption of the urogenital diaphragm or greater extension into the proximal bulbous urethra, relatively greater perineal leakage is present; when part of the membranous urethra or urogenital diaphragm remains intact, some contrast leakage into the pelvic extraperitoneal space above the urogenital diaphragm may be present, thereby simulating a Type II injury. In Sandler's series of 18 patients, 66% had Type III injuries, 16% had Type II injuries, and 16% had Type I injuries.

Both Type II and Type III injuries may present with either complete or partial ruptures. Incomplete rupture is present when urethrography shows some filling of the bladder; with a complete disruption, no such filling is present. The frequency of partial ruptures varies between 19 and 90% among the reported series; most authors suggest that approximately 25% of patients have partial ruptures. The importance of these partial injuries should not be overlooked. Although urethral strictures result from both complete and partial ruptures, strictures that are the result of partial ruptures tend to be shorter and amenable to nonoperative or endoscopic management; repair of complete ruptures usually requires formal urethroplasty.

In the past, immediate exploratory surgery in an effort to reestablish urethral continuity was the therapy of choice. In such a procedure the pelvic hematoma is evacuated and the urethra is realigned over a Foley catheter. Unfortunately, the frequency of postoperative stricture may approach 100%, as many as one-third of the patients may suffer incontinence, and the rate of impotence approaches 60%. Because of the morbidity associated with immediate reconstruction, it has been suggested more recently that delayed repair is a more desirable form of therapy. In such a procedure only a suprapubic cystostomy is placed immediately; formal urethroplasty is delayed for 4 to 6 months. By this time, the pelvic hematoma has resorbed, the prostate has redescended into the pelvis, and the pelvic fracture has stabilized. Morehouse and Mackinnon and Webster et al. report that although all patients so treated will develop a urethral stricture, there is a markedly decreased frequency of both incontinence and impotence compared with that following immediate surgical reconstruction. A combined voiding cystourethrogram and retrograde urethrogram is usually performed prior to surgery to assess the length of the resultant stricture. The typical patient with a complete Type III injury develops a stricture several centimeters long when treated by delayed repair; patients with Type II injuries generally have shorter strictures.

Question 55

Concerning blunt anterior urethral injuries,

F (A) a pelvic fracture is generally present
T (B) they result when the bulbous urethra is crushed against the inferior aspect of the symphysis pubis
F (C) on urethrography, venous intravasation of contrast material generally indicates rupture of the corpus cavernosum
F (D) a normal retrograde urethrogram generally excludes anterior urethral contusion
T (E) leakage of contrast material into the scrotum or perineum indicates disruption of Buck's fascia

Blunt injuries of the anterior male urethra occur when the patient falls astride a blunt object, crushing the bulbous urethra and surrounding

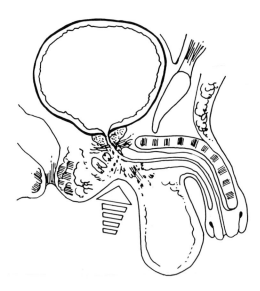

Figure 11-13. Mechanism of straddle injury. The bulbous urethra is crushed between a blunt object (arrow) and the inferior aspect of the symphysis pubis, resulting in complete or partial disruption of the anterior urethra below the urogenital diaphragm.

corpus spongiosum between the object and the inferior aspect of the symphysis pubis **(Option (B) is true)** (Figure 11-13). They are usually not associated with pelvic fracture **(Option (A) is false).** The injury may result in anterior urethral contusion or in partial or (infrequently) complete urethral disruption. If Buck's fascia remains intact, the injury is limited to the space between Buck's fascia and the tunica albuginea of the corpus spongiosum. If Buck's fascia is disrupted, however, the hematoma may spread into the scrotum, the perineum, or the anterior abdominal wall within the confines of Colles' fascia (Figure 11-14). This may result in the so-called "butterfly hematoma" on physical examination (Figure 11-15). As with posterior urethral injuries, blood is generally present at the urethral meatus.

Anterior urethral contusion is said to be present when there are clinical features of an anterior urethral injury but the result of urethrography is normal **(Option (D) is false).** Most contusions heal without sequelae, although some urologists recommend that a follow-up urethrogram be performed 6 months after the injury to exclude the possibility that a silent urethral stricture has formed.

Partial urethral rupture is the most common form of straddle injury and can be diagnosed on urethrography when contrast material leaks

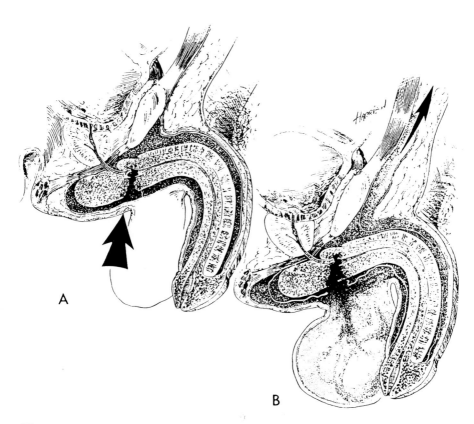

Figure 11-14. Urethral rupture inferior to the urogenital diaphragm. (A) Urethral rupture with intact Buck's fascia. The extent of blood and urine leakage is limited. (B) Urethral rupture with disruption of Buck's fascia. Blood and urine can extend from Colles' fascial attachments at the perineal body and enter the scrotum, as well as into the anterior abdominal wall beneath Scarpa's fascia. (Reprinted with permission from Petero PC, Bright TC III. Management of trauma to the urinary tract. Longmire WP Jr (ed), Advances in surgery, vol 10. Chicago: Yearbook Medical Publishers; 1976:197–244.)

from the bulbous urethra but the continuity of the urethra is maintained. Venous intravasation is common and does not imply concomitant rupture of the corpus cavernosum **(Option (C) is false).** If Buck's fascia has been disrupted, contrast material may be present in the scrotum, perineum, or anterior abdominal wall within the confines of Colles' fascia **(Option (E) is true).** With complete anterior urethral rupture, the continuity of the urethra is disrupted and no contrast material is present in the more proximal bulbous urethra. Both partial and complete urethral injuries may result in an anterior urethral stricture. As with posterior urethral

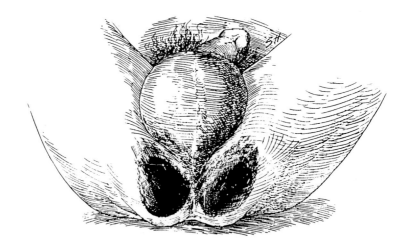

Figure 11-15. Drawing of perineum demonstrating the appearance of the "butterfly hematoma" that may result when anterior urethral injury is associated with disruption of Buck's fascia. (Reprinted with permission from Peters PC, Sagalowsky AI. Genitourinary trauma. In: Walsh PC, Gittes RF, Perlmutter AD, Stamey TA (eds), Campbell's urology, 5th ed. Philadelphia: WB Saunders; 1986:1192–1246.)

injuries, many urologists suggest that anterior urethral injuries also be treated by immediate suprapubic diversion.

Rupture of the corpus cavernosum ("fracture of the penis") is an infrequent injury that generally results when the erect penis is traumatized from strenuous sexual activity rather than from blunt perineal trauma. On urethrography, a filling defect in the corpus cavernosum, which represents a hematoma at the site of injury, may be found.

Carl M. Sandler, M.D.

SUGGESTED READINGS

1. Colapinto V, McCallum RW. Injury to the male posterior urethra in fractured pelvis: a new classification. J Urol 1977; 118:575–580
2. McAninch JW. Traumatic injuries to the urethra. J Trauma 1981; 21:291–297
3. Morehouse DD, Mackinnon KJ. Management of prostatomembranous urethral disruption: 13-year experience. J Urol 1980; 123:173–174
4. Palmer JK, Benson GS, Corriere JN Jr. Diagnosis and initial management of urological injuries associated with 200 consecutive pelvic fractures. J Urol 1983; 130:712–714

5. Pierce JM Jr. Management of dismemberment of the prostatic-membranous urethra and ensuing stricture disease. J Urol 1972; 107:259–264
6. Pontes JE, Pierce JM Jr. Anterior urethral injuries: four years of experience at the Detroit General Hospital. J Urol 1978; 120:563–564
7. Sandler CM, Harris JH Jr, Corriere JN Jr, Toombs BD. Posterior urethral injuries after pelvic fracture. AJR 1981; 137:1233–1237
8. Theros EG (ed). Genitourinary tract disease syllabus. Chicago: American College of Radiology; 1973:124–130
9. Webster GD, Mathes GL, Selli C. Prostatomembranous urethral injuries: a review of the literature and a rational approach to their management. J Urol 1983; 130:898–902

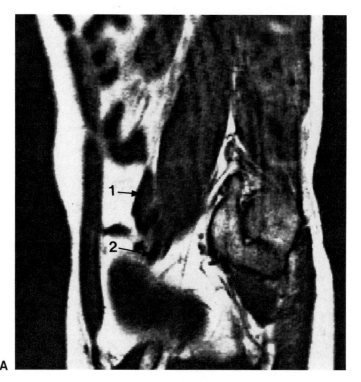

SE 500/17

Figure 12-1. This 43-year-old man has bilateral nonpalpable testes. You are shown left parasagittal (A) and coronal (B) T1-weighted MR images and a transverse T2-weighted MR image (C) (1.0 T) of the pelvis.

Case 12: Undescended Testes

Questions 56 through 60

For each of the numbered arrows (Questions 56 through 60), select the *one* lettered structure (A, B, C, D, or E) that is MOST closely associated with it. Each lettered structure may be used once, more than once, or not at all.

56. Arrow 1
57. Arrow 2
58. Arrow 3
59. Arrow 4
60. Arrow 5

    (A) Undescended testis
    (B) Iliac vein
    (C) Iliac artery
    (D) Bowel loop
    (E) Lymph node

The left parasagittal T1-weighted MR image (Figure 12-1A) includes the broad psoas muscle and the lateral portion of the bladder (see Figure 12-2A). There are multiple ill-defined structures anterior to the psoas muscle with locations characteristic of bowel loops. There are several elongated structures immediately adjacent (anterior and inferior) to the psoas muscle. The largest of these elongated structures (arrow 1) is the undescended left testis **(Option (A) is the correct answer to Question 56).** The other two elongated structures show signal voids characteristic of flowing blood in the iliac vessels. The iliac vein (arrow 2) is posterior to the iliac artery at this level **(Option (B) is the correct answer to Question 57).**

The coronal T1-weighted MR image (Figure 12-1B) at the level of the anatomic internal inguinal ring shows the flow void of the external iliac artery (arrow 3) exiting from the pelvis lateral to the slightly larger external iliac vein (Figure 12-2B) **(Option (C) is the correct answer to Question 58).** There are several bowel loops throughout the pelvis,

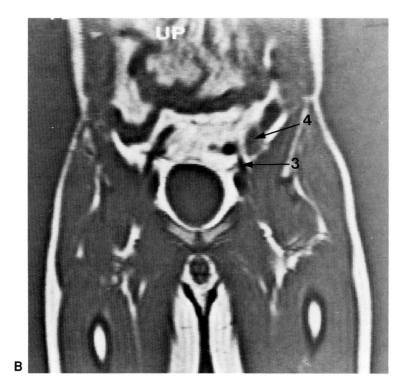

B

SE 700/28

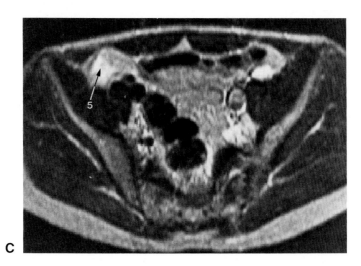

C

SE 1,500/90

Figure 12-1 (Continued)

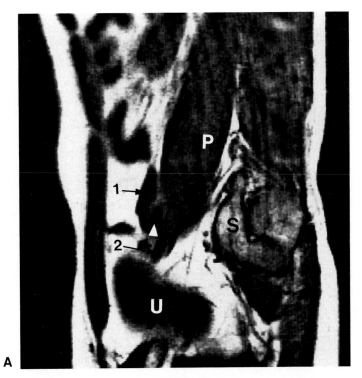

A

SE 500/17

Figure 12-2 (Same as Figure 12-1).   Undescended testis. (A) Left para-sagittal MR image showing the low signal intensity of an elongated intra-abdominal testis (arrow 1) located in close proximity to the external iliac vein (arrow 2), external iliac artery (arrowhead), and psoas muscle (P). On T1-weighted images, testicular tissue has a signal intensity similar to that of muscle. U = urinary bladder; S = sigmoid colon. (B) Coronal MR image showing an oval structure (arrow 4), which correlates with the intra-abdominal testis in panel A. The iliac artery (arrow 3) and iliac vein (V) lie medial to the testis. U = urinary bladder. (C) Transverse MR image showing the high signal intensity of the left intra-abdominal testis (straight arrow) located anterior to the left psoas muscle (P) and imme-diately lateral to the external iliac artery (curved arrow). Arrow 5 indi-cates a fluid-filled bowel loop, which has heterogeneous bright signal.

some intermediate in signal intensity, similar to muscle, and some showing long-T1 characteristics corresponding to fluid. There is an oval, intermediate-intensity structure (arrow 4) located just above the internal inguinal ring (lateral to the left iliac vessels) that corresponds to the same structure identified as the undescended left testis in Figure 12-1A **(Option (A) is the correct answer to Question 59).**

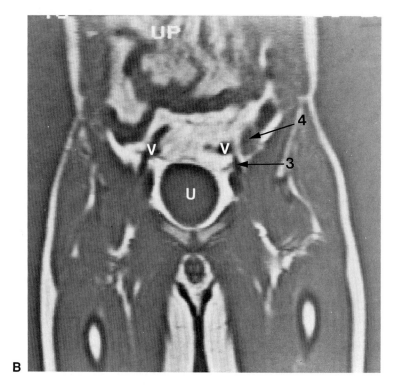

SE 700/28

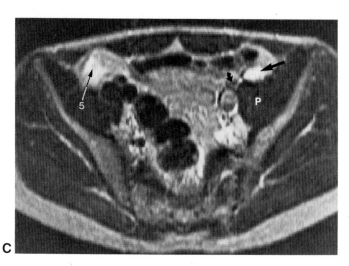

SE 1,500/90

Figure 12-1C shows a transverse T2-weighted MR image of the pelvis, demonstrating the low to intermediate signal intensity of the pelvic muscles. Immediately anterior to the left iliopsoas muscle is an oval structure with long-T2 characteristics that corresponds to the undescended left testis identified in Figures 12-1A and B. Fluid-filled loops of bowel (arrow 5, for example) may also show T2 lengthening, but bowel fluid appears less homogeneous than the testis. The sigmoid colon and other bowel loops are shown as low- to intermediate-intensity structures, many of which are connected **(Option (D) is the correct answer to Question 60).**

The right testis also showed long-T2 characteristics and was readily identified anterior to the psoas muscle at a level higher in the pelvis. Therefore, the right undescended testis is not visible on the views selected to show the left testis.

Question 61

Concerning undescended testes,

(A) the frequency in full-term neonates is about 10%
(B) 10 to 12% of patients with testicular cancer have an undescended testis
(C) those within the pelvis are found in the adventitia of the bladder
(D) 80% are below the internal inguinal ring

An undescended testis is defined as any testis not in its normal scrotal location and is categorized according to its anatomic position. A high scrotal testis is less than 4 cm below the pubic tubercle; this definition includes an intracanalicular testis that can be manipulated distal to the external ring. An obstructed testis is a morphologically normal testis that exits from the external ring and migrates cephalad to take a position superficial to the aponeurosis of the external oblique muscle because of an obstruction in the pathway of descent. An ectopic testis is one that migrates to a position remote from the path of normal descent such as the perineum, thigh, or suprapubic and penile areas. Testes in the above categories are palpable and account for 60 to 66% of undescended testes. The intracanalicular or emergent testis is one that has started along the pathway of descent and is lying within the inguinal canal between the internal and external inguinal rings. It is often elusive to the examining fingers, and the aponeurosis of the external oblique muscle may prevent palpation. Approximately 16 to 20% of undescended testes are intracanalicular. Thus, the high scrotal, ectopic, and intracanalicular testes account for more than 80% of undescended testes **(Option (D) is true)**. The least common undescended testis is the intra-abdominal testis, which is usually found just above the internal inguinal ring in close proximity to the iliopsoas muscle and iliac vessels but is occasionally enveloped within the peritoneum **(Option (C) is false)**. Even more uncommon than the intra-abdominal testis is the absent testis secondary to either incomplete development or atresia as a result of a noxious intrauterine event.

The weight of the newborn is a more accurate indicator of maturity than calendar age. In fetuses weighing less than 1,000 g, the testes are usually undescended. In those weighing less than 2,500 g, the frequency of undescended testes is 30.3%, and in those weighing more than 2,500 g the frequency is approximately 3%. The frequency is 2 to 4% for full-term infants weighing more than 3,500 g **(Option (A) is false)**. The majority of undescended testes will descend spontaneously within the first 3 months of life, lowering the frequency at 1 year of age to 0.8%; the frequency further decreases to about 0.3% in adult men. There is a hereditary tendency exhibited by abnormal testicular descent, with a familial history in 3 to 5% of cases. The trait is thought to be passed on by an autosomal dominant gene but with incomplete penetrance. There is a preponderance of bilateral involvement in premature infants. In adults, the ratio of unilateral to bilateral involvement reportedly ranges from 3:1 to 10:1.

The testis develops from the gonadal ridge, and the entire epididymis and vas deferens form from a separate source: the mesonephros and the mesonephric duct. Testicular and ductal development are variable and abnormal in 30 to 40% of undescended testes, especially those that are intracanalicular or intra-abdominal. These abnormalities are characterized by various degrees of detachment between the epididymis and testis, but by far the most commonly encountered abnormality is an elongated epididymis. These structural abnormalities of the vas deferens and epididymis confound imaging because a looped epididymis or vas deferens may resemble a blind-ending spermatic cord or atrophic testis when, in fact, the testis lies more proximal in the abdomen.

Descent relates to two critical periods: 7 weeks and 7 months postconception. During the period from 5 to 7 weeks postconception, the developing gonad on the ventral medial aspect of the urogenital ridge becomes contiguous with the gubernaculum and attaches to the caudal epididymis to form a single unit. The events by which the testes come to be at the internal inguinal ring are termed transabdominal migration and are believed to result from rapid growth of the abdominal cavity, with the remainder of the mesonephros (kidney) retracting to the retroperitoneum.

During the seventh month postconception, there is sudden swelling of the gubernaculum and extension of the processus vaginalis into the scrotum. At this time, the gubernaculum degenerates, and this is followed by rapid descent of the epididymis and testes through the inguinal canal into the scrotum. The controlling factors of this final stage of descent are not yet known, but gonadotropins, androgens, and the epididymal and gubernacular changes are all believed to play a role. At about 32 weeks, the testes enter the scrotum and the inguinal canal retracts around the spermatic cord (Figure 12-3).

Men with a history of cryptorchidism have an increased risk of testicular cancer. The analyses of 506 patients by Giwercman et al. show that this relative risk is approximately 4 to 5 times higher instead of the 10 to 40 times previously reported. Approximately 10 to 12% of patients with testicular cancer have an undescended testis **(Option (B) is true).** In such patients, tumor histologic types are pure seminoma (43%), embryonal cell carcinoma (28%), teratocarcinoma (27%), and choriocarcinoma (2%), a distribution similar to that seen in males with normally descended testes. The incidence peak of malignancy of undescended testes, as for testicular cancer in general, occurs in the third and fourth decades of life, whether the testis is in the abdomen, groin, or scrotum and irrespective of modes of correction. Nonseminomatous tumors are more likely to occur if the testis is in the scrotum after late spontaneous descent or orchiopexy. An altered environment, hormonal imbalance and testicular dysgenesis, and atrophy have been implicated as possible oncogenic factors. It is unlikely that the abdominal position of the testis is a significant factor since early orchiopexy does not eliminate the risk of malignancy, and cancer of the normally descended contralateral testis occurs more frequently in those with cancer of the undescended testis.

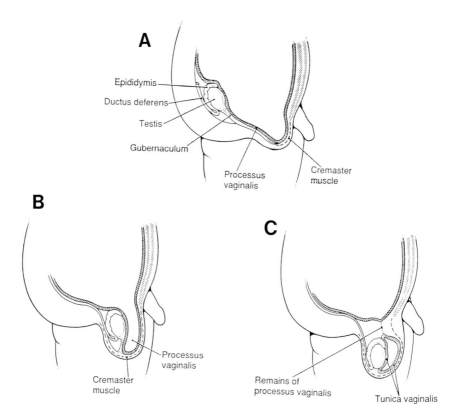

Figure 12-3. Descent of the testicle. (A) The developing gonad becomes contiguous with the gubernaculum. (B) At 7 months postconception, swelling of the gubernaculum and extension of the processus vaginalis into the scrotum occur. (C) At 32 months, the testicle is in the scrotum. The inguinal canal retracts around the spermatic cord. The processus vaginalis degenerates so that the tunica vaginalis is separated from the peritoneal cavity. (Reprinted with permission from Graham SD Jr. Surgery of the testicle. In: Droller MJ (ed), Surgical management of urologic disease: an anatomic approach. St. Louis: CV Mosby; 1992:962–984.)

Question 62

Concerning imaging of undescended testes,

(A) ultrasonography is more accurate than CT for detection of this condition
(B) the signal intensity of testes on T1-weighted MR images is similar to that of muscle
(C) lymph nodes are less echogenic than undescended testes on ultrasonography
(D) identification of the internal inguinal ring is crucial for differentiating intra-abdominal from intracanalicular testes
(E) most intra-abdominal testes are found at the aortic bifurcation

There are a number of imaging modalities available to localize non-palpable testes. The most commonly used methods are ultrasonography, CT, and MRI.

Reports based on imaging the nonscrotal testis by ultrasonography have shown varying success rates. Although 70% of low-lying and palpable testes are detected by ultrasonography, only 13% of nonpalpable testes can be localized (Figure 12-4). In general, ultrasonography is ineffective for detection of testes above the internal inguinal ring **(Option (A) is false).** Lymph nodes, which are usually less echogenic than undescended testes in the inguinal canal **(Option (C) is true),** occasionally simulate undescended testes.

CT is more sensitive than ultrasonography, but it too has limitations. It exposes the patient to ionizing radiation, is unable to separate testes from spermatic cord structure or fluid, and frequently cannot detect a testis less than 1 cm in diameter.

MRI is the latest technique used to evaluate undescended testes. Several reported series have shown the utility of this technique; however, difficulties have been encountered by some investigators in identifying nonpalpable testes. The primary advantage of MRI is its ability to produce multiplanar images without ionizing radiation. It can also produce a more detailed image, separating associated hernia fluid from testis and identifying testicular remnants.

In some instances the undescended testes may have undergone regressive changes, presumably on the basis of incomplete fusion of the gonad and ductal system or a vascular accident resulting in a vas deferens that ends blindly in a fibrous scar. Such scars are often also associated with hemosiderin deposition or calcification, supporting the contention that they are the site of a testis that has been ablated as the result of a noxious event. A portion of the epididymis may remain, but the seminiferous tubules and germ cells are usually entirely eliminated.

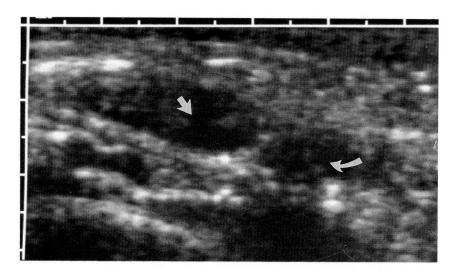

Figure 12-4. Undescended testis. Longitudinal sonogram of the right groin shows an intracanalicular testis (curved arrow) as an elongated structure with homogeneous echogenicity. Note the associated inguinal hernia (straight arrow) demonstrated with heterogeneous echogenicity.

MRI of the undescended testis is performed with a head or body coil, depending on patient size. Transverse or coronal images are obtained initially in evaluation of the undescended testis; the imaging field should extend from the perineum inferiorly to the iliac crest superiorly. Continuous 4- to 6-mm-thick sections with minimal interslice gaps are necessary because the undescended testis is frequently smaller than the normally descended contralateral testis. Since the intracanalicular testis is more elliptical in configuration than a normal testis, the coronal plane is ideal for depicting the testis in the canal. The sagittal plane should cover an area from the external inguinal ring to beyond the internal inguinal ring laterally (Figure 12-2A).

A long-TR, long-TE sequence is obtained in the transverse plane followed by short-TR, short-TE sequences in the sagittal plane. Since short-TR, short-TE images do not differentiate between the low signal intensities of hernia fluid and testis, it is occasionally necessary to obtain the coronal view with T2 weighting. With low-field magnets, long-TR, long-TE sequences of the testis may show signal intensity similar to that of fat because of the crossover of intensities. At high field, the same parameter (long-TR, long-TE) will show good contrast differential since the testis has a higher signal intensity than that of fat (Figure 12-2C). The low signal intensity of the testis on T1-weighted MR images at both

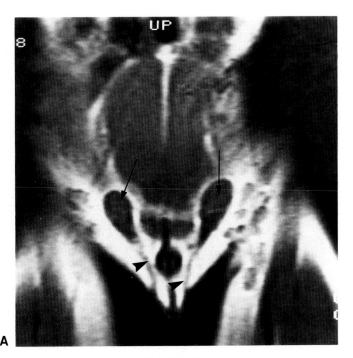

A

SE 1,000/17

Figure 12-5. Conditions mimicking undescended testes on MR images. (A) Coronal MR image (1.0 T) showing low-intensity oval structures (arrows) in the inguinal canals, consistent with bilateral inguinal hernias. Note the normal-appearing spermatic cord (arrowheads) extending beyond the hernias. Additional views showed normally descended intrascrotal testes bilaterally. (B) Transverse MR image (1.0 T) showing the high signal intensity of fluid in inguinal canals (arrows). These bilateral structures could be mistaken for the high signal intensity of undescended testes if other views were not carefully evaluated.

low and high field strength is similar to that of muscle **(Option (B) is true).**

Small undescended testes may be difficult to identify, and the appearance of testicular remnants with imaging is still unfamiliar to radiologists. If no testis is found in the usual pathway, an obstructed or ectopic location should be suspected, such as the anterior abdominal wall, femoral triangle, perineum, thigh, or the root of the penis. Since inguinal hernias are often associated with undescended testes, it is important to recognize that the hernia can mimic an intracanalicular testis (Figure 12-5). Intra-abdominal testes are commonly located close to the internal inguinal ring **(Option (E) is false).** These testes are in close association

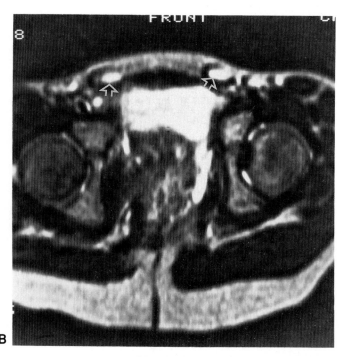

SE 2,000/80

with the lateral bladder wall, psoas muscle, iliac vessels, and peritoneum. Since nonpalpable testes may be absent or remain only as remnants, identification of distinct spermatic cord structures, even without the testis, provides important preoperative information.

The testicular location is categorized as normal scrotal, high scrotal, obstructed, ectopic, intracanalicular, and abdominal. The deep inguinal ring is used to distinguish the last two categories. It can be identified on MR images as being immediately lateral to the inferior epigastric vessels and slightly lateral to the mid-inguinal point. The mid-inguinal point is located halfway between the anterior superior iliac spine and the symphysis pubis. The deep inguinal ring is also anterior to the external iliac-femoral arterial junction (Figure 12-6). Gonads located at or above the ring are considered intra-abdominal **(Option (D) is true)**. Testes with high signal intensity on T2-weighted images are characteristic. The histologic evaluation of a structure with a long T2 indicates the presence of at least some testicular germ cell types, i.e., seminiferous tubules, germ cells, or Leydig or Sertoli cells. Tissue with these basic testicular cell types showing high signal intensity on T2-weighted images may be atrophic and contain fibrosis. Although low-signal-intensity testes have

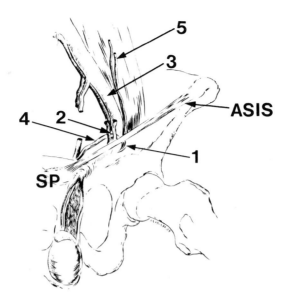

Figure 12-6. Artist's depiction of important anatomic landmarks for differentiation of intracanalicular from intra-abdominal testes. The deep inguinal ring (1) is located slightly lateral to the midpoint between the anterior superior iliac spine (ASIS) and symphysis pubis (SP). The inferior epigastric vessels (2) and external iliac artery (3) are reliable landmarks for identification of the deep inguinal ring. The vas deferens (4) and testicular vessels (5) are also in the immediate vicinity.

previously been suggested to be fibrotic, recent histologic evaluation shows that various amounts of fibrosis are present even when the signal intensity is high.

Low signal intensity on T2-weighted images is expected when the intact testis is absent. Structures with low signal intensity on T2-weighted images have been correlated histologically with sites of testicular regression containing remnant structures (vas deferens and vessels), often with an associated fibrotic nodule containing hemosiderin-laden macrophages and calcifications.

Although the spermatic cord structures may be identified on MR images, it must be remembered that the vas deferens has been noted to loop ahead of the testis during its descent. This may lead the radiologist to look for the testis too far distally or to read this study falsely as negative, since the testis may actually be present higher in the pathway of descent. The mediastinum testis is occasionally identified as a low-intensity structure eccentrically placed in the high signal intensity of the

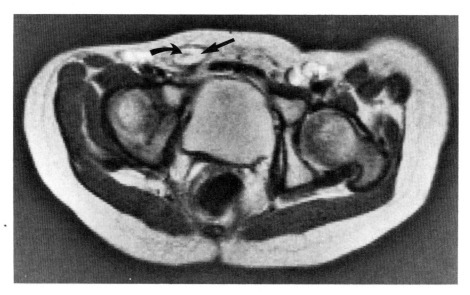

SE 1,700/70

Figure 12-7. Undescended testis. Transverse MR image (1.0 T) showing the high signal intensity of an intracanalicular testis (straight arrow). Note the low signal intensity of the mediastinum testis (curved arrow), which is confirmatory for testicular tissue but is inconsistently visualized.

testis (Figure 12-7). Identification of the mediastinum testis has been described as helpful in confirming that a visualized structure is indeed a testis. However, the infrequency with which it is identified limits its usefulness.

The size and shape of a nonpalpable gonad may be misleading. It is generally accepted that an undescended testis in the inguinal canal will be oval. Intra-abdominal testes and testicular remnants, regardless of position, are quite often rounded. Therefore, an oval shape cannot be considered a required diagnostic feature, except for testes in the canal.

MRI is especially attractive for evaluation of undescended testes because it can reliably localize both undescended testes and remnants of testicular regression. Neither CT nor ultrasonography has any reported experience in identifying testicular remnants, and ultrasonography has the added limitation of being ineffective for detection of testes above the canal. The advantage of MRI over CT is its ability to produce multiplanar images without ionizing radiation. The radiologist must be aware of the expected pathway of testicular descent and of both typical and atypical MR characteristics of such testes. Precise triangulation of structures on all views, however, is also needed for accurate diagnosis.

Question 63

Which *one* of the following is MOST likely to be associated with an undescended testis?

(A) Seminoma
(B) Infertility
(C) Inguinal hernia
(D) Prune belly syndrome
(E) Intersex disorders

In male neonates, there is often a persistent opening of the processus vaginalis, an outpouching of the peritoneum, which leads to inguinal hernias. In patients with undescended testes, there is an associated 70% incidence of inguinal hernias because there is always a persistent opening of the processus vaginalis **(Option (C) is correct).**

Anorchia, defined as the absence of the testis, reportedly occurs in 3 to 5% of all males having surgery for an undescended testis. The cause of anorchia is either a failure of the testis to develop from the original gonadal mass or a loss of blood supply, such as by torsion of the testis during fetal or neonatal life. The vas deferens and a rudimentary epididymis are usually present and may have descended into the canal or upper portion of the scrotum. Unilateral anorchia is of no clinical significance since fertility is unlikely to be affected and the opposite testis may undergo compensatory hypertrophy. Bilateral absence of the testes has serious consequences and requires hormonal replacement at puberty.

Besides having less volume, an undescended testis also has histologic differences from a normal testis. Abnormal development of germ cells begins very early in life, perhaps *in utero*. In children with a unilateral undescended testis, the normally descended testis has more germ cells than the undescended testis but has fewer than a normal testis in age-matched controls. In nearly 40% of cases of unilateral undescended testis, the combined germ cell count of both testes does not exceed that for bilateral undescended testes, suggesting a germ-cell deficiency of both testes. The mean number of germ cells and the size of the seminiferous tubules in an undescended testis show asymmetry from the opposite descended testis, and there are increasing differences at 18 to 24 months of age, with initiation of peritubular hyalinization and fibrosis. This pattern leads to the infertility (Option (B)) seen in older cryptorchid men, particularly if the condition was bilateral. In a group of men who had late spontaneous descent of previous bilateral undescended testes, only 33% were found to have a normal semen analysis, whereas 47%

were classified as being sterile or having severely reduced fertility. Pre-
and postoperative biopsies in patients undergoing orchidopexy have
shown either moderate or marked improvement in spermatogenesis in
52% of the patients. Because of the histologic changes that take place
near 2 years of age, orchidopexy by 18 months of age is advocated to
maximize fertility.

The final testicular descent is aided by an increase in intra-abdominal
pressure from the growth of the abdominal wall musculature and the
enclosed viscera. Therefore, it is common for patients with prune belly
syndrome (Eagle-Barrett syndrome) (Option (D)) to have associated
undescended testes that are intra-abdominal in location. The prune belly
syndrome is an uncommon disorder, however, and thus it is not the most
likely association with undescended testis among the conditions listed
in this question.

The germ cells migrate to the testis from the dorsal mesentery of the
hindgut during week 6 of embryonic development. Abnormalities associated with hermaphrodites (Option (E)), in whom both the testicular and
ovarian gonads are present, suggest an abnormality occurring early in
the stage of differentiation, and these gonadal structures commonly do
not descend in a normal manner. Patients with hypospadias, the mildest
expression of an abnormality of the urogenital sinus, have associated
undescended testes. Again, the relative infrequency of these intersex
conditions makes them less likely to be associated with undescended
testis than with hernia.

As was noted above, men with a history of cryptorchidism have an
increased risk of testicular cancer, usually seminoma (Option (A)). This
relative risk is only 4 to 5 times higher instead of the 10 to 40 times
previously reported, and testicular cancer is certainly not as commonly
associated as hernia. Intra-abdominal testes are more likely to undergo
malignant degeneration than are inguinal testes. This difference has
been attributed primarily to the 1.5 to 2.0°C increase in temperature
within the abdominal cavity. Although there are no data demonstrating
that orchidopexy decreases this potential for malignant degeneration,
current thinking suggests that the testis be placed in the scrotum to
minimize degenerative changes and allow for early palpation of any
tumor.

Peggy J. Fritzsche, M.D.

SUGGESTED READINGS

EMBRYOLOGY, TESTICULAR DESCENT, AND ANATOMY

1. Beltran-Brown F, Villegas-Alvarez F. Clinical classification for undescended testes: experience in 1,010 orchidopexies. J Pediatr Surg 1988; 23:444–447
2. Kogan SJ. Cryptorchidism. In: Kelalis PP, King LR, Gelman AB (eds), Clinical pediatric urology, 2nd ed. Philadelphia: WB Saunders; 1985:864–888
3. Marshall FF, Shermeta DW. Epididymal abnormalities associated with undescended testis. J Urol 1979; 121:341–343
4. Moore KL. The developing human, 3rd ed. Philadelphia: WB Saunders; 1982
5. Moul JW, Belman AB. A review of surgical treatment of undescended testes with emphasis on anatomical position. J Urol 1988; 140:125–128
6. Romanes GJ. Cunningham's textbook of anatomy, 11th ed. Oxford: Oxford University Press; 1972:351
7. Scorer MD, Farrington GH. Congenital anomalies of the testes. In: Harrison JH, Gittes RF, Perlmutter AD, Stamey TA, Walsh PC (eds), Campbell's urology, vol 2, 4th ed. Philadelphia: WB Saunders; 1978:1549–1561

CANCER

8. Batata MA, Whitmore WF Jr, Chu FC, et al. Cryptorchidism and testicular cancer. J Urol 1980; 124:382–387
9. Brown LM, Pottern LM, Hoover RN. Testicular cancer in young men: the search for causes of the epidemic increase in the United States. J Epidemiol Community Health 1987; 41:349–354
10. Campbell HE. The incidence of malignant growth of the undescended testicle: a reply and reevaluation. J Urol 1959; 81:663–668
11. Chilvers C, Dudley NE, Gough MH, Jackson MB, Pike MC. Undescended testis: the effect of treatment on subsequent risk of subfertility and malignancy. J Pediatr Surg 1986; 21:691–696
12. Giwercman A, Grindsted J, Hansen B, Jensen OM, Skakkebaek NE. Testicular cancer risk in boys with maldescended testis: a cohort study. J Urol 1987; 138:1214–1216
13. Martin DC. Germinal cell tumors of the testis after orchiopexy. J Urol 1979; 121:422–424

FERTILITY

14. Bremholm Rasmussen T, Ingerslev HJ, Høstrup H. Bilateral spontaneous descent of the testis after the age of 10: subsequent effects on fertility. Br J Surg 1988; 75:820–823
15. Gilhooly PE, Meyers F, Lattimer JK. Fertility prospects for children with cryptorchidism. Am J Dis Child 1984; 138:940–943
16. Hadziselimovic F. Cryptorchidism, management and implications. New York: Springer-Verlag; 1983:71–81
17. Hedinger E. Histopathology of undescended testes. Eur J Pediatr 1982; 139:266–271

18. Huff DS, Hadziselimovic F, Duckett JW, Elder JS, Snyder HM. Germ cell counts in semithin sections of biopsies of 115 unilaterally cryptorchid testes. The experience from the Children's Hospital of Philadelphia. Eur J Pediatr 1987; 146(Suppl 2):S25–S27
19. Puri P, O'Donnell B. Semen analysis of patients who had orchidopexy at or after seven years of age. Lancet 1988; 2:1051–1052

IMAGING OF UNDESCENDED TESTES

20. Fritzsche PJ, Hopkins R. Nonpalpable testes and testicular remnants: MR findings with surgical and pathologic correlation. AJR (submitted)
21. Fritzsche PJ, Hricak H, Kogan BA, Winkler ML, Tanagho EA. Undescended testis: value of MR imaging. Radiology 1987; 164:169–173
22. Kier R, McCarthy S, Rosenfield AT, Rosenfield NS, Rapoport S, Weiss RM. Nonpalpable testes in young boys: evaluation with MR imaging. Radiology 1988; 169:429–433
23. Landa HM, Gylys-Morin V, Mattrey RF, Krous HF, Kaplan GW, Packer MG. Magnetic resonance imaging of the cryptorchid testis. Eur J Pediatr 1987; 146(Suppl 2):S16–S17
24. Lee JK, Glazer HS. Computed tomography in the localization of the nonpalpable testis. Urol Clin North Am 1982; 9:397–404
25. Weiss RM, Carter AR, Rosenfield AT. High resolution real-time ultrasonography in the localization of the undescended testis. J Urol 1986; 135:936–938

Notes

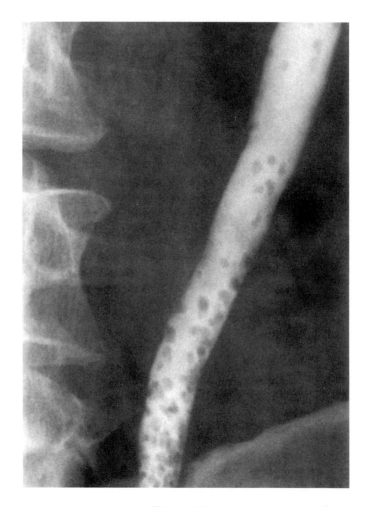

Figure 13-1

Case 13: Ureteral Lesions

Questions 64 through 68

For each numbered image (Questions 64 through 68), select the *one* lettered diagnosis (A, B, C, D, or E) that is MOST likely. Each lettered diagnosis may be used once, more than once, or not at all.

A 64. Figure 13-1
E 65. Figure 13-2
C 66. Figure 13-3
D 67. Figure 13-4
B 68. Figure 13-5

      (A) Ureteritis cystica
      (B) Transitional cell carcinoma
      (C) Pseudodiverticulosis
      (D) Mucosal edema
      (E) Blind-ending ureteral bud

Multiple, sharply defined filling defects are seen in the ureter in Figure 13-1. Those along the sides of the ureter can be seen arising from the ureteral wall. This is the classic appearance of ureteritis cystica **(Option (A) is the correct answer to Question 64).** Transitional cell carcinoma (TCC) is often multifocal but would not be so uniform in appearance. Vascular impressions create extrinsic compression defects rather than the intrinsic defects seen with ureteritis cystica.

In Figure 13-2, there appears to be a second ureter overlying the ilium. However, this "duplicated" ureter ends quickly and does not ascend to the kidney. This is a blind-ending branch of a ureteral bud or a ureteral diverticulum, and it ascends for only a few centimeters **(Option (E) is the correct answer to Question 65).** The blind-ending ureter fills by reverse peristalsis; fluoroscopy will show this process and hence confirm the diagnosis.

Multiple small outpouchings from the opacified ureteral lumen are present in the midportion of the left ureter in Figure 13-3, and the ureter appears mildly narrowed but not obstructed. These tiny ureteral diver-

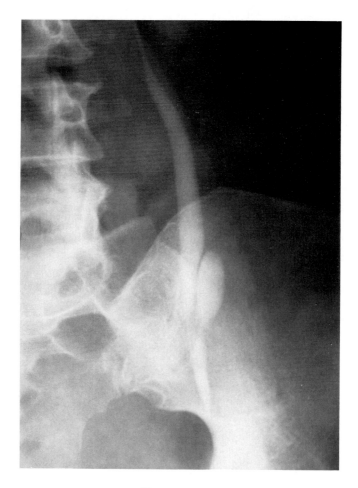

Figure 13-2

ticula are much smaller than the blind-ending ureteral bud illustrated in Figure 13-2 and are characteristic of pseudodiverticulosis **(Option (C) is the correct answer to Question 66).**

The filling defects in the right renal pelvis and ureter in Figure 13-4 are small but have a more linear configuration than those seen in the patient with ureteritis cystica (Figure 13-1). Mucosal ridges are especially well seen in the renal pelvis. This appearance is typical of mucosal edema **(Option (D) is the correct answer to Question 67).** Irregularity of the urothelium is also seen with TCC. However, it produces focal masses rather than this linear configuration.

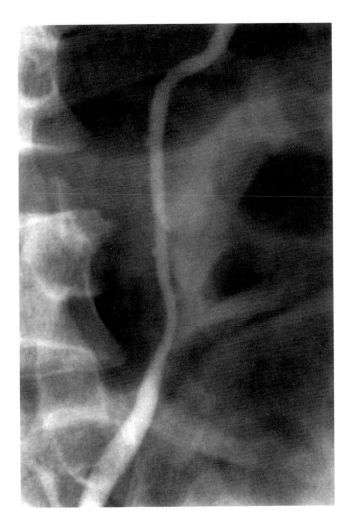

Figure 13-3

A relatively large filling defect is seen in the retrograde pyelogram depicted in Figure 13-5. This defect partially obstructs the ureter, as is evidenced by the mild ureteral dilatation proximal to the filling defect. The differential diagnosis for this appearance includes a lucent stone, blood clot, ureteral neoplasm, and sloughed papilla, which is being passed down the ureter. The characteristic feature seen in the figure is dilatation of the ureter distal to the filling defect (goblet sign). This is seen in primary TCC of the ureter but not in other entities **(Option (B) is the correct answer to Question 68).**

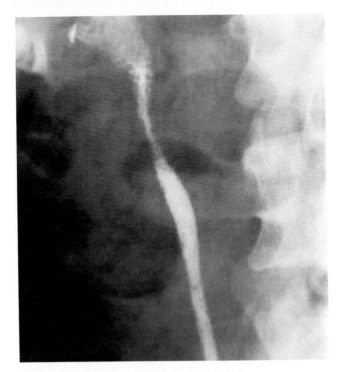

Figure 13-4

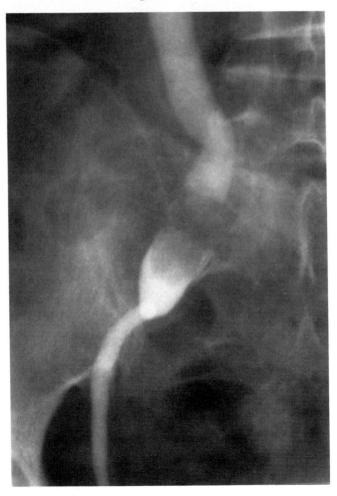

Figure 13-5

Question 69

Concerning ureteritis cystica,

F (A) multiple small, contrast-filled diverticula project from the ureteral wall
T (B) most patients have a history of chronic urinary tract infections
T (C) it is more common in the proximal than the distal ureter
T (D) it often involves the renal pelvis and bladder
F (E) it is associated with transitional cell carcinoma

Ureteritis cystica is an uncommon abnormality that may be seen throughout the urothelium. When it occurs in the renal pelvis it is called pyelitis cystica, whereas when it occurs in the bladder it may be referred to as cystitis cystica. In patients with ureteritis cystica, multiple small, subepithelial cysts form in the wall of the ureter and project into the lumen. The cysts are probably formed by degeneration and cavitation of Brunn's cell nests. The walls are composed of immature epithelium, and the cysts contain a clear proteinaceous fluid.

Most patients with ureteritis cystica have a history of chronic urinary tract infections, and the cysts may form as a result of this continued inflammatory irritation **(Option (B) is true).** Once formed, the cysts do not regress.

The radiographic appearance of ureteritis cystica is characteristic. Opacification of the collecting system by excretory urography or antegrade or retrograde pyelography reveals multiple small, sharply circumscribed, smooth filling defects that project into the ureteral lumen **(Option (A) is false).** Their number varies from only a few to innumerable, and they may affect only a portion of the ureter or the entire collecting system. Involvement of the proximal ureter is more common than involvement of the distal ureter **(Option (C) is true).**

The changes of ureteritis cystica are not limited to the ureter. A similar appearance may be seen in the renal pelvis (pyelitis cystica), and the whole process may be called pyeloureteritis cystica. Among 23 patients reported by Loitman and Chiat, 17 had ureteritis cystica and 6 had pyelitis cystica. Four patients had involvement of both the ureter and renal pelvis (pyeloureteritis cystica). The changes also occur in the bladder (cystitis cystica); these changes cannot be recognized on imaging studies since they are too small, but they can be detected by direct visual inspection by cystoscopy **(Option (D) is true).**

Ureteritis cystica is a benign condition with no malignant potential. There is no association with TCC **(Option (E) is false).** The differential diagnosis of ureteritis cystica includes multiple papillary TCCs, suburothelial hemorrhage, and ureteral involvement by tuberculosis. However, the appearance of multiple well-defined, small filling defects is characteristic and allows the diagnosis of ureteritis cystica to be made in most cases.

Question 70

Concerning transitional cell carcinoma,

T (A) the frequency of occurrence in the renal pelvis, ureter, bladder, and urethra is proportional to the surface area of the urothelium in these structures

F (B) a negative urinary cytologic test makes it an unlikely diagnosis

F (C) obstruction of the collecting system is rare

T (D) dilatation of the ureter distal to a filling defect is much more commonly seen with this condition than with a ureteral stone

T (E) the risk of spreading the tumor along the catheter tract contraindicates percutaneous nephrostomy for tumor in the upper urinary tract

TCC is the most common primary cancer of the urothelium, accounting for over 90% of all cancers of the renal pelvis or ureter. Its frequency of occurrence at specific sites is roughly proportional to the surface area of the urothelium, such that 1 primary ureteral tumor is seen for every 3 tumors arising in the renal pelvis and every 60 tumors in the bladder **(Option (A) is true).** Most of the remaining primary cancers of the pelvicalyceal system and ureter are squamous cell carcinomas; less than 1% are adenocarcinomas.

There are several recognized causes of TCC. Many patients have a history of chronic urinary tract infection or renal stones resulting in chronic mucosal irritation. Textile workers, as well as those in the rubber and plastics industries, may be exposed to aminophenols, which are carcinogenic. Bladder tumors are more common in these patients because there is a longer exposure to the urothelium from the urine-filled bladder. The increased incidence of renal pelvic tumors seen in phenacetin abusers is presumably due to the aminophenols that are degradation products of phenacetin.

Smoking pseudotics

TCC of the renal pelvis or ureter usually occurs in older patients. The average age at diagnosis is 65 years. Men predominate by a ratio of 4:1, and hematuria is the most common presentation. Flank pain, which may be due to obstruction of the ureter or ureteropelvic junction by the tumor, occurs in approximately 25% of patients.

Urinary cytologic tests can be quite helpful in making the diagnosis of TCC, but a negative result does not exclude the tumor **(Option (B) is false).** The frequency of a positive urinary cytologic test increases with increases in either the grade or stage of the tumor. The grade of the tumor is a histologic description ranging from grade I, which shows only slight anaplasia, to grade IV, which has marked anaplasia. The tumor stage reflects the degree of invasion. Stage A has no invasion, stage B is superficially invasive, and stage C involves the muscularis, whereas stage D extends to the adventitial surface. Nocks et al. reported positive urinary cytologic tests in no patients with grade I tumors, 29% with grade II tumors, and 79% with grade III tumors of the renal pelvis. They found positive cytologic tests ranging from 14% in patients with stage A disease to 89% in patients with stage D disease. The method of collecting urine for cytologic evaluation is also important. Voided urine is least likely to give positive results. Urine collected passively by catheter is better than voided urine but is not as likely to give positive results as that obtained by lavage. The highest accuracy of these passive techniques is found with samples obtained by repeated washing (barbotage). If fluoroscopy is available, however, brush biopsy, which is the most sensitive technique, may be performed.

The imaging study by which the diagnosis of TCC of the renal pelvis or ureter is made most often is the excretory urogram. The most common finding is one or more filling defects. The filling defects are usually irregular, as TCCs grow in a frondlike manner, allowing contrast material into the interstices of the tumor (Figure 13-6). However, about 15% of TCCs are of the nonpapillary type and have a smooth contour (Figure 13-7). For TCCs within the ureter, the frequency of nonpapillary tumors rises to approximately 40%.

TCCs may obstruct the collecting system, and high-grade obstruction may prevent opacification of the affected portion. A "phantom calyx" results from nonopacification due to calyceal or infundibular obstruction. Obstruction leading to ipsilateral nonfunction is even more common when the tumor is in the ureter. Anderstrom et al. reported nonfunction in 21 of 49 patients (43%) **(Option (C) is false).**

A unique feature of the papillary tumor is dilatation of the ureter distal to the filling defect (Figure 13-5). This "goblet sign" reflects the appearance of the contrast-filled distal ureter and is best demonstrated on retrograde pyelography. The sign is relatively specific, as it is not seen with ureteral stones **(Option (D) is true).** Coiling of a retrograde catheter in the dilated portion of the ureter distal to the ureteral tumor is termed Bergman's sign.

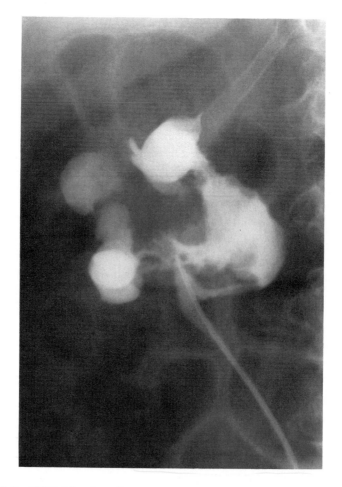

Figure 13-6. TCC. The frondlike pattern of the tumor allows contrast material into the interstices and results in an irregular filling defect. (Reprinted with permission from Dunnick et al. [1].)

The treatment of TCC of the ureter is nephroureterectomy with resection of a cuff of bladder. If the distal ureter is left, it may be the site of recurrent tumor (Figure 13-8). Ureteral resection may be adequate for superficial tumors. However, it is important to examine the entire ureteropelvicalyceal system carefully for multifocal tumors before attempting a limited resection.

TCCs tend to spread along the path of urine flow. They may also spread along a catheter tract. Thus, suprapubic catheterization is contraindicated in patients with bladder tumors and percutaneous nephrostomy is

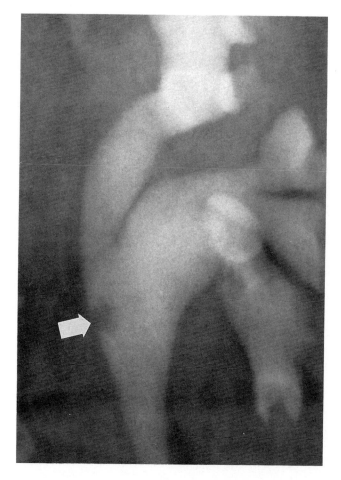

Figure 13-7. TCC. This tumor, which arises from the medial wall of the renal pelvis (arrow), has a smooth contour, typical of the nonpapillary type.

contraindicated in patients with TCC of the upper tracts **(Option (E) is true).**

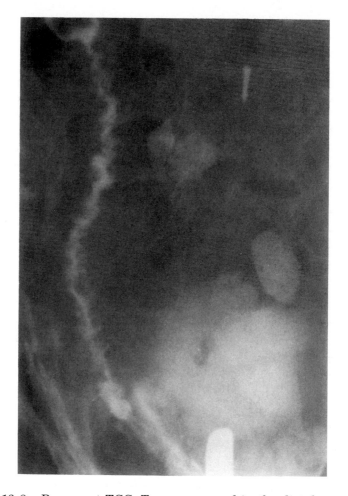

Figure 13-8. Recurrent TCC. Tumor recurred in the distal ureter after a nephrectomy had been performed for TCC. Retrograde ureterogram demonstrates multiple irregular filling defects in the distal ureter.

Question 71

Concerning pseudodiverticulosis,

F (A) it is due to a series of congenital defects in the ureteral wall
T (B) most patients have a history of chronic urinary tract infections
T (C) it is most common in the upper and middle portions of the ureter
F (D) radiographically it is indistinguishable from ureteritis cystica
T (E) it is associated with an increased incidence of transitional cell carcinoma

Ureteral pseudodiverticulosis is the manifestation of a proliferative response to focal inflammation, which results in buds of epithelium projecting into the ureteral wall. These pouch-like invaginations measure 1 to 3 mm and project into the loose connective tissue of the lamina propria. Since all layers of the ureter are not involved, the lesions are not true diverticula.

The development of multiple pseudodiverticula is most probably a manifestation of chronic infection and inflammation leading to reactive hyperplasia of the urothelium, and thus pseudodiverticulosis is an acquired lesion rather than a consequence of a congenital abnormality **(Option (A) is false)**. Most patients with pseudodiverticulosis have a history of chronic urinary tract infection **(Option (B) is true)**.

The multiple ureteral pseudodiverticula seen in patients with pseudodiverticulosis are located within the ureteral wall and thus are neither congenital (true) nor acquired (false) diverticula. A congenital or true diverticulum is an outpouching of the entire wall. It is usually much longer than it is wide and may be a blind-ending ureteral bud. Acquired or false diverticula are the result of defects in the ureteral wall and are often traumatic in origin. The ureteral mucosa protrudes through the defect, which may be in any portion of the ureter. True diverticula are more common in the distal ureter. Pseudodiverticulosis more commonly involves the middle and upper portions of the ureter **(Option (C) is true)**. Involvement may be bilateral in as many as two-thirds of cases.

The pseudodiverticula are protrusions of urothelium into the ureteral wall. They may be visualized by excretory urography or antegrade or retrograde pyelography when they are opacified by contrast material. The affected segment of the ureter often appears slightly narrowed but is not obstructed. The cystic lesions of ureteritis cystica protrude into the ureteral lumen. Thus, pseudodiverticulosis and ureteritis cystica are clearly distinguishable radiographically **(Option (D) is false)**.

Cellular atypism is often seen in patients with pseudodiverticulosis, and these patients are at increased risk of developing TCC **(Option (E)**

is true). Cochran et al. reported TCC of the bladder in 7 of 10 patients with ureteral pseudodiverticulosis. One of these patients also had a synchronous TCC of the ureter. TCC was found in 4 of 15 patients (27%) reported by Wasserman et al. and in 2 of 6 patients (33%) reported by Parker et al. Thus, ureteral pseudodiverticulosis may be a useful marker of epithelial dysplasia that may become malignant.

Question 72

Concerning a blind-ending ureteral bud,

T (A) it may arise from the ureter or the bladder
T (B) a common sheath surrounds both the ureter and the bud
T (C) the blind-ending ureter fills by retrograde peristalsis
F (D) most patients present with symptoms of urinary tract infection
F (E) it is more common in men than in women

The blind-ending ureteral bud, a form of ureteral diverticulum, is a branch of the ureter, and the wall of the blind-ending bud has the same components as the normal ureteral wall. It is at least twice as long as it is wide and joins the ureter at an acute angle. The blind-ending bud is almost always oriented with the blind end directed cranially. It usually arises from the ureter but may arise from the bladder **(Option (A) is true).** Blind-ending ureteral buds that arise from the bladder are the result of a late-forming ureteral bud coming from the Wolffian duct. The bud fails to induce the metanephric blastema, and there is no connection with the kidney.

Occasionally, a fibrous cord may extend from the blind-ending ureteral bud to the kidney. Although a common sheath surrounds both the ureter and the blind-ending bud **(Option (B) is true),** they may be widely separated. There is a common arterial supply to both the ureter and the associated ureteral bud.

The blind-ending ureteral bud fills by reflux in the same manner as a bifid ureter. Peristalsis is initiated in the renal pelvis or in a major infundibulum and moves down the ureter to the junction with the ureteral bud. Peristalsis then proceeds up the blind-ending ureter in a retrograde manner **(Option (C) is true).** This can sometimes initiate a "yo-yo" effect, with alternating antegrade and retrograde peristalsis.

The blind-ending ureteral bud may contain a ureteral calculus or

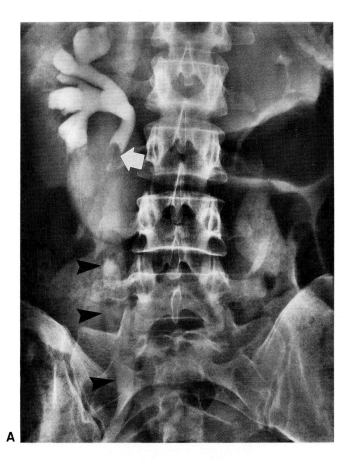

Figure 14-2 (Same as Figure 14-1). (A) The 1-hour radiograph from an excretory urogram shows a dilated collecting system with a filling defect (arrow) caused by a blood clot. The distal ureter is also dilated (arrowheads) due to an additional obstructing clot near the ureterovesical junction. (B) Arterial phase of selective right renal arteriogram in 5° left posterior oblique projection reveals a group of tortuous vessels of varying caliber (arrows). The density projected over the mid-kidney laterally is costal cartilage.

no signal because of a flow void associated with vessels. This was confirmed at subsequent angiography (Figure 14-4B).

The presence of hematuria and abnormal vasculature is common in patients with renal cell carcinoma (Option (A)). There is no mass effect on the collecting system or extending from the renal contour in the test patient. A mass, as well as abnormal vessels, is usually also apparent on arteriography (Figure 14-5B). Hence, renal cell carcinoma is less likely than vascular malformation.

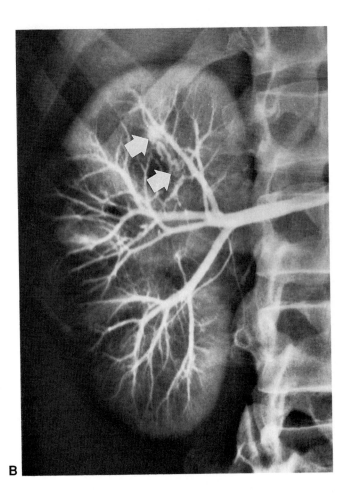

B

The "nutcracker" phenomenon (Option (B)) may cause hematuria, but it is purely a venous lesion, which is not visible in the arterial phase of a renal angiogram. The angiographic findings are primarily perihilar and periureteral (Figure 14-6). Moreover, the nutcracker phenomenon is an abnormality of the left renal vein, whereas the abnormality in the test case is right-sided.

Transitional cell carcinoma (Option (D)) arises from the uroepithelium and is commonly associated with hematuria. The lack of a mucosal lesion in association with the vascular abnormality of the test patient is strong evidence against this diagnosis. Images of a patient with transitional cell carcinoma are shown in Figure 14-7. The retrograde pyelogram (Figure 14-7A) shows the obstructing tumor at the ureteropelvic junction. The arteriogram (Figure 14-7B) reveals encasement of the proximal

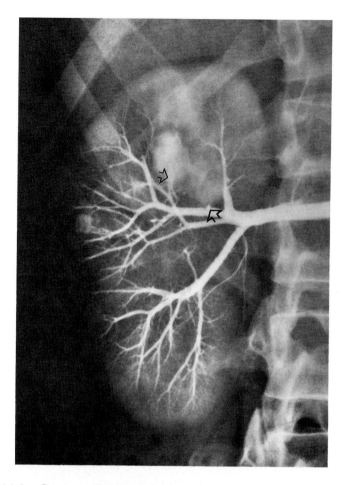

Figure 14-3. Same patient as in Figures 14-1 and 14-2. Vascular malformation. Selective right renal arteriogram obtained after embolization of the feeding vessels to the vascular malformation shows persistent stain due to parenchymal stasis following occlusion of the supplying vessels (arrows).

vessels by this infiltrating lesion. In addition, fine neovasculature is demonstrated in the renal pelvis at the level of the obstructing lesion shown on the retrograde pyelogram.

Substance abuse (Option (E)) causes a necrotizing angiitis that involves the renal vasculature in a diffuse manner in most patients. The test patient has a localized lesion with otherwise normal vascular anatomy.

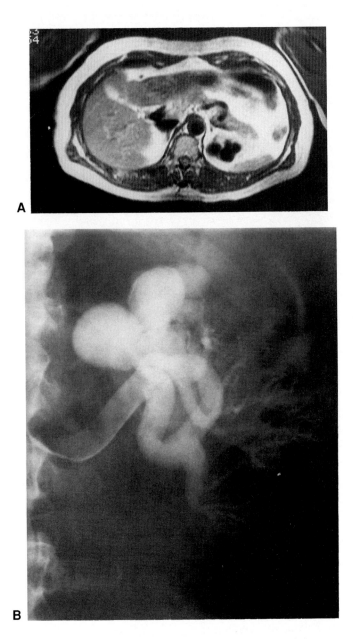

Figure 14-4. Large renal vascular malformation. (A) T1-weighted MR image demonstrates a signal void due to the presence of rapidly flowing blood in the lobulated, medial left upper-pole mass. (B) Selective left renal arteriogram confirms the vascular nature of the mass.

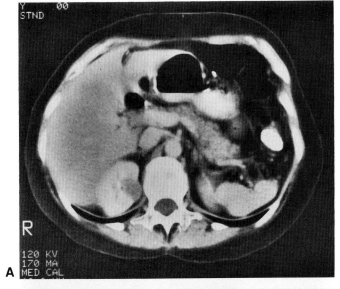

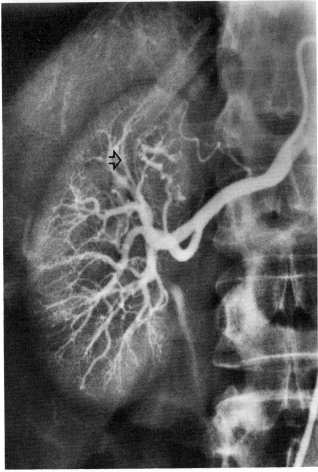

Figure 14-5. Renal cell carcinoma. (A) CT scan shows a 3-cm mixed-attenuation mass extending from the medial aspect of the upper pole of the right kidney. (B) Selective renal arteriogram in the early arterial phase shows several tortuous, ectatic vessels at the medial upper pole. Displacement of adjacent normal vessels (arrow) indicates the presence of a mass.

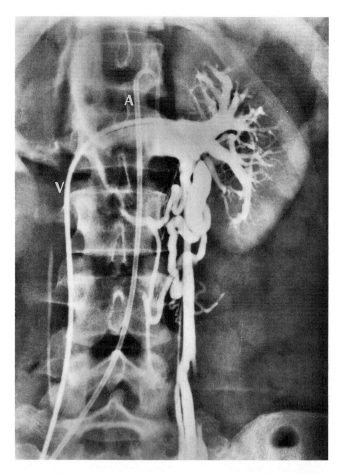

Figure 14-6. Nutcracker phenomenon. Left selective renal venogram demonstrates large variceal vessels in the perihilar and periureteral locations. A 10-mm-Hg gradient was present between the proximal renal veins and the inferior vena cava due to compression of the renal vein between the superior mesenteric artery and the aorta. A catheter is present in the aorta and renal artery (A). A venous catheter is also present (V).

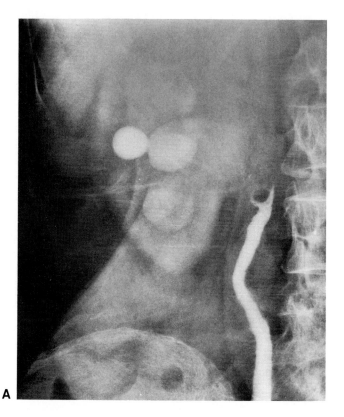

A

Figure 14-7. Transitional cell carcinoma. (A) Retrograde pyelogram shows a filling defect at the level of the right ureteropelvic junction causing proximal hydronephrosis. The ureter just below the obstruction has a characteristic goblet shape. (B) Selective renal arteriogram demonstrates several proximal vessels to be narrowed as a result of tumor encasement (arrows). Fine tumor vascularity is also present (open arrow).

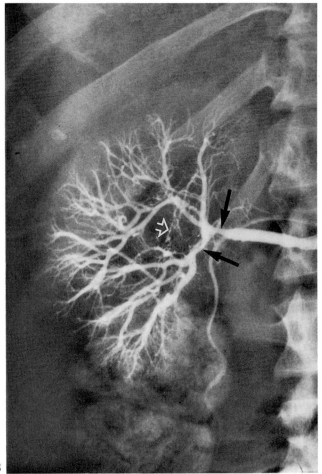

B

Question 74

Concerning renal cell carcinoma,

 T (A) embolotherapy is not indicated for small tumors
 F (B) sonography is preferred for staging
 T (C) alcohol embolization should be performed through a balloon-occlusion catheter
 F (D) the 5-year survival rate with renal vein involvement is 10%
 F (E) 50% of patients have renal vein involvement at presentation

The most widely used staging system for renal cell carcinoma is that proposed by Robson as follows:

Stage I   The tumor is confined within the renal capsule.

Stage II   The tumor extends through the renal capsule into the perinephric fat but remains confined by the renal (Gerota's) fascia. Ipsilateral adrenal involvement may occur in this stage.

Stage IIIA   The tumor involves the renal vein or the inferior vena cava.

Stage IIIB   The tumor involves regional lymph nodes.

Stage IIIC   Both regional lymph nodes and venous structures are involved.

Stage IVA   The tumor extends through the renal fascia to involve adjacent organs.

Stage IVB   Distant metastases are present.

The goal of radiologic staging of renal cell carcinoma is accurate prediction of the pathologic stage of the lesion so that treatment will be optimal. Sonography does not demonstrate the perinephric fat and renal fascia as separate structures; thus, stage I and stage II lesions cannot be differentiated. CT and MRI do demonstrate these structures, and so they are preferred for radiologic staging **(Option (B) is false)**. Sonography also fails to show the central retroperitoneum in patients with overlying intestinal gas; thus, nodal involvement and renal vein involvement may be missed. CT and MRI show these areas with good reliability. Comparison of the pathologic stage with the radiologic stage demonstrates accuracies of 80 to 90% for CT and 75 to 95% for MRI.

Involvement of the main renal vein occurs in 21 to 35% of cases at presentation, and involvement of the vena cava occurs in 5 to 10% of cases at presentation **(Option (E) is false)**. The clinical significance of renal vein and vena cava involvement has been disputed. Some investigators have shown that these patients survive as long as stage II patients provided that the surgery includes en bloc resection of the tumor thrombus. Other investigators contend that venous involvement shortens survival. Stage III includes patients with either venous or lymph node involvement. Even though the significance of venous involvement is controversial, it is agreed that nodal involvement shortens survival in the overall stage III group.

Renal vein and vena cava involvement are associated with the formation of many retroperitoneal collateral veins. These vessels are often seen on CT and MRI and are of importance in that the surgeon must deal with them during nephrectomy. Tumor thrombus may extend from the renal vein into the vena cava and right atrium. Obstruction of the hepatic veins due to tumor thrombus has also been reported as a rare complication.

McNichols et al. followed 499 patients and reported survival rates according to Robson's classification. They found that the 5-year survival rate is 67% for stage I patients, 51% for stage II, 33.5% for stage III **(Option (D) is false),** and 13.5% for stage IV. The 10-year survival rate is 56% for stage I, 28% for stage II, 20% for stage III, and 3% for stage IV.

Surgery is the primary method of therapy. Embolotherapy is not indicated for small localized lesions that are easily managed surgically **(Option (A) is true).** At present, the embolization of renal cell carcinoma is performed most often as a preoperative maneuver to make surgical resection of larger lesions feasible without excessive blood loss. Preoperative embolotherapy can be particularly useful for large right-sided lesions in which a transabdominal approach is required. Using this route, the surgeon identifies the renal vein and inferior vena cava before seeing the more posterior renal artery. If the kidney has been adequately embolized prior to the surgery, the renal vein can be ligated before the artery without the sequela of kidney distension. In this way, the surgeon can safely retract the inferior vena cava from the renal pedicle and more easily identify the artery. Embolotherapy may also be used to control renal hemorrhage associated with large unresectable or recurrent renal cell carcinomas.

A variety of embolic materials have been used to embolize renal cell carcinomas. In general, materials such as Gelfoam are quite adequate, particularly for preoperative treatment. Gelfoam or other agents may be used 1 to 2 hours before surgery to prevent most of the flank pain and fever that occur during the 12 to 48 hours following embolization of the kidney. Absolute alcohol has become a popular method of quickly obliterating the entire renal tumor vasculature in large lesions. Alcohol should always be injected through a balloon-occlusion catheter **(Option (C) is true)** (Figure 14-8). When standard angiographic catheters are used, reflux of alcohol into the aorta is a source of potential complication. There have been cases reported in which the alcohol refluxes into the aorta and then enters the inferior mesenteric artery and causes left colon infarction.

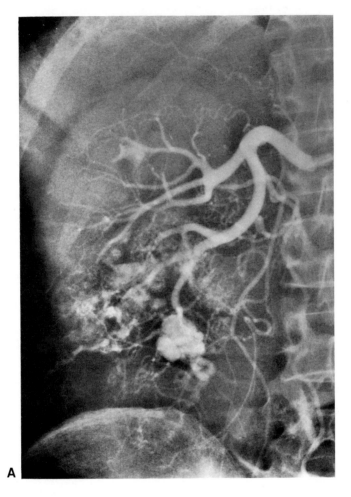

A

Figure 14-8. Alcohol embolization of renal cell carcinoma. (A) Selective right renal arteriogram shows a large hypervascular tumor of the lower half of the kidney. (B) Spot film demonstrating the inflated occlusion balloon (arrow). A small amount of contrast material has been injected to confirm cessation of flow following injection of 12 mL of absolute alcohol.

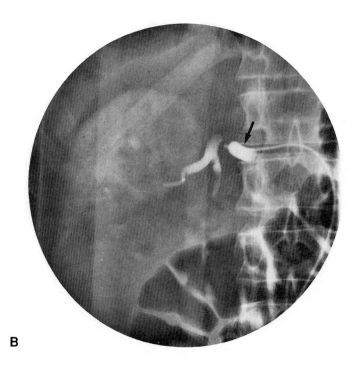

B

Question 75

Concerning the "nutcracker" phenomenon,

F (A) the frequency of right and left renal involvement is the same
T (B) it causes hematuria
T (C) a pressure gradient exists in the renal vein
F (D) embolization is the treatment of choice

The nutcracker phenomenon may be defined as compression of the left renal vein **(Option (A) is false)** as it passes between the superior mesenteric artery and aorta, resulting in a pressure gradient between the renal vein and the inferior vena cava **(Option (C) is true).** This proximal left renal vein hypertension results in the formation of renal collateral veins that have a peripelvic and periureteric distribution as they drain inferiorly to connect with the hypogastric veins (Figure 14-6). In normal individuals, there is no gradient observed as pullback pressure measurements are made from the veins at the renal hilum into the inferior vena cava. In patients with the nutcracker phenomenon, gradients of 6 to 10 mm Hg have been demonstrated. Some investigators consider gradients as small as 3 mm Hg to be abnormal. It is thought that the small forniceal veins of the kidney rupture into the calyces as a result of the elevated renal venous pressure. The resultant hematuria **(Option (B) is true)** may account for some cases of so-called "essential" hematuria. There are no good surgical or radiologic data on the number of cases of such unexplained hematuria that are due to the nutcracker phenomenon.

The treatment of hematuria due to the nutcracker phenomenon is difficult. Embolotherapy of the arterial system has no role in this condition, because the hematuria is of venous origin **(Option (D) is false).** Surgical ligation of the peripelvic and periureteric varicosities serves no logical purpose since these vessels are functioning as collateral drainage from the compressed renal vein. In fact, one would expect such ligation to worsen the problem. Procedures that address the physiologic abnormality and would control the significant gross hematuria include renal vein bypass or reimplantation. Autotransplantation of the kidney may represent a viable choice in this era in which many large medical centers have expert renal transplant teams.

Question 76

Which *one* of the following is MOST important in embolizing a renal vascular malformation?

(A) Occluding the nidus
(B) Occluding all visible feeding vessels
(C) Eliminating the arteriovenous shunting
(D) Use of a permanent coil
(E) Use of a balloon-occlusion catheter

Renal vascular malformations that are treated by embolization should be completely obliterated if possible to avoid recurrence of the lesion and hematuria. Most vascular malformations have more than one feeding vessel. Small feeding vessels that are not apparent at initial angiography will often be recruited as new sources of supply to the malformation once larger feeding vessels are occluded. Thus, occluding the initial visible feeding vessels (Option (B)) as they enter the malformation may ultimately fail as a permanent method of obliterating the malformation. One must permanently occlude the nidus of the malformation **(Option (A)**

is correct). The nidus may be considered that portion of the malformation where the supplying, abnormal, and draining vessels interconnect. Arteriovenous shunting, when present, will be obliterated by treatment (Option (C)) of the central nidus. Permanent obliteration can be achieved with glue such as bucrylate or by injection of absolute alcohol into the nidus through one of its feeding branches. Although a balloon-occlusion catheter is recommended when using alcohol, it is not the most important facet of treatment (Option (E)). Permanent obliteration can also be effected by nonabsorbable particles such as polyvinyl alcohol foam (PVF). In the test patient, several feeding branches of the malformation were embolized with PVF. Complete angiographic obliteration of the lesion was achieved (Figure 14-3). This patient's hematuria ceased after embolization with PVF, and, at the time of this writing, the patient remains free of symptoms 3 years following embolotherapy. The use of metallic coils is not indicated in treating most malformations (Option (D)). These devices are too large and will occlude feeding vessels too proximal to the nidus. This creates a situation in which the malformation may be supplied from other arterial feeders, resulting in a recurrence. A coil in a proximal feeding vessel also has the drawback of restricting access to the lesion should future treatment be necessary.

Takebayashi et al. reported their experience using absolute alcohol embolization to treat seven patients with renal arteriovenous malformations and massive hematuria. Total occlusion of the malformation was achieved in three patients, whereas partial occlusion occurred in four cases. Two of the patients with partial alcohol occlusion had supplementary Gelfoam embolization. No serious complications were encountered. Long-term follow-up of 12 to 40 months revealed no further hematuria in six patients. One patient had recurrent minor hematuria that did not require treatment. These investigators concluded that alcohol ablation of renal arteriovenous malformations was safe and efficacious.

Question 77

Concerning renal vascular disease associated with substance abuse,

T (A) methamphetamine is a cause
T (B) LSD is a cause
T (C) microaneurysms are a typical feature
T (D) hypertension is a common feature
F (E) associated gastrointestinal vascular lesions are rare

A necrotizing angiitis has been described in association with drug abuse. These patients present clinically with hypertension **(Option (D) is true)**, renal failure, or pulmonary edema. Methamphetamine is a common drug used by patients with this necrotizing angiitis **(Option (A) is true)**, but other illicit drugs have been implicated, including heroin and LSD **(Option (B) is true)**. Since many drug abusers use multiple drugs, it is often difficult to identify which drug is most responsible. Some workers have postulated that a drug contaminant is a possible cause of the renal damage.

Addicts often have circulating antibody-antigen complexes, which, with complement activation, can damage blood vessels. Pathologically, the process begins as edema and inflammation of small and medium-sized arteries. The kidney is the most common site of involvement, but gastrointestinal vessels are also frequently involved **(Option (E) is false)**. Thrombosis of the inflamed vessels is accompanied by fragmentation of the internal elastic lamina. The weakness in the vessel wall leads to the formation of microaneurysms **(Option (C) is true)** (Figure 14-9). The combination of vessel obliteration and microaneurysm formation produces an angiographic pattern that may be indistinguishable from that of polyarteritis nodosa. Patients with these vascular lesions often progress to renal failure. Citron et al. studied 14 drug abusers with various symptoms by means of angiography. The findings of necrotizing angiitis indistinguishable from polyarteritis were reported. Renal failure, hypertension, pulmonary edema, and pancreatitis were encountered in this group. Four patients died from renal failure. Treatment in these patients consists of withdrawing the offending drugs and treating the renal lesions by means of anti-inflammatory agents.

A nephropathy associated with heroin abuse has also been described. Pathologically, a focal glomerulosclerosis is present. Immune complex deposition is demonstrated in renal biopsies. Massive proteinuria and uremia develop in such patients. Another cause of massive proteinuria in intravenous drug abusers is renal amyloidosis. The deposition of

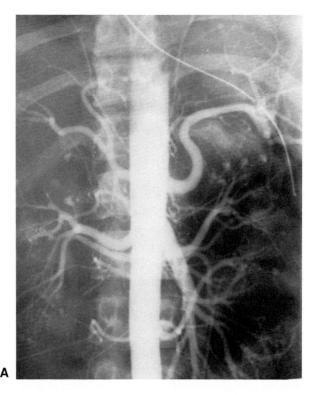

A

Figure 14-9. Angiogram in an intravenous-heroin abuser. (A) Aorto-gram. Microaneurysms involving the renal arteries and branches of the celiac and superior mesenteric arteries are present. (B) Selective right renal arteriogram. Multiple microaneurysms, as well as narrowed and attenuated arterial branches, can be seen. (Courtesy of Roger Naravel, M.D., Greater Baltimore Medical Center, Baltimore, Md.)

amyloid is thought to be due to the chronic suppurative skin infections that are found in many intravenous drug abusers. The kidneys are enlarged, with increased echogenicity on sonographic examination. Angiography shows no specific changes in patients with renal amyloidosis.

Harold A. Mitty, M.D.

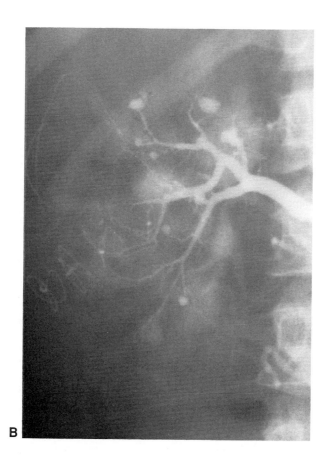

B

SUGGESTED READINGS

RENAL VASCULAR MALFORMATION

1. Cho KJ, Stanley JC. Non-neoplastic congenital and acquired renal arterio-venous malformations and fistulas. Radiology 1978; 129:333–343
2. Gloviczki P, Hollier LH. Arteriovenous fistulas. In: Haimovici H (ed), Haimo-vici's vascular surgery, 3rd ed. East Norwalk, CT: Appleton & Lange; 1989:709–711
3. Takebayashi S, Hosaka M, Ishizuka E, Hirokawa M, Matsui K. Arteriovenous malformations of the kidneys: ablation with alcohol. AJR 1988; 150:587–590
4. Yakes WF, Hass DK, Parker SH, et al. Symptomatic vascular malformations: ethanol embolotherapy. Radiology 1989; 170:1059–1066

RENAL CELL CARCINOMA

5. Bosniak MA. The small (less than or equal to 3.0 cm) renal parenchymal tumor: detection, diagnosis, and controversies. Radiology 1991; 179:307–317
6. Cox GG, Lee KR, Price HI, Gunter K, Noble MJ, Mebust WK. Colonic infarction following ethanol embolization of renal-cell carcinoma. Radiology 1982; 145:343–345
7. Goncharenko V, Gerlock AJ Jr, Kadir S, Turner B. Incidence and distribution of venous extension in 70 hypernephromas. AJR 1979; 133:263–265
8. Levine E. Malignant renal parenchymal tumors in adults. In: Pollack HM (ed), Clinical urography. Philadelphia: WB Saunders; 1990:1221–1224, 1239–1256
9. McNichols DW, Segura JW, DeWeerd JH. Renal cell carcinoma: long-term survival and late recurrence. J Urol 1981; 126:17–23
10. Robson CJ, Churchill BM, Anderson W. The results of radical nephrectomy for renal cell carcinoma. J Urol 1969; 101:297–301

"NUTCRACKER" PHENOMENON

11. Bagley DH, Allen J. Flexible ureteropyeloscopy in the diagnosis of benign essential hematuria. J Urol 1990; 143:549–553
12. Beinart C, Sniderman KW, Saddekni S, Weiner M, Vaughan ED Jr, Sos TA. Left renal vein hypertension: a cause of occult hematuria. Radiology 1982; 145:647–650
13. Kumon H, Tsugawa M, Matsumura Y, Ohmori H. Endoscopic diagnosis and treatment of chronic unilateral hematuria of uncertain etiology. J Urol 1990; 143:554–558
14. Nishimura Y, Fushiki M, Yoshida M, et al. Left renal vein hypertension in patients with left renal bleeding of unknown origin. Radiology 1986; 160:663–667

SUBSTANCE ABUSE

15. Balthazar EJ, Lefleur R. Abdominal complications of drug addiction: radiologic features. Semin Roentgenol 1983; 18:213–220
16. Cintron BP, Halpern M, McCarron M, et al. Necrotizing angiitis associated with drug abuse. N Engl J Med 1970; 283:1003–1011
17. Jacobs IG, Roszler MH, Kelly JK, Klein MA, Kling GA. Cocaine abuse: neurovascular complications. Radiology 1989; 170:223–227
18. Streiter ML, Bosniak MA. The radiology of drug addiction: urinary tract complications. Semin Roentgenol 1983; 18:221–226
19. Subramanyam BR, Balthazar EJ, Horii SC, Hilton S. Abdominal lymphadenopathy in intravenous drug addicts: sonographic features and clinical significance. AJR 1985; 144:917–920

Notes

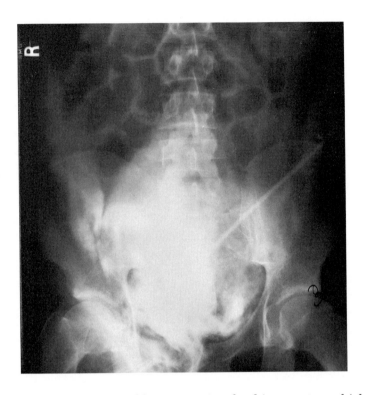

Figure 15-1. This 20-year-old man was involved in a motor vehicle accident and sustained a pelvic fracture. You are shown a radiograph from a cystogram performed through a percutaneously placed suprapubic catheter.

Case 15: Extraperitoneal Bladder Rupture

Question 78

Which *one* of the following is the MOST likely diagnosis?

- (A) Intraperitoneal bladder rupture
- (B) Extraperitoneal bladder rupture
- (C) Combined intraperitoneal and extraperitoneal bladder rupture
- (D) Combined intraperitoneal bladder and urethral rupture

Figure 15-1 is a radiograph from a cystogram performed after placement of a suprapubic cystostomy. The bladder margin (straight arrows, Figure 15-2) is straightened on the left side because of compression of its margin by extraperitoneal fluid. Obvious leakage of contrast material is seen in the pelvis, overlying the right inferior pubic ramus and hip, and along the right anterior abdominal wall extending between the lateroconal and transversalis fascias (curved arrow, Figure 15-2). The extravesical contrast material has an irregular, streaky configuration and does not appear to flow freely within the abdomen. There is no contrast material outlining bowel loops, as would be expected if some of the contrast were intraperitoneal (Figure 15-3). The findings are therefore most consistent with a complex extraperitoneal bladder rupture **(Option (B) is correct).** A CT scan of the pelvis performed on the test patient approximately 30 minutes following the cystogram demonstrates contrast material surrounding the bladder in the pelvic extraperitoneal space (Figure 15-4). Extension of the contrast material into the anterior abdominal wall (arrow) is also seen. There is no contrast material in the peritoneal space, a finding that confirms the diagnosis of extraperitoneal bladder rupture. Because no intraperitoneal component is present, both intraperitoneal bladder rupture (Option (A)) and combined intraperitoneal and extraperitoneal bladder rupture (Option (C)) are not likely. Combined intraperitoneal bladder and urethral rupture (Option (D)) is

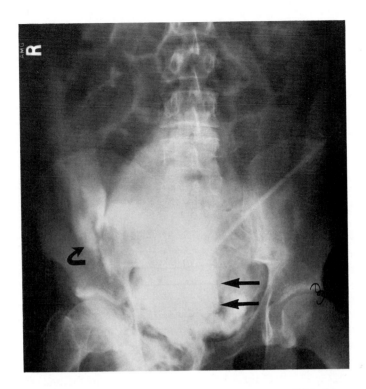

Figure 15-2 (Same as Figure 15-1). Extraperitoneal bladder rupture. The left margin of the bladder (straight arrows) is straightened and compressed by an extraperitoneal fluid collection. There is extensive leakage of contrast material into the pelvic extraperitoneal space; this contrast is seen overlying the right hip and right pubic ramus and extending into the retroperitoneal fat that makes up the flank stripe between the lateroconal and transversalis fascias (curved arrow). There is no contrast material outlining bowel loops or the intraperitoneal viscera. The injury demonstrated, therefore, is a complex extraperitoneal bladder rupture.

unlikely for the same reason; in addition, this diagnosis can be established only by retrograde urethrography combined with a cystogram performed through a suprapubic cystostomy if there is a complete urethral disruption.

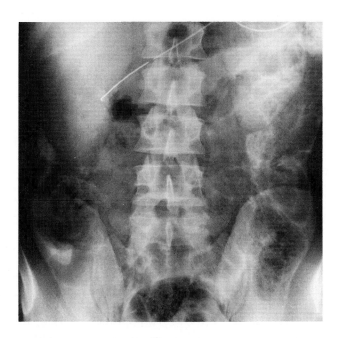

Figure 15-3. Intraperitoneal bladder rupture. Contrast material is present medial to the flank stripe and outlines multiple small bowel loops.

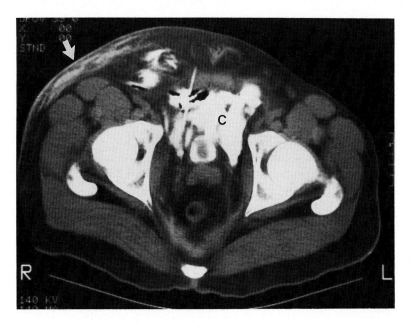

Figure 15-4. Same patient as in Figures 15-1 and 15-2. Extraperitoneal bladder rupture. CT scan of the pelvis performed several minutes after the cystogram shown in Figure 15-1. Contrast material leakage in the pelvic extraperitoneal space is present (C). Extension of the contrast material into the subcutaneous tissues of the anterior abdominal wall is evident (white arrow). Air is present in the soft tissues along the suprapubic catheter tract.

Question 79

Concerning intraperitoneal bladder rupture following blunt trauma,

F (A) the mechanism of injury is secondary to a laceration of the dome of the bladder by a bone spicule

T (B) it is the most common form of major bladder injury in children

T (C) it generally occurs in patients with a distended bladder at the time of injury

F (D) contrast-enhanced CT is the diagnostic procedure of choice

F (E) return of urine through a Foley catheter usually excludes the diagnosis

Intraperitoneal bladder rupture occurs when there is a sudden rise in intravesicular pressure as a result of a blow to the lower abdomen (Figure 15-5) in a patient with a distended bladder **(Option (C) is true).** The injury results in an approximately horizontal tear along the peritoneal-ized portion of the bladder wall (the dome). It is here, according to Oliver and Taguchi, who experimented on cadavers, that the bladder dome is most susceptible to this type of injury because this area of the wall is the least well supported by adjacent structures **(Option (A) is false).** Because distension at the time of injury is necessary for intraperitoneal bladder rupture to occur, the injury is common in alcoholics or as a result of an automobile injury from a seat belt or steering wheel. A pelvic fracture need not be present, but in one series a fracture was found in approximately two-thirds of patients in whom intraperitoneal bladder rupture was secondary to blunt trauma. Because urine may continue to drain through a Foley catheter in a patient with an intraperitoneal bladder rupture **(Option (E) is false),** the injury, if not suspected, may go undiagnosed. This can result in hyperkalemia, uremia, and acidosis as urine is reabsorbed from the peritoneal cavity. Intraperitoneal bladder rupture is the most common form of bladder injury in children because the bladder is an intraperitoneal organ before the age of puberty **(Option (B) is true).** By the age of 20 years, however, the bladder descends into its adult position in the true pelvis. With this exception, reports of the relative proportion of intraperitoneal and extraperitoneal bladder rupture vary among the published series; in one series of nearly 100 patients with bladder rupture secondary to blunt trauma, Sandler found that intraperitoneal ruptures made up approximately one-third of the cases.

CT has gained increased acceptance for the evaluation of patients suffering from blunt abdominal and pelvic trauma, leading to much recent interest in the value of CT for the initial evaluation of bladder injuries. Mee et al. demonstrated that CT-cystography performed utilizing excreted contrast material after intravenous injection was unreliable in

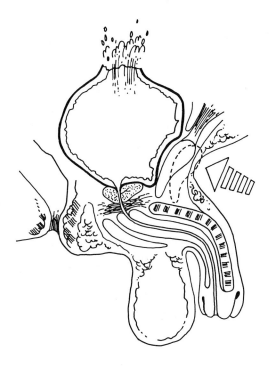

Figure 15-5. Mechanism of intraperitoneal bladder rupture. There is a sudden rise in intravesicle pressure secondary to a blow to the lower abdomen which results in rupture of the dome of the bladder.

detecting acute bladder injuries when compared with conventional cystography **(Option (D) is false)**. Mee et al. postulated that this failure was related to the variable degree of bladder distension that occurs from excretion of contrast material. Their findings were not surprising because it is well known that the cystographic phase of an excretory urogram is also unreliable for the detection of major bladder injuries, as demonstrated by Brosman and Paul in 1976. Subsequently, Lis and Cohen found that CT-cystography performed with retrograde filling of the bladder with diluted contrast material was as accurate as conventional cystography. It must be emphasized that this method of evaluating the bladder is appropriate only for patients in whom CT is to be performed for another purpose. In patients with no other indication for CT, conventional cystography remains the most cost-effective and reliable method of diagnosis.

Question 80

Concerning extraperitoneal bladder rupture following blunt trauma,

F (A) on cystography, leakage of contrast material beyond the pelvic extraperitoneal space in men generally indicates an associated urethral injury

F (B) the bladder injury is most often found adjacent to the area of pelvic fracture

T (C) most cases can be managed nonoperatively

F (D) a false-negative cystogram occurs in at least 25% of cases

Extraperitoneal bladder rupture is the most common form of major bladder injury, making up one-half to two-thirds of the cases in most of the reported series. The classically described mechanism for extraperitoneal bladder rupture is laceration of the base of the bladder by a bone spicule in conjunction with a fracture or fractures of the bony pelvis (Figure 15-6). Extraperitoneal bladder rupture may also occur when stress is applied to the iliac wings or the puboprostatic ligaments, causing a tear of the bladder wall. This mechanism has been postulated to be responsible for extraperitoneal bladder injury found in association with diastasis of the symphysis pubis or separation of the sacroiliac joints.

Recently, these classically described mechanisms for extraperitoneal bladder injury have been questioned. Carroll and McAninch reported that only 35% of the bladder lacerations in their series were adjacent to a bony fracture, and Corriere and Sandler reported a similar experience following analysis of cystograms in 82 patients with extraperitoneal bladder rupture **(Option (B) is false)**. Wolk et al. reported three patients in whom extraperitoneal bladder rupture occurred without a pelvic fracture; the authors speculated that in such cases a compressive mechanism, analogous to that which results in intraperitoneal rupture, was responsible for the injury. In such cases, or when the site of injury is remote from the location of the fracture, local factors such as the degree of bladder distension or the site and severity of the injury result in an extraperitoneal bladder rupture in which the pelvic fracture is presumed to be associated rather than causative. Cass believed that 24% of the cases of extraperitoneal bladder rupture in his series were secondary to a compressive injury rather than to laceration by a bone spicule.

When leakage of contrast material on cystography is confined to the pelvic extraperitoneal space, the injury is referred to as simple extraperitoneal bladder rupture. The typical radiographic finding in such cases is that of flame-shaped areas of contrast leakage surrounding the bladder in the true pelvis. With complex extraperitoneal bladder rupture, leakage of contrast material extends beyond the pelvic extraperitoneal space.

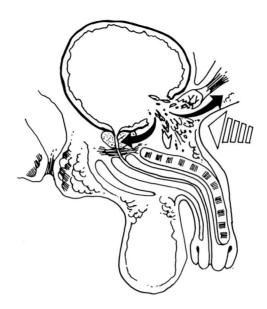

Figure 15-6. The classically described mechanism of an extraperitoneal bladder rupture is a laceration of the base of the bladder by a bone spicule in conjunction with a pelvic fracture.

Such leakage may extend into the scrotum, the hip joint, the perineum, the penis, or the anterior abdominal wall. With large amounts of leakage, the typical streaky appearance of retroperitoneal contrast material may be lost, and thus confusion with other injuries is possible. For example, when contrast leakage extends into the perineum as a result of disruption of the superior fascia of the urogenital diaphragm, confusion of an extraperitoneal bladder rupture with a posterior urethral injury is possible **(Option (A) is false).** Similarly, when the leakage extends into the anterior abdominal wall, confusion of an extraperitoneal bladder rupture with combined intraperitoneal and extraperitoneal rupture, as in the test case, is possible. In addition, the contrast material may dissect upward in the retroperitoneum and be detected by CT in the anterior pararenal, perinephric, or postpararenal space.

Combined intraperitoneal and extraperitoneal bladder rupture (Figure 15-7) is the least common form of major bladder injury and occurs as a result of lacerations in both the base and the dome of the bladder. In most of the reported series, combined bladder rupture makes up between 1 and 10% of the cases. A pelvic fracture has been present in all cases of combined bladder rupture reported to date.

Most authorities continue to believe that the diagnosis of bladder rupture is best established by static cystography. In such a study, both

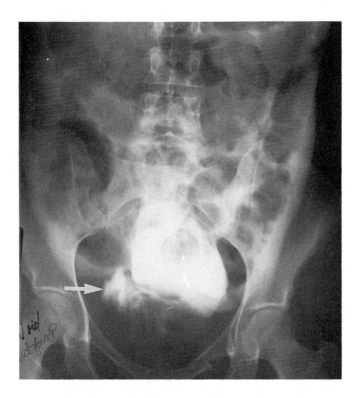

Figure 15-7. Combined intraperitoneal and extraperitoneal bladder rupture. The extraperitoneal component is indicated by the arrow. The intraperitoneal component is outlining bowel loops on the left.

the degree of opacification and the volume to which the bladder is distended can be controlled. Multiple studies have demonstrated that a well-performed static cystogram has a sensitivity of 85 to 100% for the diagnosis of bladder rupture **(Option (D) is false).** The majority of false-negative diagnostic studies occur with penetrating injuries, especially those secondary to small-caliber bullet wounds. It is postulated that cystograms in such patients are falsely negative because the wound is sealed by surrounding tissues or because edema of the bladder wall renders the wound self-sealing. Carroll and McAninch point out that if strict attention to proper film sequence and cystographic technique had not been followed, the sensitivity of cystography would have fallen from 100 to 79% in their series. Proper bladder distension requires filling of the bladder with contrast material to a minimum volume of 300 to 350 mL; proper technique requires that a minimum of three radiographs, including a postdrainage radiograph, be obtained in every case. In

Sandler's 1986 series, 3 of 21 cases of simple extraperitoneal rupture could be diagnosed only on the postdrainage radiograph.

The standard method of treatment of an intraperitoneal bladder rupture is surgical repair of the laceration, since there is believed to be a great risk of peritonitis with nonoperative management. In the past, surgery has also been advocated for treatment of extraperitoneal rupture. More recent experience, however, has demonstrated that bladder drainage is the only form of therapy necessary except in the rare patient in whom a bone spicule is actually found to have remained within the bladder following injury **(Option (C) is true)**. Corriere and Sandler report that of 41 patients with extraperitoneal bladder rupture from blunt trauma, treated with either Foley catheter or suprapubic cystostomy drainage, all eventually healed without complication. The majority (87%) of such cases were found to be healed on follow-up cystograms performed 10 days after injury; the remainder healed with variable periods of drainage, ranging up to 30 days. Thus, the importance of differentiating intraperitoneal rupture from extraperitoneal rupture is reemphasized.

Carl M. Sandler, M.D.

SUGGESTED READINGS

1. Bonavita JA, Pollack HM. Trauma of the adult bladder and urethra. Semin Roentgenol 1983; 18:299–306
2. Brosman SA, Paul JG. Trauma of the bladder. Surg Gynecol Obstet 1976; 143:605–608
3. Carroll PR, McAninch JW. Major bladder trauma: the accuracy of cystography. J Urol 1983; 130:887–888
4. Carroll PR, McAninch JW. Major bladder trauma: mechanisms of injury and a unified method of diagnosis and repair. J Urol 1984; 132:254–257
5. Cass AS, Luxenberg M. Features of 164 bladder ruptures. J Urol 1987; 138:743–745
6. Cass AS, Luxenberg M. Management of extraperitoneal ruptures of bladder caused by external trauma. Urology 1989; 33:179–183
7. Corriere JN Jr, Sandler CM. Management of the ruptured bladder: seven years of experience with 111 cases. J Trauma 1986; 26:830–833
8. Corriere JN Jr, Sandler CM. Mechanisms of injury, patterns of extravasation and management of extraperitoneal bladder rupture due to blunt trauma. J Urol 1988; 139:43–44
9. Corriere JN Jr, Sandler CM. Management of extraperitoneal bladder rupture. Urol Clin North Am 1989; 16:275–277
10. Flancbaum L, Morgan AS, Fleisher M, Cox EF. Blunt bladder trauma: manifestation of severe injury. Urology 1988; 31:220–222

11. Kane NM, Francis IR, Ellis JH. The value of CT in the detection of bladder and posterior urethral injuries. AJR 1989; 153:1243–1246
12. Lis LE, Cohen AJ. CT cystography in the evaluation of bladder trauma. J Comput Assist Tomogr 1990; 14:386–389
13. Lowe FC, Fishman EK, Oesterling JE. Computerized tomography in diagnosis of bladder rupture. Urology 1989; 33:341–343
14. Mee SL, McAninch JW, Federle MP. Computerized tomography in bladder rupture: diagnostic limitations. J Urol 1987; 137:207–209
15. Oliver JA, Taguchi Y. Rupture of the full bladder. Br J Urol 1964; 36:224–225
16. Sandler CM. Bladder trauma. In: Pollack HM (ed), Clinical urography. Philadelphia: WB Saunders; 1990:1505–1521
17. Sandler CM, Hall JT, Rodriguez MB, Corriere JN Jr. Bladder injury in blunt pelvic trauma. Radiology 1986; 158:633–638
18. Sandler CM, Phillips JM, Harris JD, Toombs BD. Radiology of the bladder and urethra in blunt pelvic trauma. Radiol Clin North Am 1981; 19:195–211
19. Wolk DJ, Sandler CM, Corriere JN Jr. Extraperitoneal bladder rupture without pelvic fracture. J Urol 1985; 134:1199–1201

Notes

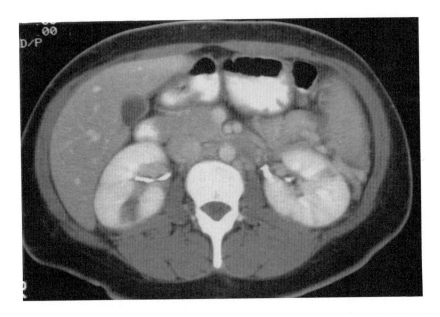

Figure 16-1. This 27-year-old woman presented with acute flank pain. You are shown a contrast-enhanced abdominal CT scan.

Case 16: Renal Infarction

Question 81

Which *one* of the following is the MOST likely diagnosis?

(A) Acute tubular necrosis
(B) Renal infarction
(C) Acute bacterial pyelonephritis
(D) Lymphoma
(E) Renal vein thrombosis

The kidneys are well opacified during the bolus phase of this contrast-enhanced CT examination (Figure 16-1). Excretion of the contrast agent into the collecting systems is seen bilaterally. The calyces are delicately cupped and show no evidence of ureteral obstruction. However, parenchymal defects are present in both kidneys. These nonopacified areas have straight margins, are wedge shaped, and exhibit a thin peripheral rim of parenchyma with normal opacification (Figure 16-2). This appearance is characteristic of segmental renal infarction **(Option (B) is correct).**

In acute tubular necrosis (Option (A)), the kidneys are also densely opacified by intravascular contrast material, but renal function is impaired and contrast material would not be seen in the collecting systems. Furthermore, focal perfusion defects are not a feature of acute tubular necrosis, and flank pain is not a likely symptom.

In acute bacterial pyelonephritis (Option (C)) the kidney is swollen and edematous. Renal opacification and function are diminished. There is often inhomogeneous parenchymal enhancement as a result of areas of poor intrarenal perfusion. When discrete focal defects are present, the peripheral rim opacification seen in images of segmental renal infarction is not present in images of acute bacterial pyelonephritis.

Figures 16-1 and 16-2 are reprinted with permission from Dunnick et al. (2).

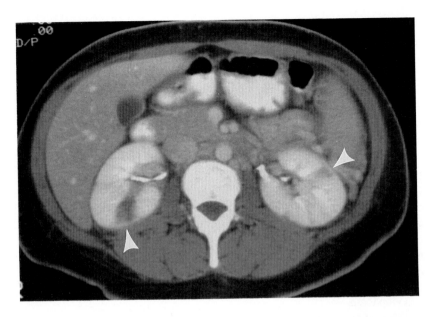

Figure 16-2 (Same as Figure 16-1). Renal infarctions. A postcontrast abdominal CT examination demonstrates wedge-shaped defects in both kidneys. The margins of these lesions are straight, and a thin periphery of cortex (arrowheads) is preserved by collateral flow from capsular vessels.

Involvement of the kidney by malignant lymphoma (Option (D)) may result in either diffuse infiltration or, more commonly, one or more focal renal masses. However, the masses are rounded and do not have straight edges or the wedge shape seen with renal infarctions. Renal enlargement is common, and associated retroperitoneal lymphadenopathy is often present. Acute flank pain would not be common in uncomplicated renal lymphoma.

The affected kidney is globally enlarged and poorly functioning in renal vein thrombosis (Option (E)). The thrombus can often be visualized as a region of low density within an enlarged renal vein. Focal renal perfusion defects do not occur unless there is secondary arterial thrombosis.

Question 82

Concerning acute tubular necrosis,

(A) it is less likely to occur after the use of a nonionic than of an ionic contrast agent
(B) it is usually reversible
(C) the nephrogram is diminished in intensity
(D) sonography can distinguish it from obstruction
(E) recovery is hastened by diuretic therapy

Acute intrinsic renal failure, or acute tubular necrosis (ATN), is most commonly the result of renal ischemia. Specific etiologies include shock from traumatic injury, burns, surgery, hemorrhage, an allergic reaction, or severe dehydration. Vascular surgery in which the arterial supply to the kidney is compromised is a frequent cause of ATN. There is a wide spectrum in the renal response to hypoperfusion ranging from prerenal azotemia to complete cortical necrosis. The effect on the kidney is more closely related to the severity of the ischemia than to the specific etiology of the hypoperfusion.

A variety of chemical toxins, including aminoglycosides, amphotericin, heavy metals, cyclosporine, myoglobin, iodinated contrast agents, and methoxyflurane anesthesia, may also produce ATN. The risk of ATN is increased in patients with preexisting renal failure, especially those with diabetes mellitus. Although nonionic contrast agents cause fewer adverse reactions than ionic agents, a decreased risk of contrast-induced renal failure has not been proven **(Option (A) is false).** For example, Steinberg et al. studied the nephrotoxic effects of low-osmolar agents versus conventional high-osmolar agents in 1,004 patients. The incidence of nephrotoxicity was similar when judged by changes in serum creatinine and creatinine clearance.

The effects of ATN begin immediately after the insult with oliguria. The serum creatinine level becomes elevated within 24 hours. Renal function reaches its nadir at approximately 3 days after the insult but usually returns to normal in 7 to 12 days **(Option (B) is true).** Fluid and electrolyte balance must be maintained until renal function returns.

The kidney is diffusely enlarged in ATN. The parenchyma is uniformly thickened, and the cortical margin is smooth. A dense, prolonged nephrogram is demonstrated on excretory urography or CT (Figure 16-3). A poor or absent nephrogram indicates that contrast material is not reaching the kidney and is not seen in uncomplicated ATN **(Option (C) is false).** There is often very little excretion of contrast material into the collecting

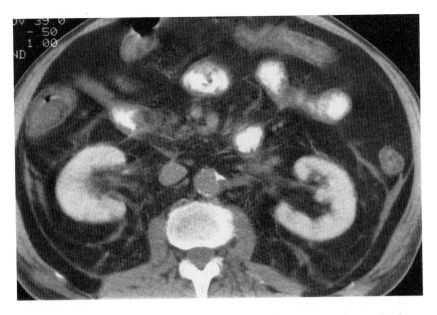

Figure 16-3. Acute tubular necrosis. This CT examination, which was obtained 1 day after intravenous administration of contrast agent, reveals dense kidneys without contrast excretion. This is contrast-induced renal failure from a study performed the previous day.

system. When excretion does occur, the collecting system is thin and attenuated by the swollen parenchyma.

Sonography may be used to distinguish ATN from ureteral obstruction **(Option (D) is true).** The kidneys are enlarged and have normal or decreased echogenicity, reflecting edema. In patients with acute renal failure due to ethylene glycol poisoning, calcium oxalate deposition in the tubules may create an increase in echogenicity. The collecting system is thin, reflecting the very small urine volume and compression by the enlarged kidney.

The precise mechanism of ATN is uncertain, but tubular damage may be caused by a variety of mechanisms, including ischemia and a direct toxic effect of agents such as contrast media. The tubular damage leads to tubular obstruction. Passive leak of filtrate into the renal interstitium results in renal failure. An alternate theory argues that the primary insult is preglomerular ischemia. Renal failure would be due to reduced glomerular filtration rather than to leakage of filtrate across damaged tubular cells. Thus, dehydrated patients, in whom there is greater contact of the toxin with the tubular cells, have more severe damage.

Although numerous risk factors, such as preexisting renal insufficiency, diabetes mellitus, dehydration, cardiovascular disease, multiple myeloma, hypertension, and hyperuricemia, have been identified for contrast-induced renal failure, the most significant is preexisting renal failure. Routine measurement of the serum creatinine level before any intravenous contrast agent injection is probably unnecessary, but it is recommended in patients with known or suspected renal disease.

Once the damage has occurred, hydration or forced diuresis with fluids and a diuretic is beneficial. Patients treated with a diuretic recover more quickly **(Option (E) is true).** However, it is important to monitor the electrolyte levels and overall fluid balance during such treatment, because the usual homeostatic control of both is impaired in patients with ATN or other renal diseases.

Question 83

Concerning renal infarction,

F (A) the initial reaction of the kidney to occlusion of the renal artery is a decrease in size
F (B) the combination of a normal nephrogram with no contrast excretion is typical
T (C) calyceal blunting is not seen
F (D) a patent main renal artery excludes this diagnosis
T (E) segmental renal infarction usually causes cortical scarring

When the main renal artery is occluded, the viability of the kidney depends upon collateral circulation. Therefore, both the clinical and radiographic manifestations depend upon the speed with which the occlusion occurs and upon the ability to develop collateral vessels.

Acute thrombosis of the renal artery usually occurs as the result of abdominal trauma, either blunt or penetrating. Thromboembolism of the renal artery is usually associated with cardiac disease, such as atrial fibrillation, rheumatic valvular disease, or a ventricular aneurysm. Other causes of acute renal artery occlusion include acute dissection of an aortic aneurysm and rupture of a renal artery aneurysm; it may also occur as a complication of renal artery angioplasty.

The clinical findings are often obscured by injury to adjacent organs. However, most patients have flank pain and hematuria (generally microscopic). Fever and leukocytosis are often present but are nonspecific.

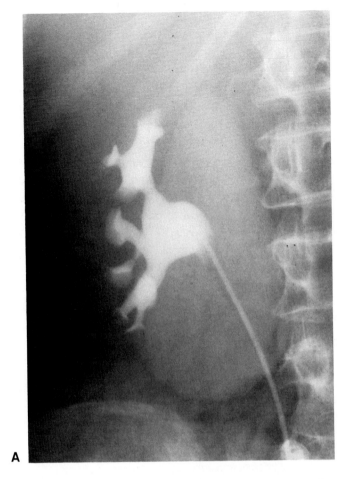

A

Figure 16-4. Renal emboli. (A) The retrograde pyelogram demonstrates a normal collecting system. (B) Two discrete emboli are seen (arrows) in the major branch renal arteries.

Acute anuria suggests bilateral renal artery occlusion but could be due to severe volume depletion.

With acute occlusion of the main renal artery, the kidney becomes edematous and enlarges **(Option (A) is false).** Experimental studies show that the kidney becomes darker in color, reflecting an increase in the number of erythrocytes in the glomerular and intertubular capillaries.

Excretory urography demonstrates absent function on the affected side. Neither a nephrogram nor contrast agent excretion into the col-

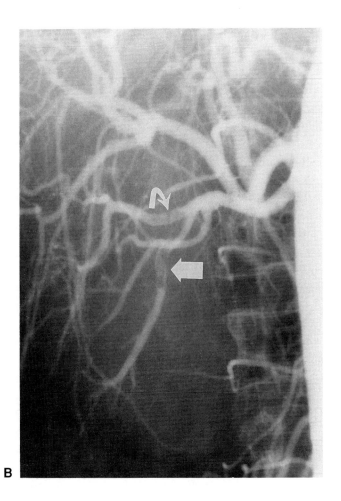

B

lecting system will be visible because contrast material does not reach the kidney **(Option (B) is false).**

Retrograde pyelography may be performed to exclude ureteral obstruction. If retrograde pyelography is performed, the calyces remain delicately cupped (Figure 16-4A) **(Option (C) is true).** There may be attenuation of the collecting system by the edematous kidney.

Sonography demonstrates an enlarged kidney but does not show a textural change from the normal kidney. The main value of sonography is to exclude obstruction, but subtle calyceal changes in acute obstruction may be difficult to detect.

CT is often performed in patients with suspected renal infarction because of its ability to identify pathologic changes in adjacent organs. The renal enlargement and poor contrast enhancement are well demonstrated. A thin parenchymal rim preserved by cortical vessels, which receive collateral flow via the capsular circulation, is usually seen.

If only a branch renal artery is occluded, only a portion of the kidney will be infarcted. These segmental renal infarctions are seen as wedge-shaped areas of low attenuation. They are sharply marginated and often demonstrate a 2- to 4-mm cortical rim of preserved renal parenchyma.

Arteriography demonstrates the renal artery occlusion directly and can often define the etiology, such as embolism, aortic dissection, or renal artery aneurysm (Figure 16-4B). A patent main renal artery does not exclude renal infarction, since the occlusion may be in one or more of the branch vessels **(Option (D) is false).**

Chronic renal artery occlusion is often due to gradual stenosis of the renal artery by vascular disease such as atherosclerosis or fibromuscular dysplasia. Patients with this condition are asymptomatic unless there is an acute event, such as sudden thrombosis of a high-grade renal artery stenosis.

The treatment of acute renal artery thrombosis is anticoagulation. Heparin is given intravenously and is followed by oral agents. In cases of bilateral embolization or embolization to a solitary kidney, surgical intervention or selective intra-arterial thrombolytic therapy may be considered. However, thrombolysis is more successful in acute thrombosis than in embolism and is most successful when thrombosis is due to a renal artery stenosis, which can be dilated after the clot has been lysed.

The late effect of renal infarction is fibrosis and scarring. Hilton et al. demonstrated the progression of a focal infarct to a depressed cortical scar by using serial CT scans. If the infarction is segmental, a focal scar can be demonstrated in an otherwise normal kidney **(Option (E) is true).**

Question 84

Concerning the radiologic features of acute bacterial pyelonephritis,

- (A) the nephrogram is diminished
- (B) the collecting system is attenuated
- (C) the kidney appears normal on sonography
- (D) a striated nephrogram is often seen on CT
- (E) perfusion of the periphery of the kidney by capsular vessels is more common with pyelonephritis than with infarction

Patients presenting with a urinary tract infection are treated with antibiotics. When they respond well, recovery is complete and imaging studies are unnecessary. If they fail to respond, imaging studies are warranted.

Acute bacterial pyelonephritis may be diffuse, involving the entire kidney, or may be focal, i.e., confined to one or more renal "lobes." This acute focal bacterial pyelonephritis is being recognized more often now that cross-sectional imaging techniques, especially CT, are being used with greater frequency. However, the changes of acute bacterial pyelonephritis can be seen by other imaging modalities.

Excretory urography is still commonly performed in patients with a urinary tract infection resistant to antibiotic therapy. Renal stones may be detected on the preliminary radiograph, especially when it is combined with nephrotomography. Abnormal gas collections, as well as perinephric fluid collections, may be seen. After intravenous contrast medium injection, early (1-minute) nephrotomograms should be obtained. The nephrogram is diminished, reflecting the interstitial edema **(Option (A) is true)**. When the process is focal, the nephrogram will be patchy. Contrast medium excretion is variable, depending upon the degree of involvement of the kidney. When contrast agent excretion is visualized, the collecting system is attenuated by the parenchymal edema **(Option (B) is true)**.

Sonography is often used to evaluate patients with suspected acute bacterial pyelonephritis in order to exclude ureteral obstruction. The kidney is diffusely hypoechoic owing to the generalized edema. In focal pyelonephritis a mass that disrupts normal corticomedullary differentiation may be detected. These echogenic masses tend to be poorly defined as compared with a frank renal abscess, which has a better-defined margin with the renal parenchyma **(Option (C) is false)**.

The earliest finding on CT is an inhomogeneous nephrogram (Figure 16-5). Linear or wedge-shaped areas that enhance poorly with intrave-

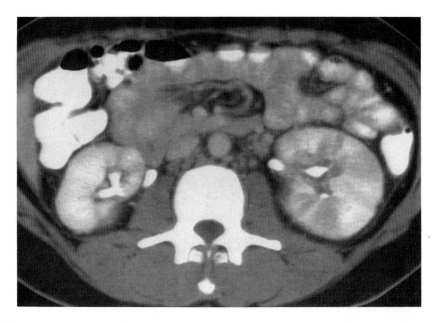

Figure 16-5. Acute bacterial pyelonephritis. This postcontrast abdominal CT examination demonstrates the striated nephrogram typical of acute bacterial pyelonephritis. The more severely affected left kidney is considerably enlarged.

nous contrast material often alternate with normal-appearing areas of renal parenchyma, giving a characteristic striated nephrogram **(Option (D) is true).** These focal areas of diminished enhancement represent more-intense areas of inflammation. If the patient is able to overcome the infection, the kidney may return to normal. However, if the tissue destruction has been too great, liquefaction will occur and may progress to frank abscess formation.

A renal abscess is usually well defined and has local mass effect with bulging rather than linear margins. The central portion of the abscess has a low density (near that of water) and does not show contrast enhancement.

Renal infarction may mimic acute bacterial pyelonephritis both clinically and radiographically. Patients with either entity may present with fever and acute flank pain. A diminished nephrogram can be seen on excretory urography, and the edema may result in decreased echogenicity on sonography with either entity.

With renal infarction, the capsular vessels are often spared. A rim sign is often seen, because these vessels supply the outermost cells of the renal cortex. The cells in the preserved periphery opacify normally with the un-affected renal parenchyma. This is not usually seen with acute bacterial pyelonephritis, as the inflammation extends to the cortical margin **(Option (E) is false).** The presence or absence of the rim sign thus helps to distinguish segmental renal infarction from focal pyelonephritis.

Question 85

Concerning renal vein thrombosis,

(A) infants of diabetic mothers are predisposed to it
(B) membranous glomerulonephritis is a common etiology in adults
(C) marked proteinuria is nearly always present
(D) right-sided involvement is easier to visualize on sonography than left-sided involvement
(E) it responds well to systemic anticoagulation

Renal vein thrombosis may be diagnosed by a variety of noninvasive imaging techniques, including CT, sonography, and MRI. Many patients are asymptomatic, and so the diagnosis may be an incidental finding during one of these cross-sectional imaging techniques.

There are many etiologies of renal vein thrombosis, including volume depletion, thromboembolic states, involvement of the renal pedicle by tumor, and intrinsic renal disease. Volume depletion is more commonly responsible in children than in adults and may be due to severe vomiting, diarrhea, hemorrhage, or solute diuresis consequent to maternal diabetes mellitus **(Option (A) is true).** The resulting hemoconcentration induces sludging and thrombosis. Thrombosis of the renal vein may be the result of extension from thrombosis of the pelvic veins and inferior vena cava (IVC) or may be a complication of pregnancy. However, the IVC at the level of the renal veins is usually spared because of the more rapid flow in the renal veins. Many renal diseases may be complicated by renal vein thrombosis. Both renal adenocarcinoma and Wilms' tumor may extend into the renal vein. Other tumors, including transitional cell carcinoma and metastases to the kidney, have been reported to have renal vein extension, but this is rare.

One of the most common etiologies in adults is membranous glomeru-lonephritis **(Option (B) is true).** These patients frequently present with the nephrotic syndrome. Renal vein thrombosis is seen less frequently in patients with the nephrotic syndrome due to membranoproliferative

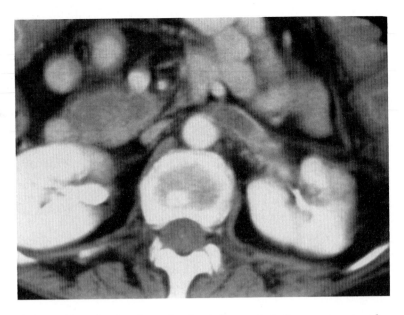

Figure 16-6. Renal vein thrombosis. A dynamic bolus contrast-enhanced abdominal CT examination reveals an enlarged left renal vein. The thrombus is seen as a nonenhancing central filling defect. Collateral flow is sufficient to preserve the function of the left kidney.

disease and is infrequent in patients with diabetic nephropathy, lupus nephritis, lupoid nephritis, and focal sclerosis.

At one time renal vein thrombosis was believed to be the cause of the nephrotic syndrome. However, ligation of the renal vein produced little or no proteinuria in experimental animals. Furthermore, humans with occlusion of the renal vein but without underlying glomerular disease do not develop the nephrotic syndrome **(Option (C) is false).** Thus, it appears that the nephrotic syndrome causes renal vein thrombosis, not vice versa.

The kidney is diffusely enlarged in acute renal vein thrombosis. Parenchymal opacification will be diminished relative to the arterial perfusion, which is reduced by the increased intrarenal pressure. On excretory urography, the collecting system is attenuated by the edematous kidney and consequent to decreased excretion, which allows more time for water resorption. If periureteral veins enlarge to serve as venous collaterals, notching of the renal pelvis or ureter may be seen.

Changes can also be seen on sonography. The kidney is enlarged, and the cortex is less echogenic than normal owing to the edema. The venous

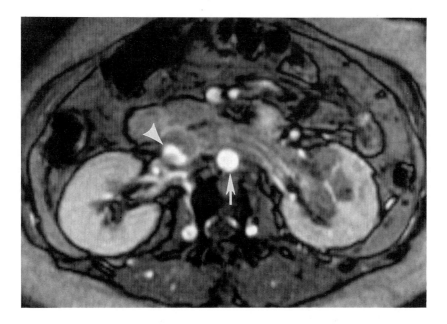

Figure 16-7. Thrombus in the left renal vein and IVC. This gadolinium-enhanced limited-flip-angle MR image demonstrates flowing blood in the aorta (arrow) but in only a portion of the IVC (arrowhead).

thrombus can be directly imaged, especially on the right side, where the liver serves as an acoustic window **(Option (D) is true).**

An abdominal CT examination enhanced with an intravascular bolus of contrast material defines the renal vein thrombus as a low-attenuation region within an enlarged renal vein (Figure 16-6). Extension into the IVC is also well imaged by this technique. Secondary CT signs of renal vein thrombosis include enlargement of the renal vein, diminished parenchymal opacification, opacified perinephric ("cobwebbing") or periureteral collateral veins, thickening of Gerota's fascia, and delayed excretion of contrast into an attenuated collecting system.

MRI is being used more often to detect renal vein thrombosis (Figure 16-7). Limited-flip-angle techniques demonstrate absence of flow. When the coronal projection is used, the precise extent of propagation of the renal vein thrombus into the IVC can often be delineated.

The treatment of renal vein thrombosis revolves around treating the underlying disease and preventing complications. In children, hydration and the maintenance of electrolyte balance alleviate the most common predisposing conditions. Anticoagulant therapy can be considered if the

IVC is also thrombosed but is seldom necessary in children if the thrombus is limited to the renal vein.

The prognosis of renal vein thrombosis in adults depends strongly on the underlying renal disease. Death has been reported, however, from massive pulmonary embolism. Anticoagulation with heparin followed by warfarin is often indicated. This arrests further extension of the thrombus within either the kidney or the IVC. Clinical response to this therapy has been good, and systemic thrombolytic treatment has seldom been tried **(Option (E) is true).**

N. Reed Dunnick, M.D.

SUGGESTED READINGS

RENAL INFARCTION

1. Coburn JW, Agre KL. Renal thromboembolism and other acute occlusive diseases of the renal arteries. In: Schrier RW, Gottschalk CW (eds), Diseases of the kidney. Boston: Little, Brown; 1988:2361–2375
2. Dunnick NR, McCallum RW, Sandler CM. A textbook of uroradiology. Baltimore: Williams & Wilkins; 1991:164–166
3. Hann L, Pfister RC. Renal subcapsular rim sign: new etiologies and pathogenesis. AJR 1982; 138:51–54
4. Hilton S, Bosniak MA, Raghavendra BN, Subramanyam BR, Rothberg M, Megibow AJ. CT findings in acute renal infarction. Urol Radiol 1984; 6:158–163

ACUTE INTRINSIC RENAL FAILURE

5. Brezis M, Rosen S, Epstein FH. Acute renal failure. In: Brenner BM, Rector FC Jr (eds), The kidney, vol 1, 4th ed. Philadelphia: WB Saunders; 1991:993–1004
6. Gomes AS, Lois JF, Baker JD, McGlade CT, Bunnell DH, Hartzman S. Acute renal dysfunction in high-risk patients after angiography: comparison of ionic and nonionic contrast media. Radiology 1989; 170:65–68
7. Lang EK, Foreman J, Schlegel JU, Leslie C, List A, McCormick P. The incidence of contrast medium induced acute tubular necrosis following arteriography. Radiology 1981; 138:203–206
8. Schwab SJ, Hlatky MA, Pieper KS, et al. Contrast nephrotoxicity: a randomized controlled trial of a nonionic and an ionic radiographic contrast agent. N Engl J Med 1989; 320:149–153
9. Steinberg EP, Moore RD, Brinker JA, et al. Nephrotoxicity of low osmolality contrast media versus high osmolality media. Invest Radiol (suppl 1) 1991; 26:S86

BACTERIAL PYELONEPHRITIS

10. Gold RP, McClennan BL, Rottenberg RR. CT appearance of acute inflammatory disease of the renal interstitium. AJR 1983; 141:343–349
11. Rauschkolb EN, Sandler CM, Patel S, Childs TL. Computed tomography of renal inflammatory disease. J Comput Assist Tomogr 1982; 6:502–506
12. Soulen MC, Fishman EK, Goldman SM, Gatewood OM. Bacterial renal infection: role of CT. Radiology 1989; 171:703–707
13. Thornbury JR. Acute renal infections. Urol Radiol 1991; 12:209–213
14. Yoder IC, Pfister RC, Lindfors KK, Newhouse JH. Pyonephrosis: imaging and intervention. AJR 1983; 141:735–740
15. Zaontz MR, Pahira JJ, Wolfman M, Gargurevich AJ, Zeman RK. Acute focal bacterial nephritis: a systematic approach to diagnosis and treatment. J Urol 1985; 133:752–757

RENAL VEIN THROMBOSIS

16. Gatewood OM, Fishman EK, Burrow CR, Walker WG, Goldman SM, Siegelman SS. Renal vein thrombosis in patients with nephrotic syndrome: CT diagnosis. Radiology 1986; 159:117–122
17. Keating MA, Althausen AF. The clinical spectrum of renal vein thrombosis. J Urol 1985; 133:938–945
18. Llach F, Koffler A, Finck E, Massry SG. On the incidence of renal vein thrombosis in the nephrotic syndrome. Arch Intern Med 1977; 137:333–336
19. Winfield AC, Gerlock AJ Jr, Shaff MI. Perirenal cobwebs: a CT sign of renal vein thrombosis. J Comput Assist Tomogr 1981; 5:705–708

CONTRAST REACTIONS

20. Katayama H, Yamaguchi K, Kozuka T, Takashima T, Seez P, Matsuura K. Adverse reactions to ionic and nonionic contrast media. A report from the Japanese Committee on the Safety of Contrast Media. Radiology 1990; 175:621–628
21. Palmer FJ. The RACR survey of intravenous contrast media reactions. Final report. Australas Radiol 1988; 32:426–428

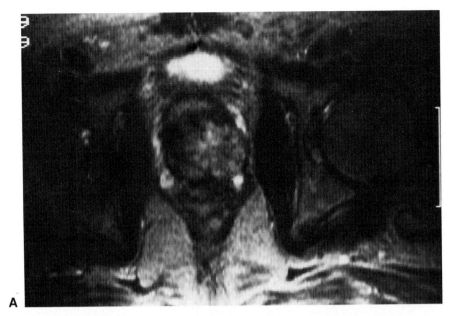

SE 2,500/90

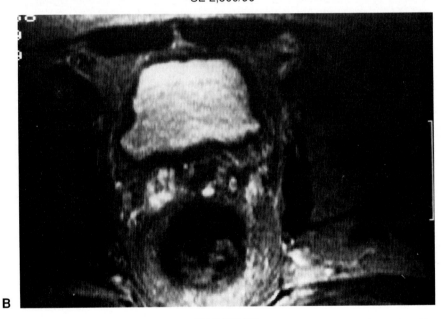

SE 2,500/90

Figure 17-1. This 64-year-old man has prostatic carcinoma. You are shown transverse T2-weighted MR images at the level of the mid-prostate (A) and above the level of the prostate (B).

Case 17: Prostatic Carcinoma

Question 86

Based on these images, which *one* of the following is the CORRECT stage of the tumor?

(A) Stage A
(B) Stage B
(C) Stage C1
(D) Stage C2
(E) Stage D

Figure 17-1A shows an enlarged prostate (P, Figure 17-2A) with heterogeneous signal throughout; the peripheral zone is not clearly delineated from the transitional zone. There is bulging of the prostatic contour on the left side, as well as abnormal signal within the left levator ani muscle and obliteration of the left periprostatic venous plexus. Figure 17-1B shows the low-intensity tumor extending superiorly and posteriorly to replace the normal high-intensity seminal vesicles centrally and in the left paracentral region (curved arrow, Figure 17-2B). There is no evidence of lymph node or bony involvement in these images. These findings indicate that the tumor has extended beyond the prostatic capsule to involve the seminal vesicles and, thus, are consistent with a stage C2 tumor **(Option (D) is correct).**

The most commonly used system for prostatic cancer staging is the Whitmore-Jewett system, which consists of four primary stages (A through D). Stage A tumors (Option (A)) are clinically unsuspected and nonpalpable cancers, usually diagnosed following a transurethral resection (TUR) of the prostate for benign prostatic hyperplasia (BPH). These stage A lesions are subdivided into stage A1 tumors, which are histologically well-differentiated lesions present on a few chips of the TUR specimen, and stage A2 tumors, which either are histologically anaplastic or, if histologically well differentiated, are present in a large portion of the surgical specimen. Stage B tumors (Option (B)) are clinically palpable lesions, which may be unilateral (stage B1) or bilateral (stage B2).

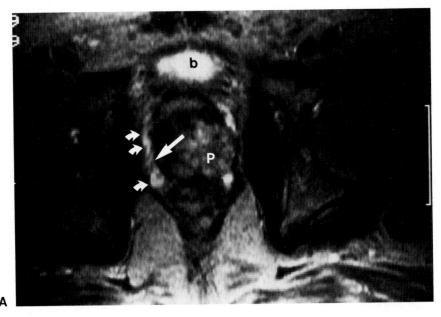

SE 2,500/90

Figure 17-2 (Same as Figure 17-1). (A) Transverse T2-weighted MR image at the level of the mid-prostate demonstrates inhomogeneous signal throughout the entire prostate (P), with loss of the normal zonal anatomy. The oval bright signal anteriorly represents fluid in the bladder (b). The periprostatic venous plexus (curved arrows) is visible on the right, with a small area at approximately 8 o'clock (straight arrow), where the neurovascular bundle is located. On the left side, the periprostatic venous plexus is interrupted by the tumor, which causes bulging of the prostatic contour and obliterates the neurovascular bundle. (B) Transverse T2-weighted MR image from the same sequence as panel A but at a higher level shows the high signal intensity of the urinary bladder anteriorly (b). The high signal intensity of the seminal vesicles is replaced centrally and in the left paracentral region (curved arrow) by tumor. The normal high signal intensity of the remaining right seminal vesicle is visible (straight arrow).

Stage C tumors are also palpable and have extended beyond the prostatic capsule. Stage C1 lesions (Option (C)) have extended into the periprostatic fat alone, whereas stage C2 tumors have extended to involve the seminal vesicles either via the ejaculatory ducts or following spread through the periprostatic fat. Stage D tumors (Option (E)) have metastasized either to regional lymph nodes (stage D1) or to distant sites, especially bone (stage D2).

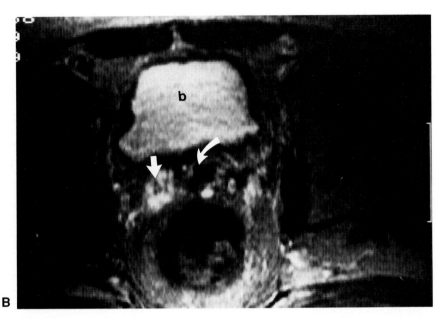

SE 2,500/90

Intraglandular focal prostatic cancer can be detected as a low-intensity area disrupting the normal high signal intensity of the peripheral zone of the prostate. Since older men often have concurrent BPH and prostatic carcinoma, the normal zonal anatomy of the prostate (Figure 17-3) may be grossly distorted consequent to benign or malignant disease (Figure 17-4). Accordingly, MRI is not considered reliable enough to be recommended for either screening or detection of prostatic cancer. It is more valuable in detecting extraglandular disease (stage C) than intraglandular disease (stages A and B).

MRI is valuable for staging prostatic carcinoma. When prostatic carcinoma extends beyond the confines of the capsule, it disrupts the normal uniform signal of the periprostatic fat. Disruption of the periprostatic fat is best seen on T1-weighted images or on the first echo of T2-weighted images. The periprostatic space also contains an extensive complex of periprostatic veins, which are normally bright on the second echo of T2-weighted sequences. Asymmetric displacement or obliteration of these veins may occur when prostatic carcinoma becomes extracapsular (Figure 17-2A). The levator ani muscle is indistinguishable from the prostatic margin laterally; therefore, displacement or interruption of this muscle is indicative of extracapsular spread of tumor or stage C disease. It is wise to confirm a suspected abnormality of the levator ani muscle

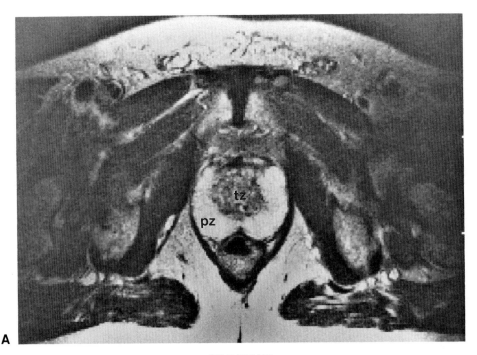

SE 2,000/70

Figure 17-3. (A) Transverse MR image demonstrates the normal zonal anatomy of the gland; the peripheral zone (pz) has high, uniform signal intensity, and the inner gland or transitional zone (tz) has inhomogeneous signal intensity. (B) Transverse MR image inferiorly at the apex of the gland. The normal high signal intensity of the peripheral zone is interrupted on the right side (open arrow) by a lower-intensity nodule. Note the continuity of the levator ani muscle (arrowheads), which matches the signal intensity of the obturator internus muscle (straight arrow).

by imaging in more than one projection or by changing the direction of the readout gradient to avoid confusion with a chemical-shift artifact. The transverse and coronal T2-weighted images are most sensitive for detection of tumor invasion of the levator ani muscle.

Tumor involvement of the seminal vesicles is best identified on T2-weighted transverse scans (Figure 17-2B) but can also be verified on coronal and sagittal views. Tumor involvement of the seminal vesicles is identified as asymmetric obliteration of the bladder-seminal vesicle angle and, on T2-weighted images, as a low-intensity tumor replacing the high signal intensity of the fluid-filled seminal vesicles (Figure 17-5).

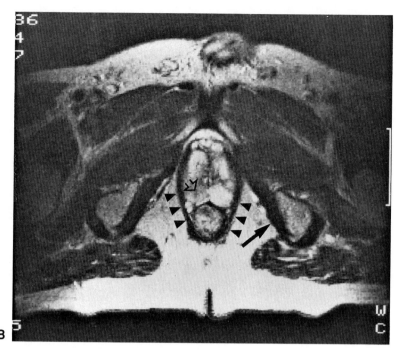

SE 2,000/70

The ability of MRI to detect lymphadenopathy is similar to that of CT, but MRI has the advantage of being able to separate lymph nodes from vascular structures without the use of contrast agents. Detection of lymph node involvement is based on increased size; even 1-cm pelvic nodes should be considered suspicious for metastasis in a patient with known prostatic carcinoma. MRI has a limitation similar to that of CT in that normal-sized nodes infiltrated by tumor cannot be identified and enlarged nodes secondary to inflammation cannot be differentiated from cancer. MRI is able to identify direct tumor extension into muscles and bones in the pelvis. However, bone scintigraphy is the best noninvasive method for determining the extent of osseous metastatic disease.

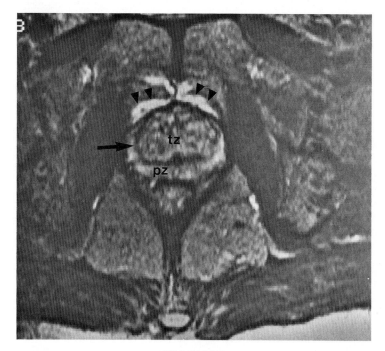

SE 1,500/95

Figure 17-4. Benign prostatic hyperplasia. Transverse MR image showing an enlarged transitional zone (tz) with compression of the usual high
signal intensity of the peripheral zone (pz). The low intensity of the
pseudocapsule (arrow) separates the enlarged transitional zone from the
peripheral zone. The periprostatic venous plexus is noted anteriorly
(arrowheads) but is obliterated laterally in this patient with BPH.

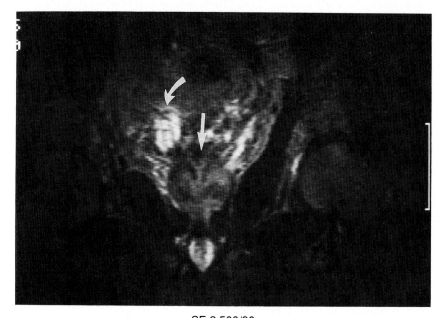

SE 2,500/90

Figure 17-5. Prostatic carcinoma. Coronal MR image of the pelvis shows
the inhomogeneous signal of the tumor throughout the prostate, obliterating the normal zonal anatomy. The low signal intensity of the tumor
extends into the seminal vesicles superiorly (straight arrow). The normal
seminal vesicle on the right (curved arrow) shows high signal intensity
typical of the fluid-filled structure.

Questions 87 through 91

For each of the following conditions related to prostatic carcinoma (Questions 87 through 91), select the *one* lettered stage (A, B, C, D, or E) that BEST describes it. Each lettered stage may be used once, more than once, or not at all.

B 87. Palpable nodule that is >1.5 cm on one side
A 88. Nonpalpable diffuse glandular involvement
C 89. Neurovascular bundle involvement
E 90. Metastasis to bone
D 91. Metastasis to pelvic lymph nodes

    (A) Stage A
    (B) Stage B
    (C) Stage C
    (D) Stage D1
    (E) Stage D2

The prognosis of prostatic carcinoma and the options for its treatment depend greatly on the stage of disease. If the tumor is confined to the prostate, it is treated by radical prostatectomy or radiation therapy. Extracapsular tumors are usually treated by radiation therapy or other palliative therapy. The exception to this treatment plan would be a stage C tumor that asymmetrically extends into the periprostatic fat but spares the neurovascular bundle on the opposite side. In these cases, nerve-sparing surgery can be performed with an approximately 30% chance of preserving potency.

Stages A and B disease are confined to the gland. A palpable nodule measuring >1.5 cm on one side of the gland would be stage B1 disease **(Option (B) is the correct answer to Question 87).** Stage A disease is clinically unsuspected and nonpalpable regardless of whether it is focal or diffuse **(Option (A) is the correct answer to Question 88).**

The prostate gland is marginated by the prostatic capsule, a fibrous membrane that is thin posteriorly and laterally and thicker anteriorly. The capsule is pierced by the paramedian ejaculatory ducts posteriorly and by the paired neurovascular bundles posterolaterally. The neurovascular bundle is best visualized in the transverse imaging plane at approximately the 4 and 8 o'clock positions. The neurovascular bundle is seen as an area of intermediate signal intensity on T2-weighted images because it is surrounded by the periprostatic fat and venous plexus. Involvement of the neurovascular bundle and its periprostatic fat is characteristic of a stage C1 lesion **(Option (C) is the correct answer to Question 89).** Prostatic carcinoma spreads in a relatively progressive

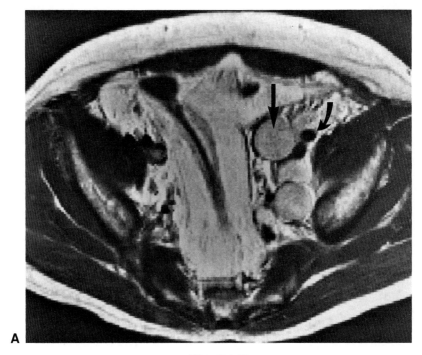

SE 2,500/70

Figure 17-6. Prostatic carcinoma. (A) Transverse MR image shows multiple rounded high- to intermediate-intensity nodules in the external iliac chain of lymph nodes (straight arrow). Note the signal void of the external iliac vessels (curved arrow). (B) Coronal MR image shows the low signal intensity of lymph nodes in the iliac region (curved arrow) and para-aortic region (straight arrow).

order from immediate extracapsular involvement to lymph nodes to bone. The tumor rarely spreads to the lymph nodes until it has extended beyond the confines of the prostatic capsule. At least one-third of patients with newly diagnosed carcinoma of the prostate have stage C or D disease at the time of diagnosis. The mortality rate increases markedly when the pelvic lymph nodes are involved. Detection by both CT and MRI relies on visualizing enlargement due to macroscopic tumor involvement of the lymph nodes. Microscopic tumor involvement is detected by either percutaneous or open biopsy. The histologic grade of Gleason's score is directly related to the likelihood of lymph node involvement; the lower scores of 1 through 3 have virtually no lymph node involvement, and the higher scores of 7 through 10 nearly always indicate involvement,

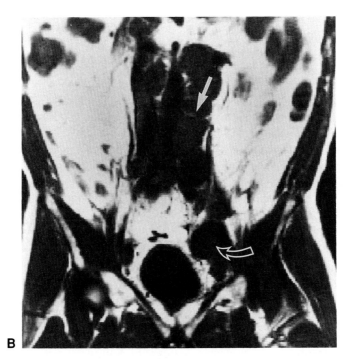

B

SE 500/17

whether it be microscopic or macroscopic. In patients with prostatic carcinoma, the medial group of external iliac nodes (also known as obturator nodes) are usually involved first and then the common iliac nodes and para-aortic nodes become involved (Figure 17-6). Involvement of nodes confined to the pelvis is considered stage D1 disease **(Option (D) is the correct answer to Question 91)**. Lymph node involvement in the para-aortic region is known as stage D2, as is metastasis to bone **(Option (E) is the correct answer to Question 90)**.

While an effective screening program for prostatic carcinoma will detect cancers at an earlier stage, it will also detect many carcinomas that would never become symptomatic. Desirable screening programs for disease should not cause patient morbidity, and treatment of asymptomatic carcinomas does carry a risk of morbidity. General agreement concerning an optimal strategy for prostatic carcinoma screening has not yet been reached.

Question 92

Concerning imaging of prostatic carcinoma,

F (A) CT is more specific than MRI for detecting stage C disease
T (B) on T2-weighted MR images, the signal intensity of tumor is low compared with that of the peripheral zone
F (C) inguinal nodes are generally involved with metastasis before iliac nodes
F (D) on transrectal ultrasonography, more than 50% of hypoechoic lesions are malignant
T (E) MRI and transrectal ultrasonography have equal specificity for evaluating seminal vesicle invasion

Significant benefits of MRI compared with other imaging techniques are its excellent contrast resolution and multiplanar imaging ability. MRI permits improved detection of bladder base and seminal vesicle involvement and the rare case of posterior extension of prostatic carcinoma to involve the rectum. CT is as good as MRI in detecting lymph node enlargement. However, the CT diagnosis of local spread depends solely on morphologic changes, since tumor and other soft tissues have similar X-ray attenuation. On MRI, detection of extraglandular spread depends not only on morphologic changes but also on signal intensity abnormalities **(Option (A) is false)**. It is acceptable for normal seminal vesicles to be asymmetric in size, preventing accurate detection of tumor based on the size of seminal vesicles as seen on CT (Figure 17-7). On MRI, tumor involvement of the seminal vesicles shows asymmetry in the signal intensity, thereby accurately detecting the tumor regardless of size.

On T1-weighted (short-TR, short-TE) images, the prostate shows a homogeneous signal of intermediate signal intensity and the anatomic zones cannot be differentiated. T2-weighted (long-TR, long-TE) sequences clearly delineate the zonal anatomy of the prostate because the lower signal intensity of the central and transitional zones is contrasted with the higher intensity of the peripheral zone. The signal intensity of a focal tumor is low compared with that of the peripheral zone on T2-weighted images **(Option (B) is true)**. The transitional and central zones have similar relaxation times and cannot be differentiated on MR images in the normal patient.

The multiplanar imaging capability of MRI is valuable in delineating prostatic anatomy. The transverse plane is the best plane for differentiating the centrally located transitional zone (sometimes referred to as the inner gland) from the peripheral zone or outer gland of the prostate. The

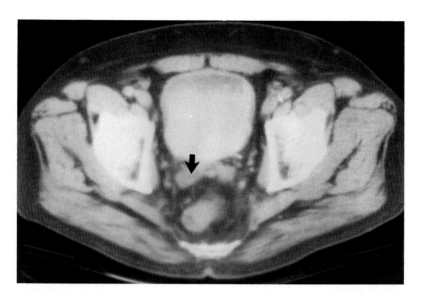

Figure 17-7. Prostatic carcinoma. Same patient as in Figures 17-1 and 17-2. Transverse CT image of the pelvis at the level of the bladder and seminal vesicles. Note that the right seminal vesicle (arrow) is larger than the left. The corresponding MR images are Figures 17-1B and 17-2B, which show the larger right seminal vesicle to be normal in signal intensity but show tumor invading centrally.

transverse plane also demonstrates the relationship of the seminal vesicles and complements the coronal plane in its demonstration of the levator ani and obturator internus muscles. Differentiation between the peripheral and central zones is most easily achieved on transverse and coronal images. The sagittal plane is the optimal choice for assessing the relationship of the prostate to the bladder, seminal vesicles, and rectum.

On MRI, focal low-intensity defects in the normally high-intensity peripheral zone are considered consistent with, but not specific for, prostatic carcinoma. The value of MRI relates to its ability to stage tumors. Its ability to visualize the bladder, seminal vesicles, and rectum in the sagittal and coronal planes is an advantage over CT, and detection of seminal vesicle and lymph node extension cannot be evaluated by transrectal ultrasonography (TRUS) but is evaluated equally well by CT and MRI.

In prostatic carcinoma, nodal metastasis occurs in the following sequence: (1) obturator nodes, (2) medial group of external iliac nodes, (3) internal iliac nodes, (4) common iliac nodes, and (5) para-aortic nodes.

Inguinal node involvement is uncommon **(Option (C) is false).** The obturator nodes are commonly considered part of the medial group of the external iliac nodes, but anomalous origin from the internal iliac chain is also recognized. Both CT and MRI rely on morphology (size) for detection of abnormal pelvic lymph nodes. A frequent problem occurring in patients with cancer of the prostate is that nodes are involved without being enlarged. When the nodes are normal in size, CT and MRI are both unable to distinguish between normal nodes and those involved with tumor. MRI is preferred over CT when surgical clips cause artifact in the region of interest.

In 1990, Rifkin et al. published the results of a cooperative multi-institutional study showing the overall staging accuracy of MRI to be 69%, with a sensitivity of 77% and a specificity of 57%. The overall staging accuracy of ultrasonography was 58%, with a sensitivity of 66% and a specificity of 46%.

On a TRUS radial view, the normal prostate appears as a symmetric, triangular, ellipsoid structure circumferentially defined by a continuous prostatic capsule that is usually clearly defined and highly echogenic. The radial transverse image demonstrates right-to-left symmetry. The longitudinally oriented image, parallel to the long axis of the body, will show the base and the apex of the prostate to best advantage. Prostate imaging by TRUS is more sensitive than specific and therefore creates problems of false-positive results. There is a much greater prevalence of benign prostatic lesions than carcinomas in both asymptomatic and symptomatic men. Furthermore, benign prostatic lesions often coexist with prostatic carcinoma. The reported probability (positive predictive value) that a peripherally located hypoechoic lesion represents a carcinoma has ranged from 0 to 50% **(Option (D) is false).** Overall, the average rate of cancer in peripherally located hypoechoic lesions is approximately 20 to 30%. Sensitivity for diagnosis of prostatic carcinoma by TRUS is 66% according to the results of the multi-institutional study reported in 1990, and the specificity is 46%. False-positive rates are high because TRUS cannot consistently differentiate benign conditions (BPH, prostatic cysts, prostatic calculi, prostatic infarcts, and prostatitis) and normal tissue structures (blood vessels and muscle) from cancer.

Sonographically, a focal prostatic carcinoma is characteristically shown as a hypoechoic lesion in the peripheral zone (Figure 17-8). In 1986, Dähnert et al. reported that 52 patients with stage A or B prostate carcinoma showed lesions on TRUS that were anechoic (54%), slightly hypoechoic (22%), and isoechoic (24%). In 1989, a group of 51 patients with prostate carcinoma was reviewed by Rifkin et al. for correlation of

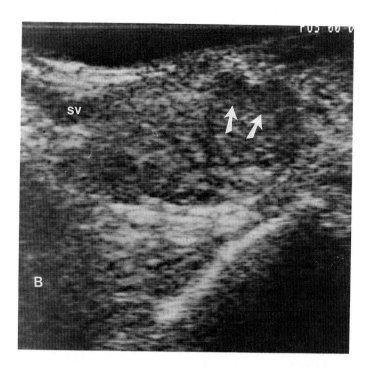

Figure 17-8. Prostatic carcinoma. Longitudinal TRUS image of the mid-prostate shows bladder (B) and seminal vesicles (sv). There are hypoechoic lesions (arrows) in the peripheral zone near the apex in this patient with prostatic carcinoma.

histologic grade and stromal fibrosis with echogenicity on TRUS. It was found that low-grade (better-differentiated) tumors correlated significantly with hypoechoic lesions. There was some overlap since some higher-grade lesions also appeared hypoechoic. However, the hyperechoic lesions were only associated with anaplastic high-grade lesions (those with a Gleason score from 8 to 10). An important consideration in TRUS of patients with prostatic carcinoma is the appearance of the prostatic capsule and seminal vesicles. The capsule is best seen on the radially displayed scans as a well-delineated circumferential margin. Tumor extension into the seminal vesicles is demonstrated by distortion of the normally hypoechoic seminal vesicles with irregular dense echoes. In the cooperative multi-institutional study, TRUS correctly classified 14 of 65 seminal vesicles involved with tumor (sensitivity, 22%) and 270 of 308 seminal vesicles free from disease (specificity, 88%). The corresponding figures for MRI were 18 of 65 (sensitivity, 28%) and 272 of 308 (specificity,

88%) **(Option (E) is true).** TRUS also provides only a limited view of the structures surrounding the gland and yields no information about lymph node status.

Question 93

Concerning prostatic carcinoma,

(A) it occurs in about 30% of men over the age of 50 years
(B) it rarely metastasizes until the primary tumor exceeds 1 cm^3 in volume
(C) elevated prostate-specific antigen values are specific for the diagnosis
(D) it arises in the peripheral zone in more than 90% of patients
(E) it occurs as often in the anterior half of the prostate as in the posterior half

Carcinoma of the prostate is the second most frequently recognized cancer in men, following carcinoma of the lung in incidence. It is also the second most lethal tumor in men in the United States. Since 1970, cancer mortality statistics show that the incidence of prostatic carcinoma has gradually increased; it is now tied with carcinoma of the colon and rectum as the second most common cause of death from cancer among men in the United States. The highest incidence rates of prostatic carcinoma are among blacks in the United States, followed by whites in North America and Scandinavia. The lowest rates are in Southeast Asia. Many aspects of prostatic cancer pathobiology are not understood. Clinical manifestations occur in fewer than 1% of the patients with the tumor, and postmortem studies have shown that one-third of men examined, of all ages, harbored asymptomatic prostate cancer **(Option (A) is true).** Approximately 50% of men over the age of 70 will have prostatic carcinoma either with or without symptoms.

The natural history of the disease suggests that the majority of prostatic carcinomas are at least moderately differentiated at first and subsequently lose differentiation. In 1966 Gleason devised a system of pathologic classification of prostatic carcinomas that combines clinical staging with histologic grading. Numerical values for staging grades are assigned to two areas of the gland and are added to yield a prognostic score. Cancers having an increased original Gleason score have an increased frequency of metastasis. Tumor volume is related to metastasis, seminal vesicle extension, capsular invasion, and histologic differentiation. It appears that metastasis is not likely to occur until the tumors are well over 1 cm^3 in volume **(Option (B) is true).**

Certain biochemical markers, i.e., prostate-specific antigen (PSA) and prostatic acid phosphatase (PAP), have been used to assist in the diagnosis and staging of prostatic carcinoma. Both PSA and PAP are nonspecific, and their levels may be elevated in BPH **(Option (C) is false).** It is also known that prostate massage, needle biopsy, and TUR will increase these levels.

Stamey et al. noted that 88% of men undergoing prostatectomy for BPH had serum PSA levels above the upper normal level of 2.5 ng/mL. At the slightly elevated levels, there was overlap of patients with BPH and stage A carcinoma, but as the PSA levels increased the predictive value for carcinoma became greater. The PSA level is increased with advanced clinical stages and is proportional to the estimated volume of the tumor. PSA is elevated in virtually all patients with stage C or D prostate carcinoma. With stage B disease, 95% of patients will have elevated PSA levels; the likelihood of elevated PSA is lower with stage A1 (38%) and stage A2 (57%) disease. PSA is more sensitive than PAP in detecting prostatic carcinoma and will probably be more useful in monitoring for post-therapeutic recurrence.

The distribution of cancer within the prostate is approximately 70% in the peripheral zone, 20% in the transitional zone, and 10% in the central zone **(Option (D) is false).** Prostatic tumors originate anteriorly nearly as often as posteriorly and are quite uniformly distributed around the entire circumference of the glands **(Option (E) is true).**

Peggy J. Fritzsche, M.D.

SUGGESTED READINGS

STAGING

1. Bezzi M, Kressel HY, Allen KS, et al. Prostatic carcinoma: staging with MR imaging at 1.5 T. Radiology 1988; 169:339–346
2. McNeal JE. Normal anatomy of the prostate and changes in benign prostatic hypertrophy and carcinoma. Semin US CT MR 1988; 9:329–334
3. Whitmore WF Jr. Natural history and staging of prostate cancer. Urol Clin North Am 1984; 11:205–220

IMAGING

4. Dähnert WF, Hamper UM, Eggleston JC, Walsh PC, Sanders RC. Prostatic evaluation by transrectal sonography with histopathologic correlation: the echopenic appearance of early carcinoma. Radiology 1986; 158:97–102

5. Fritzsche PJ, Wilbur MJ. The male pelvis. Semin US CT MR 1989; 10:11–28
6. Gevenois PA, Salmon I, Stallenberg B, van Sinoy ML, van Regemorter G, Struyven J. Magnetic resonance imaging of the normal prostate at 1.5 T. Br J Radiol 1990; 63:101–107
7. Kahn T, Bürrig K, Schmitz-Dräger B, Lewin JS, Fürst G, Mödder U. Prostatic carcinoma and benign prostatic hyperplasia: MR imaging with histopathologic correlation. Radiology 1989; 173:847–851
8. Littrup PJ, Lee F, McLeary RD, Wu D, Lee A, Kumasaka GH. Transrectal US of the seminal vesicles and ejaculatory ducts: clinical correlation. Radiology 1988; 168:625–628
9. Resnick MI. Transrectal ultrasound guided versus digitally directed prostatic biopsy: a comparative study. J Urol 1988; 139:754–757
10. Rifkin MD, Choi H. Implications of small, peripheral hypoechoic lesions in endorectal US of the prostate. Radiology 1988; 166:619–622
11. Rifkin MD, McGlynn ET, Choi H. Echogenicity of prostate cancer correlated with histologic grade and stromal fibrosis: endorectal US studies. Radiology 1989; 170:549–552
12. Rifkin MD, Zerhouni EA, Gatsonis CA, et al. Comparison of magnetic resonance imaging and ultrasonography in staging early prostate cancer. Results of a multi-institutional cooperative trial. N Engl J Med 1990; 323:621–626
13. Waterhouse RL, Resnick MI. The use of transrectal prostatic ultrasonography in the evaluation of patients with prostatic carcinoma. J Urol 1989; 141:233–239

PATHOPHYSIOLOGY

14. Ahmann FR, Schifman RB. Prospective comparison between serum monoclonal prostate specific antigen and acid phosphatase measurements in metastatic prostatic cancer. J Urol 1987; 137:431–434
15. Mulholland SG. The impact of radiology on the management of prostatic disease: a clinician's perspective. Semin US CT MR 1988; 9:335–338
16. Nadji M, Tabei SZ, Castro A, et al. Prostatic-specific antigen: an immunohistologic marker for prostatic neoplasms. Cancer 1981; 48:1229–1232
17. Stamey TA, Yang N, Hay AR, McNeal JE, Freiha FS, Redwine E. Prostate-specific antigen as a serum marker for adenocarcinoma of the prostate. N Engl J Med 1987; 317:909–916

Notes

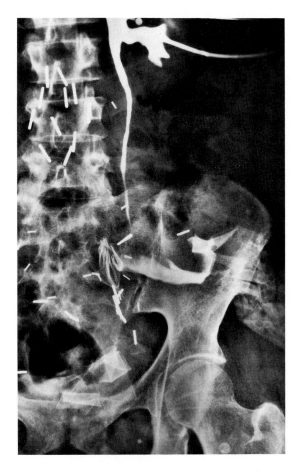

Figure 18-1. This 50-year-old woman developed persistent urine leakage from an abdominal drain 1 week after a hysterectomy and lymph node dissection for carcinoma of the cervix. You are shown a nephrostogram.

Case 18: Ureteral Fistula

Question 94

Which *one* of the following is the BEST course of action?

(A) Immediate ureteral reimplantation
(B) Transureteroureterostomy
(C) Nephrectomy
(D) Continued nephrostomy drainage
(E) Ureteral stent placement

The antegrade nephrostogram (Figure 18-1) demonstrates free flow of contrast material from the calyceal system into the ureter. There is extravasation along the drain site at the level of the sacrum. Note that both the drain and the abdominal dressing contain contrast material. There appears to be a small amount of contrast in the bladder, indicating that the ureter is not completely transected. The therapeutic goal in such a case is to control the urinary leakage while allowing the ureter to heal with an adequately sized lumen. This is most often accomplished by placement of a ureteral stent **(Option (E) is correct).** Figure 18-2 demonstrates the status of the patient following placement of a double-pigtail stent. A separate nephrostomy tube is still in place. An antegrade study now shows free flow of the contrast material into the bladder. There is no urine leakage via the drain site. The nephrostomy tube was removed 1 day later, and the patient was discharged. The double-pigtail stent was removed 2 months later.

The importance of antegrade ureteral opacification in various oblique views is demonstrated by a nephrostogram of another patient (Figure 18-3A). This markedly oblique view shows the true ureteral lumen and the site of leakage. Careful manipulation of the guide wire and catheter allowed entrance into the bladder by the guide wire so that a stent could be placed across the ureteral injury (Figure 18-3B).

Immediate ureteral reimplantation (Option (A)) is an option if a very distal ureteral transection injury is apparent at the time of surgery. In

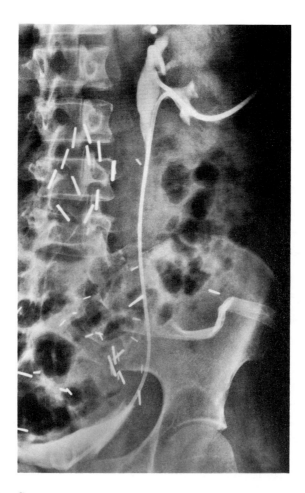

Figure 18-2. Same patient as in Figure 18-1. Nephrostogram following placement of a ureteral stent. There is free flow of contrast material into the bladder. No leakage is present at the drain site.

the postoperative period, prevention of urine leakage into the abdomen or retroperitoneum is an important primary consideration. It is often necessary to perform a percutaneous nephrostomy as the primary interventional procedure in patients with ureteral injuries recognized after surgery. Continued nephrostomy drainage (Option (D)) will control the urine leak from the injured ureter in some cases. However, in many instances some urine will continue to leak. Patients with inoperable pelvic carcinoma and vesicovaginal or ureterovaginal fistulas are usually not candidates for stent placement. Control of the leak from the ureter and/or bladder may fail because the combination of tumor and injured

A

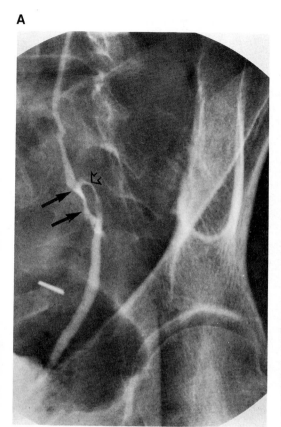

B

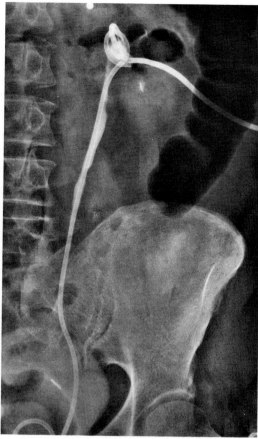

Figure 18-3. (A) Nephrostogram in a patient who sustained ureteral injury during a hysterectomy. This oblique view demonstrates the site of leakage (solid arrows) as well as the displacement of the ureter (open arrow). (B) An 8-French ureteral stent was placed after a steerable guide wire was used to traverse the deformed ureter demonstrated in panel A.

tissue does not allow healing. This problem is most severe when there has been radiotherapy to the injured area. Persistent fistulas in such patients may require ureteral occlusion. A variety of devices, including balloons, coils, clips, and plugs, have been used to effect ureteral occlusion so that drain sites and ureteral fistulas become dry, while nephrostomies provide proximal drainage.

Transureteroureterostomy (Option (B)) is a procedure in which one shortened or injured ureter is brought across the midline and anastomosed to the functionally normal ureter. This procedure carries the

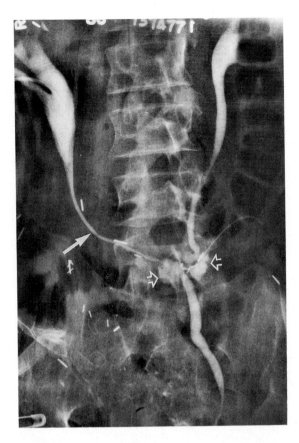

Figure 18-4. Transureteroureterostomy. Contrast material was injected through a catheter in the right ureter (solid arrow). There is filling of the left system via the anastomosis. Note the contrast material leakage (open arrows) at the anastomosis.

inherent risk associated with performing surgery on the otherwise intact and normally draining ureter. Surgical complications at the ureteroureterostomy site may result in a situation that compromises the urine drainage from both sides (Figure 18-4).

Nephrectomy (Option (C)) or total renal artery embolization will solve the problem of a fistula by ending urine production. This may be a choice when the remaining kidney is sound and when other methods of controlling ureteral leakage have failed. It is certainly not desirable to sacrifice a kidney unless there is no other viable option.

Question 95

Ureteral reimplantation with a short ureter is facilitated by:

T (A) psoas hitch
T (B) ileal interposition
T (C) Boari flap
T (D) autotransplantation

Most ureteral injuries are due to penetrating trauma (e.g., gunshot wounds) or to operative or endoscopic procedures. It is estimated that 95% of ureteral lacerations due to violence are the result of gunshot wounds. Stab wounds are only rarely associated with ureteral injury.

Surgical injuries to the ureter are most likely to occur when extensive dissection of the pelvis and retroperitoneum is necessary. Gynecologic procedures have been reported to have a risk of ureteral injury in the range of 1 to 10%. The risk is greatest in patients undergoing radical hysterectomies for carcinoma of the cervix. The number of ureteral injuries associated with obstetric procedures has diminished since high- and mid-forceps deliveries have increasingly been replaced by cesarean section. The general surgical procedures most commonly associated with ureteral injury include abdominoperineal resection and operative procedures for Crohn's disease. Surgery for abdominal aortic aneurysm and thrombo-occlusive disease of the aortoiliac vessels may place the ureters at risk. This is particularly true if there is an associated perianeurysmal fibrosis that encases the ureter.

Ureteral injury during open or endoscopic surgery may not be recognized at the time of the procedure. In the series reported by Carlton, 64% of ureteral injuries associated with open surgical procedures were not diagnosed until at least 48 hours after surgery. Similarly, although 40% of ureteral injuries associated with endoscopic procedures were diagnosed in the operating room, 40% were not recognized until more than 48 hours after the procedure. Ureteroscopic procedures have been associated with a 10 to 17% rate of ureteral injury. This frequency should decrease as the 11-French rigid ureteroscopes are replaced by the newer, smaller, flexible scopes.

The factors that determine the method of management of ureteral injury include the location and extent of injury. In large surgical series the complications of ureteral obstruction and ureteral extravasation occurred in approximately the same number of cases. Simple removal of the ligature in the case of an accidentally sutured ureter is generally not practiced since the ureteral blood supply may have been impaired

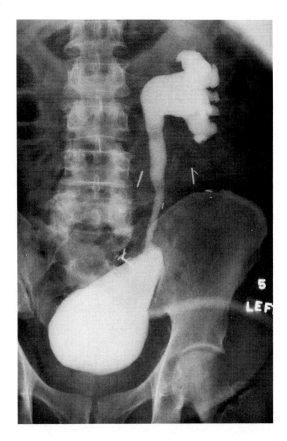

Figure 18-5. Psoas hitch. Cystogram via a cystostomy tube. The left side of the bladder has the characteristic upward angulation caused by its fixation to the psoas muscle. There is reflux into the left ureter and collecting system.

consequent to external compression by the ligature. There is then a risk of a slough of the ureter in the post-repair period. For this reason, ligated ureters are usually treated by primary surgical repair. Many ureteral injuries are distal, and so reimplantation into the bladder is preferred to ureteroureterostomy. A variety of procedures have been devised to facilitate reimplantation of a ureter shortened as a result of the external or operative trauma. The psoas hitch is a useful procedure when the ureter is minimally shortened **(Option (A) is true).** This is a procedure in which the ipsilateral posterior surface of the bladder is stretched superiorly and sutured to the psoas muscle (Figure 18-5). An antireflux reimplantation of the ureter is performed into the elevated bladder segment. The psoas hitch also has the advantage of protecting the ureteral anastomosis since the bladder cannot pull away during voiding. The radiographic appearance is characteristic.

Another useful procedure for more-extensive loss of the pelvic ureter is the bladder flap or Boari flap procedure **(Option (C) is true).** This is a method of replacing the pelvic ureter. A segment of bladder is formed into a tube and extended cephalad. The ureter is anastomosed in an antirefluxing manner into this bladder flap or tube.

Transureteroureterostomy is a method of managing ureteral injury when primary reimplantation or reanastomosis is contraindicated by the presence of pelvic inflammation, fibrosis due to radiation, or prior surgery (Figure 18-4). It is generally not employed simply to overcome a problem of ureteral shortening due to injury.

Ileal interposition is another method of solving the problem of the short ureter **(Option (B) is true).** A loop of ileum is anastomosed from the proximal ureter to the bladder. This loop of bowel is on its native vascular pedicle and is out of continuity with the remainder of the small bowel. It is an acceptable alternative when extensive surgery requires sacrificing a long segment of ureter (Figure 18-6).

Autotransplantation can be performed when there is extensive loss of the ureter **(Option (D) is true).** It has the advantage of not requiring mobilization of a loop of bowel as in the case of ileal interpositioning. Autotransplantation does require arterial and venous anastomoses as well as ureteral reimplantation. In hospitals with experienced renal transplantation surgeons, autotransplantation is a useful alternative procedure (Figure 18-7). Autotransplantation must be preceded by arteriography to ascertain the number and status of the renal arteries. The patient must also have good iliac arteries for the anastomosis to the renal artery.

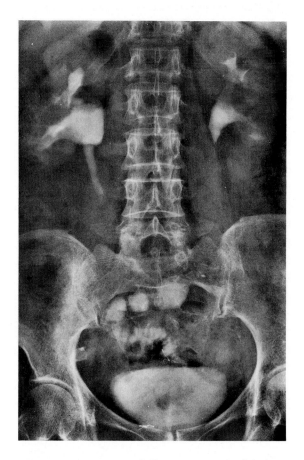

Figure 18-6. Ileal interposition following surgical injury to the right ureter. The interposed loop is well opacified, and the right collecting system is adequately drained.

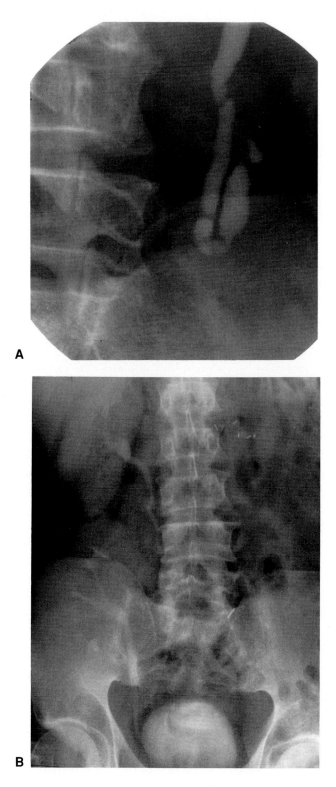

Figure 18-7. Autotransplantation following ureteroscopic injury. (A) Nephrostogram. The end of the avulsed left ureter is turned cephalad. (B) Postoperative excretory urogram demonstrates good opacification of the left kidney, which has been transplanted to the right iliac fossa.

Question 96

Concerning percutaneous nephrostomy,

T (A) the transcortical route is preferred
T (B) gas is a useful contrast agent
F (C) at least a 10-French catheter is needed for adequate drainage
F (D) major bleeding occurs in about 10% of patients
F (E) entering a lower-pole calyx facilitates subsequent ureteral stenting

The indications for percutaneous nephrostomy have expanded in recent years concurrently with the development of a number of procedures now described as interventional uroradiologic or endourologic procedures. Indications include relief of obstruction, removal of calculi, ureteral dilatation, ureteral stenting, endopyelotomies, biopsies, and urodynamic studies such as the Whitaker test.

The entrance into the kidney should avoid adjacent organs such as liver, spleen, and colon while providing safe access to the renal collecting system. In general, a site just below the twelfth rib, lateral to the paraspinal muscles and through a posterior calyx, is considered optimal. The calyx should be entered transcortically **(Option (A) is true)** and end on if possible to avoid interlobar arteries. Visualizing a posterior calyx may be difficult with the patient in the prone or prone-oblique position because the contrast material tends to collect in the dependent dilated renal pelvis. Gas injected into the collecting system will rise into the posterior calyces, facilitating their visualization and puncture **(Option (B) is true).** Gas may also be a useful contrast agent in patients with a history of severe reactions to iodinated contrast agents (Figure 18-8).

The kidney is a very vascular organ, so it is not surprising that bleeding is a potential complication. It is important to emphasize that almost all patients have some degree of gross hematuria immediately following percutaneous nephrostomy. This usually clears in 24 to 48 hours. Current techniques in which coaxial fine-needle catheter systems are used have improved the safety of the procedure so that bleeding requiring treatment such as transfusion or embolotherapy occurs in fewer than 2% of cases **(Option (D) is false).** An 8-French nephrostomy tube suffices for the routine drainage of an adult kidney **(Option (C) is false).** If there is persistent gross hematuria after nephrostomy, a larger tube (10 French to 14 French) may be used as necessary to tamponade the tract and compress the bleeding vessels.

It is important to anticipate the role of the nephrostomy in individual patient management. For example, a patient with ureteral obstruction

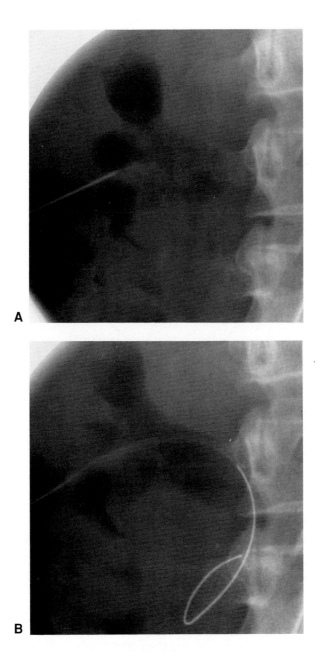

Figure 18-8. Percutaneous nephrostomy with air as a contrast agent in a patient sensitive to iodinated contrast materials. (A) The needle tip has entered a middle-posterior calyx. (B) The guide wire has been advanced into the proximal ureter.

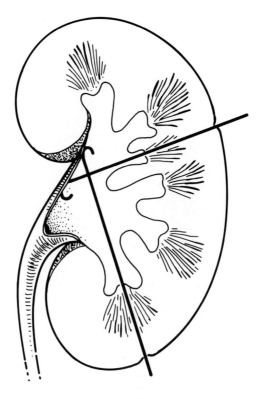

Figure 18-9. Diagram of a guide wire entering the collecting system. Note that pushing forces in a wire entering the lower pole will direct the wire to the upper pole, whereas a wire entering the middle or upper pole will be directed toward the ureteropelvic junction. Antegrade ureteral stenting is facilitated by entering the middle or upper pole of the kidney.

due to pelvic cancer may be a candidate for antegrade placement of a ureteral stent. When the percutaneous nephrostomy is performed in such a patient, a middle posterior calyx should be entered. If a ureteral stent is to be placed, a nephrostomy tract in the mid-kidney will facilitate the procedure because pushing forces will be directed toward the ureteropelvic junction. On the other hand, a nephrostomy placed in a lower-pole calyx is less well suited for stenting because pushing forces will be directed toward the upper pole **(Option (E) is false)** (Figure 18-9).

Question 97

Concerning stenting of ureteral fistulas,

F (A) the injured segment should be balloon dilated first
F (B) a 6-French stent is the largest that should be used
T (C) stents draining into an ileal conduit frequently occlude
F (D) the stent should be removed within 14 days

Ureteral stents may be placed by the retrograde (cystoscopic) or antegrade (percutaneous) route. In general, the retrograde route is preferred whenever possible so as to avoid puncturing the kidney. Retrograde ureteral stent placement is widely employed before extracorporeal shock wave lithotripsy (ESWL). An indwelling 6-French ureteral stent provides adequate renal drainage and facilitates passage of the post-ESWL stone fragments.

Retrograde stent placement for ureteral obstruction due to malignant tumor is a useful procedure. Attempts to pass stents by the retrograde route fail in about 35% of cases. These patients are then usually subjected to percutaneous nephrostomy and antegrade stent placement.

For ureteral injury with urinoma or fistula formation, ureteral stenting is often the definitive form of therapy. Careful antegrade catheterization of the ureter allows bypass of the injured ureteral segment and entry into the bladder. The injured segment should not be balloon dilated before stenting, because the damage to the ureter may be made worse **(Option (A) is false)**. Once a guide wire is in place in the bladder and across the area of extravasation, a double-pigtail stent can be passed. The stent provides a lumen for urine drainage and maintains the ureteral lumen while healing occurs. Generally, an 8-French stent is adequate for this purpose **(Option (B) is false)**. Smaller-diameter stents will provide adequate drainage, but the resultant ureteral lumen will be narrower and more likely to develop a functionally significant stricture. The duration of stenting depends on the severity of ureteral injury. Ureteral fistulas following surgical injury should be stented for 2 to 3 months **(Option (D) is false)**. Simple ureteral perforations such as by a guide wire (without fistula formation) require shorter periods of stenting (in the range of days to weeks).

In the patient with an ileal conduit, ureteral stenting requires extra care and planning. Placement of a double-pigtail stent from the kidney to the conduit is potentially dangerous. The mucosa of the conduit produces mucus, which can occlude the side holes of the stent in hours to days **(Option (C) is true)**. For this reason, it is recommended that stents placed in such cases extend from the kidney through the conduit with the distal pigtail through the stoma to drain into the collecting bag. There should be no side holes in the conduit.

Harold A. Mitty, M.D.

SUGGESTED READINGS

URETERAL FISTULAS

1. Darcy MD, Lund GB, Smith TP, Hunter DW, Castaneda-Zuniga WR, Amplatz K. Percutaneously applied ureteral clips: treatment of vesicovaginal fistula. Radiology 1987; 163:819–821
2. Gaylord GM, Johnsrude IS. Transrenal ureteral occlusion with Gianturco coils and gelatin sponge. Radiology 1989; 172:1047–1048
3. Günther RW, Klose KJ, Alken P, Bohl J. Transrenal ureteral occlusion using a detachable balloon. Urol Radiol 1984; 6:210–214
4. Lang EK. Antegrade ureteral stenting for dehiscence, strictures, and fistulae. AJR 1984; 143:795–801
5. Mitty HA, Train JS, Dan SJ. Placement of ureteral stents by antegrade and retrograde techniques. Radiol Clin North Am 1986; 24:587–600

URETERAL REIMPLANTATION

6. Carlton CE. Injuries of the kidney and ureter. In: Harrison JH, Gittes RF, Perlmutter AD, Stamey TA, Walsh PC (eds), Campbell's urology, vol 1. Philadelphia: WB Saunders; 1978:895–905
7. Kramolowsky EV. Ureteral perforation during ureterorenoscopy: treatment and management. J Urol 1987; 138:36–38
8. Lytton B, Weiss RM, Green DF. Complications of ureteral endoscopy. J Urol 1987; 137:649–653
9. Schultz A, Kristensen JK, Bilde T, Eldrup J. Ureteroscopy: results and complications. J Urol 1987; 137:865–866

PERCUTANEOUS NEPHROSTOMY

10. Coleman CC. Urinary system: nonvascular intervention. In: Kadir S (ed), Current practice of interventional radiology. Philadelphia: BC Decker; 1991:646–657
11. Ho PC, Talner LB, Parsons CL, Schmidt JD. Percutaneous nephrostomy: experience in 107 kidneys. Urology 1980; 16:532–535
12. Pfister RC, Newhouse JH. Interventional percutaneous pyeloureteral techniques. II. Percutaneous nephrostomy and other procedures. Radiol Clin North Am 1979; 17:351–363
13. Stables DP. Percutaneous nephrostomy: techniques, indications, and results. Urol Clin North Am 1982; 9:15–29

14. Cardella JF, Casteneda-Zuniga WR, Hunter DW, Hulbert JC, Amplatz K. Urine-compatible polymer for long-term ureteral stenting. Radiology 1986; 161:131–138
15. Mitty HA. Placement of ureteral stents. In: Kadir S (ed), Current practice of interventional radiology. Philadelphia: BC Decker; 1991:700–709
16. Mitty HA, Rackson ME, Dan SJ, Train JS. Experience with a new ureteral stent made of a biocompatible copolymer. Radiology 1988; 188:557–559
17. Rackson ME, Mitty HA, Lossef SV, Dan SJ, Train JS. Biocompatible copolymer ureteral stent: maintenance of patency beyond 6 months. AJR 1989; 153:783–784

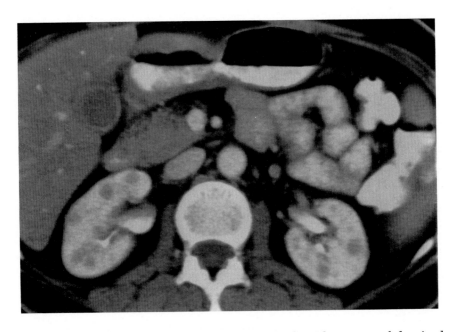

Figure 19-1. This 15-year-old girl presented with vague abdominal complaints. You are shown an enhanced CT scan.

Case 19: Burkitt's Lymphoma

Question 98

Which *one* of the following is the MOST likely diagnosis?

- (A) Burkitt's lymphoma
- (B) Candidiasis
- (C) Medullary cystic disease
- (D) Renal metastases
- (E) Leukemia

The enhanced abdominal CT scan (Figure 19-1) demonstrates multiple rounded lesions, which measure well above water density, in both kidneys. The kidneys are of normal size, there is good parenchymal opacification, and there is normal excretion of contrast material. There is no retroperitoneal lymphadenopathy or other evidence of metastatic tumor. The portions of the liver and spleen included on this image appear normal.

This appearance could be caused by metastases to the kidneys, involvement of the kidneys by malignant lymphoma, or multiple renal abscesses. Renal cysts would have a density near water, and infarcts would have a wedge-shaped appearance.

Involvement of the kidneys without other obvious evidence of metastatic disease is more common in patients with lymphoma than in those with other solid neoplasms. Renal involvement is much more common in patients with non-Hodgkin's lymphoma than in those with Hodgkin's disease. Burkitt's lymphoma is an undifferentiated non-Hodgkin's lymphoma with a propensity to involve the kidneys, and it is usually seen in young patients. It is not uncommon to see renal involvement without adjacent retroperitoneal lymphadenopathy, particularly in Burkitt's lymphoma **(Option (A) is correct).**

Although the fungus *Candida albicans* is commonly found in the gastrointestinal tract and vagina, systemic candidiasis (Option (B)) is usually limited to immunocompromised patients and those recovering from extensive burns or complicated surgical procedures. The clinical

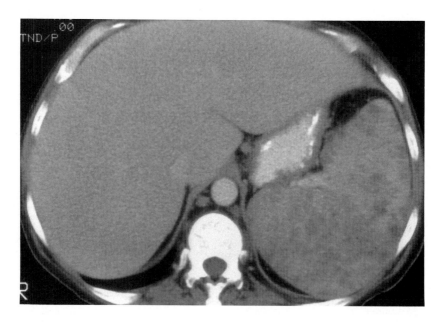

Figure 19-2. Candidiasis. Splenomegaly and multiple low-density lesions seen on this contrast-enhanced CT scan indicate involvement of the spleen in this patient with systemic candidiasis.

manifestations depend upon the severity of the infection. Immunocompromised patients often develop small abscesses in the kidneys. Involvement of the liver and spleen are also detected on enhanced abdominal CT examinations (Figure 19-2). In one series, 11% of patients with acute leukemia developed invasive candidiasis.

The kidneys are involved in approximately 90% of patients with systemic candidiasis. The diagnosis may be difficult, however, because there is no characteristic syndrome associated with the illness. Fever and chills unresponsive to antibiotic treatment are typical. Oliguria is often a presenting sign in infants. Renal parenchymal involvement is usually the result of systemic candidemia. Multiple microabscesses develop at the glomeruli. A thickened renal pelvic mucosa has been described on sonography, but this may be seen in any inflammatory condition.

Cystic lesions may be imaged by CT in patients with medullary cystic disease (Option (C)). However, the kidneys are small and the cysts have water density and a typical medullary location.

Both childhood and adult forms of medullary cystic disease occur. The childhood form of medullary cystic disease is inherited as an autosomal recessive disorder and is associated with a variety of extrarenal manifestations, including neurologic, ophthalmologic, and skeletal abnormalities and hepatic fibrosis. Retinitis pigmentosa and optic nerve atrophy are particularly common. The adult form of medullary cystic disease is inherited as an autosomal dominant disorder and does not have associated extrarenal manifestations. The pathologic findings in the kidneys are the same in both the childhood and adult forms. Patients with medullary cystic disease may present with symptoms of weakness or hyposthenuria. Children often complain of bone pain; adults may present with renal failure.

Metastases to the kidneys (Option (D)) usually appear as multiple soft tissue masses. They are often inhomogeneous and may bleed. Furthermore, there is usually evidence of metastases to other abdominal organs such as the liver, adrenal glands, or lymph nodes. The most common tumors that metastasize to the kidneys are carcinomas of the lung, breast, or gastrointestinal tract. However, these tumors are uncommon in adolescents.

Involvement of the kidneys by acute leukemia (Option (E)) is common; it is found in up to 65% of patients at autopsy. However, renal involvement usually consists of leukemic infiltrates, which are seldom seen on imaging studies. The most common renal manifestation is diffuse enlargement. A focal mass (chloroma) may be seen in patients with acute myelogenous leukemia but is uncommon. A chloroma rarely precedes the diagnosis of leukemia.

Question 99

Concerning renal lymphoma,

F (A) it is seen more often with Hodgkin's disease than with non-Hodgkin's lymphoma
F (B) it is seldom seen with Burkitt's lymphoma
F (C) renal failure is common
T (D) lymphomatous masses are usually homogeneous on CT
T (E) there is often other retroperitoneal tumor

Since the kidneys do not normally contain lymphoid tissue, primary renal lymphoma is rare. However, the kidneys are frequently involved during the course of the disease. In the series of 696 patients reported by Richmond et al., at least one kidney was involved in one-third of the patients. In 75% of the affected patients, both kidneys were involved.

Renal involvement is much more common with non-Hodgkin's lymphoma than with Hodgkin's disease **(Option (A) is false).** In the series of postmortem examinations reported by Richmond et al., 47% of patients with non-Hodgkin's lymphoma had infiltration of the renal parenchyma compared with only 13% of patients with Hodgkin's disease.

Lymphoma involves the kidneys by either direct extension or hematogenous spread. With hematogenous dissemination, multiple small foci are deposited in the cortex. Growth initially occurs by infiltration of the interstitium, and early involvement may be very difficult to detect. As the tumor grows and becomes expansile, the normal renal parenchyma may be displaced. At this stage, lymphomatous masses may be detected.

Burkitt's lymphoma is an undifferentiated form of non-Hodgkin's lymphoma. It arises from B lymphocytes and has a rapid doubling time. Burkitt's cells have a characteristic cytogenetic abnormality in which genetic material from chromosome 8 is translocated to chromosome 14. Patients from the endemic areas of equatorial Africa often have antibodies to the Epstein-Barr virus.

The clinical findings in patients in nonendemic areas, such as the United States, differ from those in endemic areas. Patients in the United States do not show the predilection for involvement of the mandible and eye seen in African patients. The gastrointestinal tract is the most common site of the tumor in North American patients. In a series of 40 patients reported by Dunnick et al., the gastrointestinal tract was involved in 13 (33%). Tumor often occurs in the kidneys and peripheral lymph nodes **(Option (B) is false).** In the series reported by Dunnick et al., renal involvement was detected by imaging studies in 5% of cases.

Patients with renal lymphoma seldom have symptoms related to the urinary tract. Renal involvement is detected most commonly during an abdominal CT scan obtained to monitor or stage the extent of disease. Renal failure may be due to diffuse infiltration, ureteral obstruction, or chemotherapy. However, lymphoma can usually be controlled, and renal failure is uncommon **(Option (C) is false).** Richmond et al. reviewed a series of 142 patients whose subsequent autopsies proved renal lymphoma. Only 23% had either clinical or biochemical changes suggesting renal involvement. Among a larger group of patients with proven malignant lymphoma, extensive renal involvement led to renal failure in only 0.5%.

Unless renal masses are large, excretory urography is usually normal. Sonography demonstrates hypoechoic masses, which may be confused with renal cysts. However, lymphomatous masses usually have internal

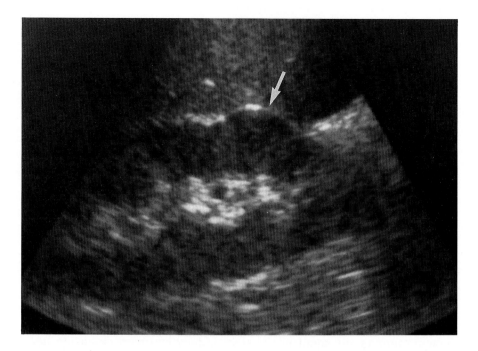

Figure 19-3. Renal lymphoma. On this longitudinal sonogram, a parenchymal mass is identified by the cortical bulge (arrow) in this patient with T-cell lymphoma.

echoes and do not demonstrate the increased through transmission seen with renal cysts (Figure 19-3).

CT is the most commonly used imaging modality for evaluating abdominal disease in patients with lymphoma. Renal lymphoma is seen as a soft tissue mass with a density similar to normal renal parenchyma on the unenhanced examination. Lymphoma does show contrast enhancement but enhances much less intensely than the renal parenchyma, which concentrates contrast material. Thus, renal lymphoma is readily detected on enhanced studies. Lymphoma is typically homogeneous in appearance, although large masses may occasionally show central necrosis **(Option (D) is true).**

Historically, renal lymphoma has been described as either diffuse infiltration or single or multiple renal masses. Cross-sectional imaging techniques, such as CT (Figure 19-4) and ultrasonography, demonstrated direct extension of tumor from para-aortic lymph notes into the perinephric space and the kidney. This was then considered a fourth manifestation of renal lymphoma. Many patients with renal lymphoma had other retroperitoneal tumor demonstrable by CT **(Option (E) is true).**

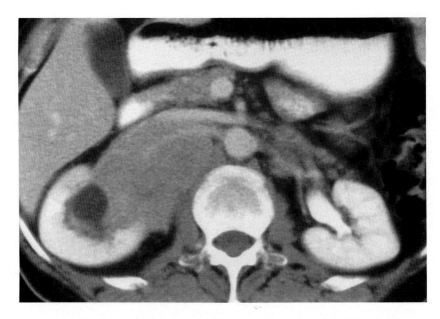

Figure 19-4. Renal lymphoma. This contrast-enhanced CT examination demonstrates involvement of the right kidney by direct extension from disease in the paracaval lymph nodes.

More recently, Cohan et al. showed that the kidneys may be involved by lymphoma without evidence of other retroperitoneal disease. In their series of 29 patients with renal lymphoma, 17 had multiple soft tissue renal masses, but only 7 (41%) of these had other retroperitoneal lymphoma detected by an enhanced abdominal CT examination. Similar results were reported by Reznek et al. Of their patients with renal lymphoma, 43% had no evidence of retroperitoneal lymph node involvement. Therefore, the absence of retroperitoneal lymphadenopathy does not preclude the diagnosis of renal lymphoma.

Question 100

Concerning medullary cystic disease,

T (A) in children, ophthalmologic abnormalities are common
F (B) in adults, renal function is seldom affected
T (C) the medullary cysts communicate freely with the renal tubules
F (D) many patients have accompanying nephrolithiasis
T (E) ultrasonography demonstrates increased parenchymal echogenicity

Medullary cystic disease is characterized by progressive renal tubular atrophy with sclerosis of the glomeruli and formation of medullary cysts. The childhood form of medullary cystic disease is inherited as an autosomal recessive disorder. There is an increased incidence of ophthalmologic disorders, especially optic nerve atrophy, which is present in 50% of patients **(Option (A) is true).** The term renal-retinal dysplasia refers to the association of medullary cystic disease and retinitis pigmentosa. Red or blond hair, hepatic fibrosis, skeletal dysplasias, and neurologic abnormalities are also associated with the childhood form.

The adult form of medullary cystic disease is inherited as an autosomal dominant disorder. The clinical onset is in young adults, and there are no associated extrarenal findings.

The diagnosis of medullary cystic disease may be made during an evaluation of growth retardation in children or progressive renal failure in adults. Children and adults may complain of lethargy, weakness, or polyuria. Laboratory studies confirm chronic renal failure in both children and adults **(Option (B) is false).** Hypokalemia occurs as a result of potassium wasting by damaged distal tubules.

The kidneys are small, with uniform parenchymal loss. There are interstitial lymphocytic infiltrates, which lead to fibrosis. The cysts are lined with simple flattened cuboidal epithelium and communicate freely with the renal tubules **(Option (C) is true).**

The abdominal radiograph is often normal, although bone changes may be seen in children. Small kidneys may occasionally be detected on the preliminary radiograph. There is no nephrocalcinosis, nor is there a tendency to form stones **(Option (D) is false).**

Excretory urography is seldom attempted because of the presence of renal failure. High-dose urography with nephrotomography may demonstrate the medullary cysts as small lucencies that do not distort the collecting system. Contrast material injected by retrograde pyelography may demonstrate dilated tubules and medullary cysts.

Sonography is used more often than urography to evaluate the kidneys in patients with medullary cystic disease. The small medullary cysts are _CRF_ easily recognized, and the parenchyma has increased echogenicity **(Option (E) is true).** In the appropriate clinical setting these sonographic findings can be used to confirm the diagnosis.

Small kidneys with a smooth cortical outline are demonstrated by CT. The medullary location of the cysts can often be appreciated.

Question 101

Concerning metastases to the kidneys,

F (A) the kidneys are sites for metastatic disease in fewer than 5% of patients with cancer

T (B) there are usually multiple lesions

T (C) they are usually asymptomatic

T (D) a solitary metastasis cannot be distinguished radiographically from a primary renal adenocarcinoma

F (E) they seldom demonstrate tumor necrosis

The kidneys may be secondarily involved by metastatic tumor either by hematogenous spread or by direct extension. The primary tumors most likely to invade the kidney directly include adrenal carcinoma (which arises within the perinephric space), malignant lymphoma, and carcinoma of the colon.

The kidneys are often involved by metastatic disease via hematogenous seeding. They receive approximately 25% of the cardiac output, and renal metastases are common. Willis found renal metastases in 8% of 600 consecutive postmortem examinations performed on patients with malignant disease, and Abrams et al. found that 13% of 1,000 patients who had died of carcinoma had renal metastases **(Option (A) is false).**

Since the metastases are hematogenously spread, it is not surprising that most patients have multiple lesions **(Option (B) is true).** In a series of 118 patients with renal metastases, Klinger found that 85 had bilateral renal metastases. Evidence of metastatic tumor in other locations is also common (Figure 19-5).

The most common sources of renal metastases are carcinomas of the lung and breast. Carcinoma of the stomach, a common source of renal metastases in earlier series, is now seen less frequently. However, there has been a significant increase in the incidence of malignant melanoma, and this is now a common source of renal metastases.

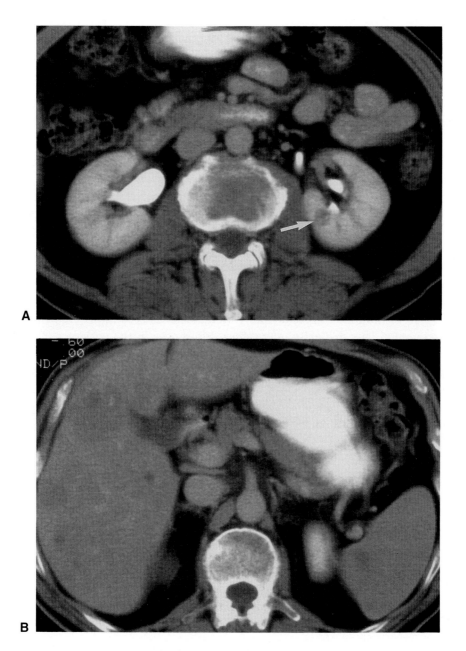

Figure 19-5. Renal metastasis. (A) A small renal metastasis (arrow) from malignant melanoma is detected on this enhanced CT examination. (B) Multiple other metastatic deposits are also seen in the liver and spleen.

Malignant lymphoma, which is rarely primary in the kidneys, often involves the kidneys secondarily. This may occur by either hematogenous dissemination or direct extension from disease in the adjacent para-aortic lymph nodes.

Metastases to the kidneys are usually asymptomatic **(Option (C) is true).** Even laboratory abnormalities are uncommon. In Klinger's series of 118 patients, only 24% had hematuria and 17% were azotemic.

For patients with a known primary tumor and a solitary renal mass, it is essential to determine whether the renal lesion is a metastasis or a second primary neoplasm. However, this distinction cannot be made on the basis of the imaging features alone **(Option (D) is true).** Renal metastases are more common than a renal carcinoma as a second primary tumor in autopsy series of patients with known cancer. However, these metastatic deposits are usually small and may not be detected by CT. Pagani and Bernardino found that a second primary renal carcinoma was detected 4.5 times as often as renal metastases.

More recently, Choyke et al. reviewed 27 patients with renal metastases. They found four times as many metastases as second primary renal carcinomas. This disparity may reflect differences in the patient populations. In advanced disease, a new renal mass is more likely to be metastatic. However, among patients in remission, a new renal mass is equally likely to be a renal carcinoma or a metastasis.

Metastases are commonly small, multicentric lesions. As they enlarge, they often outgrow their blood supply and undergo central necrosis **(Option (E) is false).** Invasion of the renal vein and inferior vena cava has been reported but is rare.

Question 102

Concerning leukemia,

F (A) the kidneys are rarely involved at autopsy

T (B) patients seldom have symptoms due to renal involvement

T (C) solid masses composed of poorly differentiated cells may occur with acute myeloblastic leukemia

F (D) accompanying retroperitoneal lymphadenopathy is seldom present

T (E) hemorrhage (intrarenal, subcapsular, or perinephric) is common

Leukemic-cell infiltrates occur most commonly in the lymph nodes, spleen, liver, and bone marrow. The kidney is the next most frequently involved organ. Kirshbaum and Preuss found renal infiltrates at autopsy in 65% of patients with leukemia **(Option (A) is false).**

Renal involvement by leukemia is usually diffuse infiltration. Although the kidneys are enlarged, renal function is preserved and the patients are asymptomatic **(Option (B) is true).**

Occasionally a focal leukemic infiltrate will occur and create a mass effect. This is most often seen with acute myelocytic leukemia **(Option (C) is true).** The focal leukemic infiltrate is composed of poorly differentiated myeloid cells and is referred to as a chloroma. Chloromas may occur in any location. Since they usually arise in a patient with known acute leukemia, their etiology is suspected. However, they may occasionally precede peripheral manifestations of the leukemia.

Renal involvement with acute leukemia is usually a histologic diagnosis. The imaging studies become abnormal when the leukemic-cell infiltration is extensive or focal. With diffuse infiltration, renal enlargement may be detected by excretory urography, sonography (Figure 19-6), or CT. Renal contours remain smooth, and the collecting system is not displaced unless a chloroma is present. Retroperitoneal lymphadenopathy is often detected by CT **(Option (D) is false).**

Radiographic studies in leukemic patients are obtained when complications are suspected. CT is especially useful in detecting retroperitoneal hemorrhage, which is often seen in leukemic patients. Common sites of hematoma formation include intrarenal, subcapsular, and perinephric locations **(Option (E) is true).**

AmL = a mass lesion

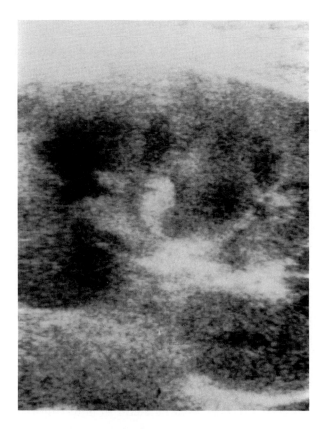

Figure 19-6. Leukemic infiltration. Sonography demonstrates an enlarged kidney but no focal masses.

Question 103

Concerning candidiasis,

(A) *Candida albicans* is seldom a pathogen in an immunocompetent host
(B) multiple small parenchymal abscesses are a feature of renal involvement
(C) papillary necrosis is rare unless the patient has underlying diabetes mellitus
(D) extension into the renal pelvis may result in a mycetoma
(E) fungus balls in the renal pelvis cannot be distinguished from tumor or blood clot by ultrasonography

Immunocompromised patients are at increased risk for developing systemic candidiasis. The urinary tract may be involved by either hematogenous spread or direct extension to the urethra and bladder from the anus. In one series, 11% of patients receiving treatment for acute leukemia developed invasive candidiasis. However, healthy adults frequently carry *Candida albicans* in the mouth, gastrointestinal tract, or vagina **(Option (A) is true).**

Since yeasts in the colon are suppressed by the normal bacterial flora, antibiotic therapy will increase the yeast count and may lead to candiduria. Glucosuria favors *Candida* growth, so poorly controlled diabetes mellitus will also contribute to *Candida* infections of the urinary tract.

Systemic fungal infections frequently involve the kidneys. In approximately 90% of patients with candidiasis, the kidneys are affected. The fungus enters the tubules, where it seems to be protected from inflammatory reaction. From the tubules, it may reinvade the renal parenchyma.

Patients with *Candida* pyelonephritis usually have flank pain, fever, and progressive uremia. Candiduria is pathologic, since fungi are not normally found in the urine. However, asymptomatic candiduria usually disappears spontaneously when the predisposing conditions are removed.

Candida pyelonephritis may create multiple small abscesses in the renal cortex **(Option (B) is true).** They are uncommon but may occur either with hematogenous dissemination or from an ascending urinary tract infection.

Renal candidiasis may also cause an infiltrating infection along the collecting tubules. Involvement of the papillary tips may lead to papillary necrosis **(Option (C) is false).** In a series of patients dying with candidiasis, Tomashefski and Abramowsky found papillary necrosis in 21%. In each patient with papillary necrosis there was other evidence of renal involvement with *Candida,* while only 2 of 16 patients with papillary necrosis had diabetes mellitus.

Fungi such as *Candida* species may form pseudomycelia. These long threads intertwine to form clusters that can aggregate into bezoars. Urinary tract bezoars (mycetomas) may be large or small and may occur as filling defects in the renal pelvis or the bladder (Figure 19-7) **(Option (D) is true).** They may be found in patients with severe *Candida* pyelonephritis or asymptomatic candiduria.

Excretory urography or retrograde pyelography may be performed to exclude urinary tract obstruction. The sonographic findings are nonspecific. A thickened urothelium with decreased echogenicity may be present but is nonspecific. A bezoar is seen as an echogenic mass within the renal pelvis. However, a bezoar cannot be distinguished from a blood clot or tumor on the basis of its sonographic appearance **(Option (E) is true).**

Lower urinary tract infections often respond to oral flucytosine, since

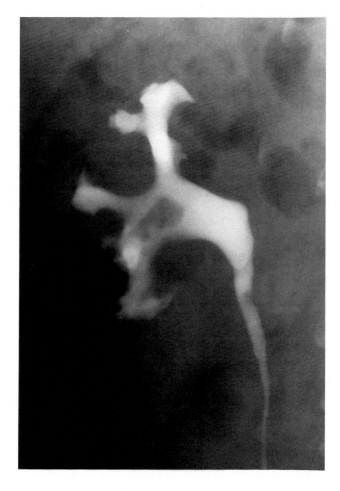

Figure 19-7. Mycetoma. A filling defect due to a mycetoma is seen on an retrograde pyelogram in this patient infected with *Candida albicans.*

it is excreted in high concentrations in the urine. Amphotericin B is the drug of choice for *Candida* pyelonephritis.

N. Reed Dunnick, M.D.

SUGGESTED READINGS

RENAL LYMPHOMA

1. Cohan RH, Dunnick NR, Leder RA, Baker ME. Computed tomography of renal lymphoma. J Comput Assist Tomogr 1990; 14:933–938
2. Dunnick NR, Reaman GH, Head GL, Shawker TH, Ziegler JL. Radiographic manifestations of Burkitt's lymphoma in American patients. AJR 1979; 132:1–6
3. Hartman DS, David CJ Jr, Goldman SM, Friedman AC, Fritzsche P. Renal lymphoma: radiologic-pathologic correlation of 21 cases. Radiology 1982; 144:759–766
4. Reznek RH, Mootoosamy I, Webb JA, Richards MA. CT in renal and perirenal lymphoma: a further look. Clin Radiol 1990; 42:233–238
5. Richmond J, Sherman RS, Diamond HD, Craver LF. Renal lesions associated with malignant lymphomas. Am J Med 1962; 32:184–207
6. Townsend RR. CT of AIDS-related lymphoma. AJR 1991; 156:969–974

CANDIDIASIS

7. Bick RJ, Bryan PJ. Sonographic demonstration of thickened renal pelvic mucosa/submucosa in mixed candida infection. JCU 1987; 15:333–336
8. Lew MA. Diagnosis of systemic *Candida* infections. Annu Rev Med 1989; 40:87–97
9. Schonebeok J. Fungal infections of the urinary tract. In: Walsh PC, Gittes RF, Perlmutter AD, Stamey TA (eds), Campbell's urology. Philadelphia: WB Saunders; 1986
10. Tomashefski JF Jr, Abramowsky CR. Candida-associated renal papillary necrosis. Am J Clin Pathol 1981; 75:190–194

MEDULLARY CYSTIC DISEASE

11. Bernstein J, Gardner KD Jr. Renal cystic disease and renal dysplasia. In: Walsh PC, Gittes RF, Perlmutter AD, Stamey TA (eds), Campbell's urology. Philadelphia: WB Saunders; 1986
12. Dunnick NR, McCallum RW, Sandler CM. A textbook of uroradiology. Baltimore: Williams & Wilkins; 1991
13. Garel LA, Habib R, Pariente D, Broyer M, Sauvegrain J. Juvenile nephronophthisis: sonographic appearance in children with severe uremia. Radiology 1984; 151:93–95
14. Rego JD Jr, Laing FC, Jeffrey RB. Ultrasonographic diagnosis of medullary cystic disease. J Ultrasound Med 1983; 2:433–436
15. Resnick JS, Hartman DS. Medullary cystic disease of the kidney. In: Pollack HM (ed), Clinical urography. Philadelphia: WB Saunders; 1990:1178–1184
16. Steele BT, Lirenman DS, Beattie CW. Nephronophthisis. Am J Med 1980; 68:531–538

RENAL METASTASES

17. Abrams HL, Spiro R, Goldstein N. Metastases in carcinoma: analysis of 1,000 autopsied cases. Cancer 1950; 3:74–85
18. Choyke PL, White EM, Zeman RK, Jaffe MH, Clark LR. Renal metastases: clinicopathologic and radiologic correlation. Radiology 1987; 162:359–363
19. Klinger ME. Secondary tumors of the genitourinary tract. J Urol 1951; 65:144–153
20. Mitnick JS, Bosniak MA, Rothberg M, Megibow AJ, Raghavendra BN, Subramanyam BR. Metastatic neoplasms to the kidney studied by computed tomography and sonography. J Comput Assist Tomogr 1985; 9:43–49
21. Nishitani H, Onitsuka H, Kawahira K, et al. Computed tomography of renal metastases. J Comput Assist Tomogr 1984; 8:727–730
22. Pagani JJ. Solid renal mass in the cancer patient: second primary renal cell carcinoma versus renal metastasis. J Comput Assist Tomogr 1983; 7:444–448
23. Pagani JJ, Bernardino ME. Incidence and significance of serendipitous CT findings in the oncologic patient. J Comput Assist Tomogr 1982; 6:268–275
24. Willis RA. Spread of tumors in the human body, 2nd ed. London: Butterworths; 1952

LEUKEMIA

25. Dunnick NR, Heaston DK. Computed tomography of extracranial chloroma. J Comput Assist Tomogr 1982; 6:83–85
26. Heiberg E, Wolverson MK, Sundaram M, Shields JB. CT findings in leukemia. AJR 1984; 143:1317–1323
27. Kirshbaum JD, Preuss FS. A clinical and pathologic study of one hundred and twenty-three fatal cases in a series of 14,400 necropsies. Arch Intern Med 1943; 71:777–792

Notes

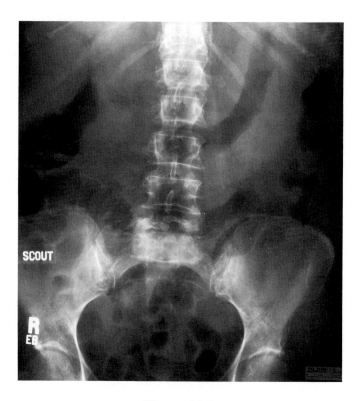

Figure 20-1

Figures 20-1 through 20-3. History withheld. You are shown a scout radiograph (Figure 20-1), a 10-minute radiograph from an excretory urogram (Figure 20-2), and a coned view of the left ureter (Figure 20-3).

Case 20: Ureteral Metastatic Disease

Question 104

Which *one* of the following is the MOST likely diagnosis?

(A) Renal artery stenosis
(B) Endometriosis
(C) Metastatic disease
(D) Primary urothelial tumor
(E) Suburothelial hemorrhage

The scout radiograph (Figure 20-1) demonstrates an air-filled stomach with an irregular lumen that appears narrowed. In addition, there is increased soft tissue density around the air-filled stomach. The appearance of the stomach on the scout radiograph is identical to its appearance on the 10-minute postinjection radiograph from the excretory urogram (Figure 20-2). This unchanging appearance of the gastric shadow in the two radiographs is highly suggestive of an infiltrative neoplastic disorder involving the gastric body and antrum. The radiograph from the excretory urogram (Figure 20-2) also demonstrates that the margin of the mid-left ureter has a scalloped appearance, which is better shown on a close-up view (Figure 20-3). Of the options listed, only metastatic disease would explain both the gastric and ureteral abnormalities **(Option (C) is correct).** Figure 20-4 is a radiograph made during an upper gastrointestinal series on the same patient; it confirms the diagnosis of linitis plastica.

Vascular impressions secondary to renal artery stenosis (Option (A)) generally involve the proximal one-third of the ureter and have a more serpiginous appearance than do the focal impressions demonstrated in Figure 20-3. Endometriosis (Option (B)) is unlikely since this lesion typically involves the ureter at the level of the pelvic brim, in the region of the uterosacral ligaments. Similarly, a primary urothelial tumor (Option (D)) most commonly involves the distal one-third of the ureter and appears as a filling defect within the ureteral lumen. Submucosal hemorrhage (Option (E)) is also unlikely as it generally causes narrowing

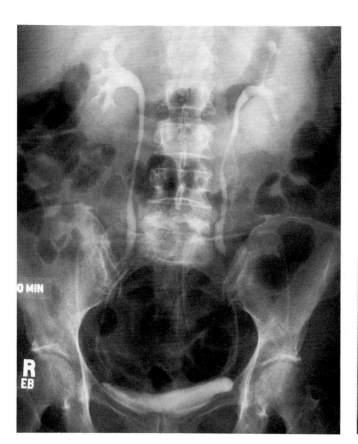

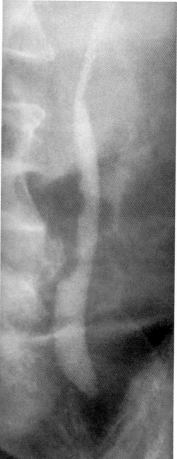

Figure 20-2   Figure 20-3

of the ureteral lumen and is typically associated with evidence of submucosal hemorrhage involving the calyces and renal pelvis.

Metastatic lesions affecting the ureter are more common than primary ureteral tumors. The ureter may be involved either as a result of direct extension of tumor from an adjacent organ or lymph node group or as a result of hematogenous spread. The majority of cases of ureteral involvement from metastatic disease occur as a result of direct extension of tumor in the pelvis from such primary sites as the cervix, prostate, ovary, colon, and bladder. In patients with lymphoma or other tumors that metastasize to retroperitoneal lymph nodes, displacement or obstruction

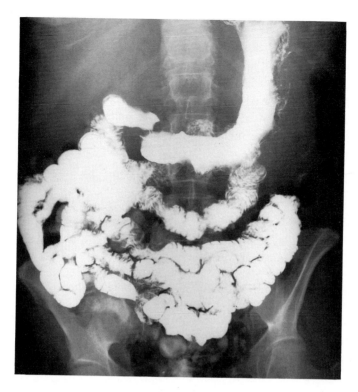

Figure 20-4. Linitis plastica. Same patient as in Figures 20-1 through 20-3. Overhead radiograph from a gastrointestinal series demonstrating luminal narrowing of the gastric antrum and body with mucosal irregularity and thickening of the gastric wall as a result of infiltrating gastric carcinoma.

of either ureter may be present. In some cases the tumor invokes an intense desmoplastic reaction in the periureteral tissues that simulates the appearance of retroperitoneal fibrosis. The frequency of ureteral obstruction approaches 40 to 75% in patients with advanced cervical carcinoma.

Ureteral involvement as a result of hematogenous metastases is considered rare; Ritchie and Ehrlich were able to document only 250 such patients reported as of 1979. In most cases, the ureteral involvement is asymptomatic and is discovered incidentally either on imaging studies performed for another purpose or at autopsy. Three types of ureteral involvement are reported: infiltration of the periureteral soft tissues, transmural involvement of the ureteral wall, and (as in the test patient) the presence of submucosal nodules. In the first two instances, the ureteral involvement may be manifest as a ureteral stricture with or without an associated soft tissue mass. Periureteral infiltration presumably results from infiltration of the adventitia by tumor cells, whereas transmural involvement suggests tumor deposition in the muscularis. Submucosal nodules are thought to represent tumor infiltration of the lamina propria. The most common sites of primary tumors reported to metastasize to the ureter include the breast, prostate, kidney, cervix, and gastrointestinal tract.

Question 105

Concerning vascular "notching" of the ureter,

(A) when it accompanies renal artery stenosis, it is usually the result of hypertrophy of the ureteral artery

(B) when it involves the proximal one-third of the ureter, it is usually arterial

(C) when it is secondary to varices of the broad ligament, it involves the right ureter more commonly than the left

(D) it occurs with occlusion of either the superior or inferior vena cava

Vascular impressions ("notching") of the ureter may result in either a focal extrinsic impression (crossing-vessel defect) or a more diffuse pattern of extrinsic serpiginous impressions along the segment of involved ureter (Figure 20-5A). The latter impressions must be present on multiple radiographs to be reliably differentiated from ureteral peristalsis. They may be either arterial or venous in origin; however, arterial impressions as reported by Williamson et al. are more common. Although there are multiple causes of such impressions (Table 20-1), the most common cause of scalloping involving the proximal one-third of the ureter is hypertrophy of the ureteral artery **(Option (B) is true)** (Figure 20-5B and C), generally in association with renal artery stenosis or occlusion. The ureteral artery extends from the renal pelvis to the bladder and generally is supplied by multiple sources, including the intrarenal dorsal and ventral branches of the renal artery; the gonadal artery; the aorta; the lumbar vessels; the internal iliac arteries directly; and the vesical, uterine, or hemorrhoidal branches of the internal iliac arteries. Flow into the ureteral artery is normally from each of the feeding vessels; however, if a renal artery stenosis is present proximal to the origin of the ureteral artery, there is reversal of flow such that the ureteral artery hypertrophies and becomes a source of blood flow to the kidney **(Option (A) is true).** Hypertrophied periureteral collaterals also may develop in patients

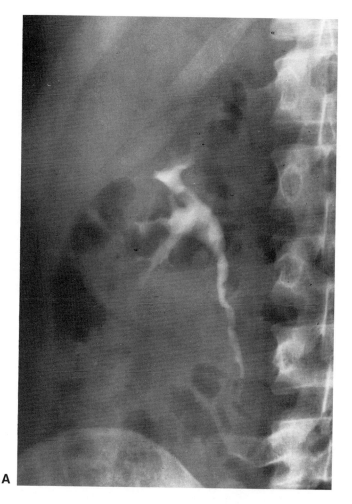

A

Figure 20-5. Ureteral notching secondary to renal artery stenosis. (A) A 10-minute postinjection radiograph from an excretory urogram demonstrates multiple serpiginous extrinsic impressions involving the renal pelvis and the proximal right ureter. (B) Midstream aortogram shows a long-segment stenosis of the right renal artery (arrow). (C) Late-phase arteriogram shows the hypertrophied ureteral artery (arrow) responsible for the serpiginous impressions demonstrated in panel A. (Courtesy of Morton Bosniak, M.D., New York University Medical Center.)

with occlusion of the infrarenal abdominal aorta or iliac artery such that the ureteral artery is a source of collateral blood flow to the lower extremities. Similar changes may occur in patients with large renal tumors or arteriovenous malformations with parasitized blood supply from ureteral collateral channels.

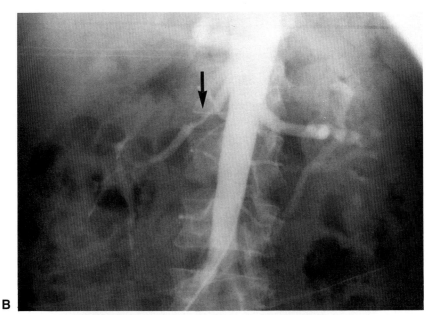

B

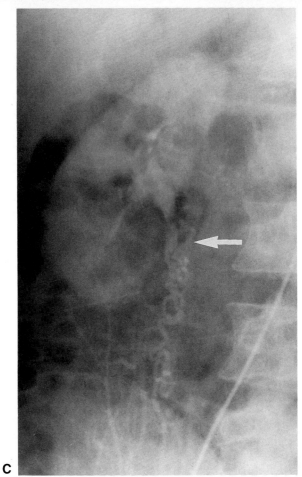

C

346

Table 20-1. Causes of ureteral notching

Arterial
  Renal artery stenosis
  Renal tumors with parasitized blood supply
  Renal arteriovenous malformations
  Aortic or iliac artery occlusion
Venous
  Congenital varicosities
  Renal vein thrombosis
  Occlusion of the azygous vein
  Occlusion of the superior or inferior vena cava
  Portal hypertension
  Carcinoma of the pancreas

Solitary venous impressions secondary to the gonadal vessels may be present in two places: first, just distal to the ureteropelvic junction, and second, at the level of S1 just proximal to the characteristic oblique impression made where the ureter crosses anterior to the iliac artery. Diffuse venous impressions associated with varicoceles in men or varicosities of the broad ligament in women most commonly occur on the left ureter **(Option (C) is false).** There are multiple theories to explain this left-sided predominance; most researchers believe that it occurs as a result of pressure on the left renal vein where it is compressed between the aorta posteriorly and the superior mesenteric artery anteriorly. The resulting "nutcracker" phenomenon causes increased venous pressure in the gonadal and ureteral vessels, which freely communicate with the renal vein.

Renal vein thrombosis and inferior vena cava obstruction are the most common venous causes of ureteral notching. In such patients, increased flow rates in renal capsular, ureteral, and lumbar venous collaterals all contribute to ureteral notching. Patients with obstruction of the superior vena cava or azygos vein also develop venous notching; this occurs as a result of transmission of increased venous pressure to the ascending lumbar system and then to periureteral and gonadal collaterals via the inferior vena cava **(Option (D) is true).** In patients with portal hypertension, spontaneous splenorenal, gastrorenal, or mesenteric renal anastomoses may decompress the increased pressure within the portal system. Similar decompressive mechanisms may occur in patients with carcinoma of the head of the pancreas who have occlusion of the splenic vein. Venous collaterals in the retroperitoneum may be demonstrated

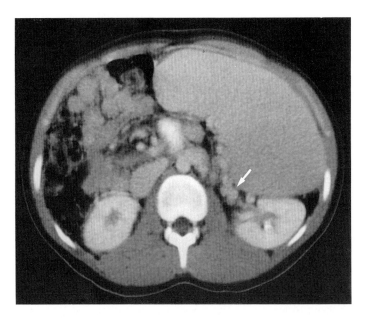

Figure 20-6. Portal hypertension. Multiple curvilinear densities adjacent to the renal pelvis (arrow) represent dilated venous collaterals in a patient with splenomegaly and portal hypertension.

on CT as multiple curvilinear or circular densities, adjacent to the renal pelvis and ureter, which enhance following administration of contrast material (Figure 20-6). Both arterial and venous collaterals are also well demonstrated by angiography.

Question 106

Concerning ureteral endometriosis,

(A) the typical radiographic appearance is that of extrinsic compression
(B) the lesion is usually located just above the level of the sacroiliac joint
(C) CT is the imaging study of choice to assess the extent of ureteral involvement
(D) nearly all patients also have endometrial implants involving the sigmoid colon

Endometriosis is a condition in which endometrial tissue is found outside of the uterine cavity. Most patients with endometriosis are between 30 and 35 years of age. The ectopic tissue is commonly located in the ovaries, the fallopian tubes, the pelvic peritoneum, and the gastrointestinal tract. The urinary tract is reported to be involved in approximately 1% of patients with endometriosis. The most common site of urinary tract involvement is the bladder, followed by the ureter; involvement of the kidneys is least common.

There are three principal theories about the etiology of endometriosis: the embryonic, the metaplastic, and the migratory theories. Proponents of the embryonic theory believe that the disease develops because of the occurrence of embryonic rests of Wolffian or Müllerian tissue. The metaplastic theory suggests that hormonal stimulation or inflammation results in the transformation of endothelial cells of the peritoneum into endometrial cells. Experimental data, however, support the migratory theory, which states that the disease occurs because of the migration of endometrial tissue into the pelvis or abdominal cavity via the fallopian tubes as the result of retrograde menstruation. Dissemination outside of the pelvis may then occur as a result of vascular or lymphatic spread of the ectopic tissue. Thus endometriosis may affect the ureter either by direct extension from disease within the pelvis or by "metastasizing" via hematogenous or lymphatic routes. Iatrogenic implantation has also been suggested as a mechanism of spread to the urinary tract in patients who have undergone previous surgery. Although ureteral involvement generally occurs in patients with widespread pelvic disease, ureteral endometriosis as the initial manifestation of the disease process may occur and is unrelated to endometrial implants involving the gastrointestinal tract **(Option (D) is false).**

The clinical findings in patients with ureteral endometriosis are relatively nonspecific but include flank pain and hematuria that may or may not coincide with the menstrual cycle. Although ureteral obstruction secondary to endometriosis has traditionally required surgical resection and/or percutaneous decompression, in recent years medical management of such patients with danazol has been reported but is not always successful.

Two forms of ureteral endometriosis have been described. In the intrinsic form, the ureter is involved by lymphatic or vascular dissemination of disease; in the extrinsic form, the ureter is secondarily affected by direct extension of endometriosis involving the pelvic organs. Pathologically, extrinsic involvement is characterized by the presence of endometrial elements in the adventitia of the ureter whereas intrinsic involvement is characterized by the presence of the endometrial tissue within the lamina propria or muscularis of the ureter. The extrinsic form is four times more common than the intrinsic variety. The simultaneous

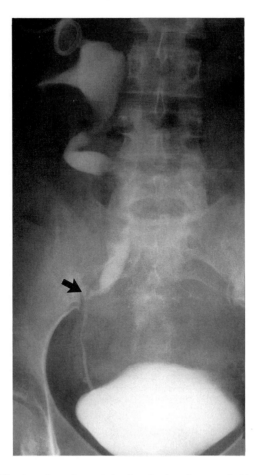

Figure 20-7. Ureteral endometriosis. Lateral angulation of the ureter (arrow) with proximal hydroureteronephrosis.

occurrence of both intrinsic and extrinsic disease in the same patient has also been described.

The radiographic features of ureteral endometriosis have been described by Pollack and Wills. There is a short to medium-length ureteral stricture (generally less than 2.5 cm in length), which affects the distal one-third of the ureter, usually within 3 cm of the inferior aspect of the sacroiliac joint in the region of the uterosacral ligaments (Figure 20-7) **(Option (B) is false).** The stricture is characteristically smooth but abruptly tapered, suggesting extrinsic compression **(Option (A) is true).** There may be sharp medial or, less commonly, lateral angulation in the region of the narrowed segment, particularly in patients with the extrinsic form of involvement (Figure 20-7). It is usually not possible, however, to differentiate intrinsic involvement from extrinsic disease on the basis of the radiographic appearance of the stricture. Because there is typically severe hydronephrosis and resulting impairment of contrast material excretion on urography and/or contrast-enhanced CT, the radiologic features of the stricture are usually best demonstrated by retrograde pyelography **(Option (C) is false).** Indeed, approximately one-half of patients have irreversible loss of renal function at the time of initial presentation. In patients with extrinsic endometriosis, sonography, MRI, and CT may be used to demonstrate both the size of the soft tissue mass that envelops the ureter and the extent of pelvic disease.

Question 107

Concerning primary ureteral neoplasms,

(A) about 75% are found in the proximal one-third of the ureter
(B) between 5 and 10% of patients with transitional cell carcinoma of the ureter have a concurrent or antecedent transitional cell tumor of the bladder
(C) between 5 and 10% of patients with a primary transitional cell tumor of the bladder will develop transitional cell carcinoma of the ureter
(D) they are twice as common in men as in women

Primary tumors of the ureter are rare, accounting for approximately 1% of all urinary tract tumors and only 6% of upper urinary tract tumors. They can be either epithelial (75%) or nonepithelial (mesodermal) (25%) in origin. They usually present in patients aged 50 to 80 years, with men being affected twice as often as women **(Option (D) is true).** Most non-epithelial tumors are benign. The most common of them is the fibro-epithelial polyp, which is also called a benign fibrous polyp.

The symptoms of a primary ureteral tumor are nonspecific, but they include flank pain, hematuria, frequency, and dysuria. There is no known pattern of familial inheritance.

Transitional cell carcinoma accounts for 75% of the cases of primary epithelial ureteral tumors, with squamous cell carcinoma (10%), adeno-carcinoma, and benign epithelial tumors accounting for the remainder. Transitional tumors are most commonly (75%) found in the distal one-third of the ureter **(Option (A) is false)** and have several known predisposing risk factors, including tobacco smoking, industrial chemical exposure, and phenacetin abuse, which in itself carries a 40-fold increase in risk. Balkan nephropathy is a disorder that develops in inhabitants of certain regions of some of the Balkan states (especially Bulgaria, Rumania, and Yugoslavia) and that is associated with a slowly progressive interstitial nephritis leading to renal failure and a high incidence of transitional cell carcinoma of the renal pelvis or ureter. The incidence of upper tract tumors in several reported series varies between 10 and 50%; in 10% of cases, the renal tumors are bilateral but tend to be of low biologic aggressiveness. More recently, an increased incidence of transitional cell tumors of the bladder has also been reported. The precise cause of the disorder is not known, but attention has been directed toward an environmental carcinogen, perhaps in the drinking water, as a more likely explanation than a genetic predisposition toward the illness. Other investigators have suggested an autoimmune mechanism or viral infection as being the most likely explanation for the disease.

Transitional cell carcinomas are divided into two histologic types, papillary and nonpapillary. Papillary lesions are more common and tend to be multicentric, whereas nonpapillary lesions tend to be solitary. An associated transitional cell carcinoma of the bladder is found in 25% of patients with transitional cell carcinoma of the ureter; however, as many as 70% of patients with transitional cell carcinoma of the ureter have a history of an antecedent transitional cell carcinoma of the bladder or a subsequent urothelial lesion elsewhere within the urinary tract (**Option (B) is false**). The majority of such metachronous lesions develop within an 18- to 24-month period. In contrast, only 5 to 10% of patients with primary transitional cell carcinoma of the bladder will develop a transitional cell carcinoma of the ureter (**Option (C) is true**). Transitional cell carcinomas develop in the bladder, renal pelvis, and ureter with a relative frequency of 50:3:1.

As many as 40% of the papillary and nearly all of the nonpapillary lesions have extended into the periureteral tissues at the time of presentation. Metastases to regional lymph nodes or hematogenous metastases to the liver, lungs, or bones may also occur. Because of the rich lymphatic drainage of the ureter, lymph node metastases tend to occur early in the course of the disease.

Approximately half of the patients with transitional cell carcinoma of the ureter present with a nonfunctioning kidney on urography because of long-standing ureteral obstruction. If sufficient excretion of contrast material is present, the lesion is demonstrated as a solitary filling defect in the ureter or a series of discrete polypoid masses within the lumen separated by what appears to be normal ureteral mucosa. Solitary lesions frequently demonstrate slight dilatation of the ureter distal to the lesion

(Bergman's sign), which is said to be due to the distal migration of the lesion as a result of ureteral peristalsis. This sign helps to differentiate the lesion from such benign solitary filling defects as blood clots and stones. On retrograde pyelography, transitional cell carcinomas produce a localized expansion of the ureter that resembles a wine "goblet." CT is useful in the characterization of such lesions because it demonstrates the soft tissue extent of the tumor and is also helpful in differentiating filling defects caused by radiolucent stones from those caused by transitional cell tumors.

Squamous cell carcinoma is the most malignant of the epithelial lesions of the ureter. These carcinomas constitute approximately 10% of malignant ureteral tumors and are generally associated with chronic urinary tract infections and the presence of calculi. Phenacetin abuse has also been associated with an increased incidence of squamous cell carcinoma. The lesion typically presents as a solitary filling defect within the ureter, and there is frequent periureteral invasion at the time of initial presentation. Adenocarcinoma of the ureter is extremely rare. The lesion is thought to arise from the cells of the nests of von Brunn, the basal layer of the urothelium.

Question 108

Which *one* of the following is MOST closely associated with suburothelial hemorrhage?

(A) Analgesic abuse
(B) Hemophilia
(C) Collagen vascular disease
(D) Trauma
(E) Anticoagulant therapy

Retroperitoneal hemorrhage involving the urinary tract is associated with a number of conditions, including renal trauma, analgesic abuse, renal neoplasms, blood dyscrasias, aortic aneurysms, and anticoagulant therapy. Such bleeding may be intrarenal, subcapsular, or perinephric when associated with the renal parenchyma or may be intramural when associated with the renal collecting system, ureter, or bladder. Intramural hemorrhage has been variously termed suburothelial, submucosal, subepithelial, and intramural bleeding and is typically associated clinically with the sudden onset of flank pain and hematuria. Among the

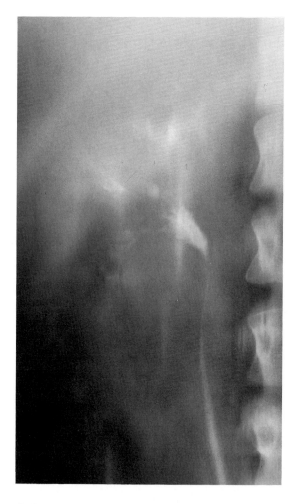

Figure 20-8. Suburothelial hemorrhage. Tomogram from an excretory urogram shows multiple irregular contour defects in the right renal pelvis, extrinsic compression of the major calyxes, and a medium-length area of narrowing of the proximal ureter secondary to submucosal hemorrhage in a patient receiving warfarin.

reported cases, suburothelial bleeding has most often been described in patients receiving anticoagulant therapy **(Option (E) is correct).**

On urography, multiple irregular linear filling defects and mucosal striations are found (Figure 20-8). Although the urographic findings in themselves are nonspecific (such findings may be present in urothelial tumors, ureteritis cystica, malacoplakia, and leukoplakia, among other conditions), they are virtually diagnostic of suburothelial hemorrhage when combined with a clinical history of anticoagulant therapy. On CT, a soft tissue density replaces the fat normally found in the renal sinus and compresses the calyces and renal pelvis. The attenuation of the soft tissue density has been found to vary between 10 and 40 Hounsfield units because it represents admixture of blood with the normally present retroperitoneal fat. A soft tissue density surrounding the proximal ureter, associated with compression of its lumen, may also be seen. In cases reported with follow-up, the findings resolved spontaneously within a few weeks.

Submucosal hemorrhage of the renal collecting system was originally reported by Antopol and Goldman in 1948. These authors reported seven patients, all of whom were treated by nephrectomy since it was believed that the lesion could not be reliably differentiated from tumor. In a more recent report, Levitt and co-workers described the histologic findings of suburothelial hemorrhage in a patient treated by partial nephrectomy. They reported that on light microscopy the hemorrhage was found in the lamina propria of the calyx. On electron microscopy, irregular wrinkling of the basement membranes of the glomerular capillaries was present. The authors suggested that a fragile pelvic capillary bed contributed to the bleeding in their patient, who had been taking analgesics but was not on anticoagulant therapy.

Carl M. Sandler, M.D.

SUGGESTED READINGS

GENERAL

1. Dunnick NR, McCallum RW, Sandler CM. Textbook of uroradiology. Baltimore: Williams & Wilkins; 1991:287–318
2. Williamson B Jr, Hartman GW, Hattery RR. Multiple and diffuse ureteral filling defects. Semin Roentgenol 1986; 21:214–233

URETERAL TUMORS

3. Ambos MA, Bosniak MA, Megibow AJ, Raghavendra B. Ureteral involvement by metastatic disease. Urol Radiol 1979; 1:105–112
4. Kenney PJ, Stanley RJ. Computed tomography of ureteral tumors. J Comput Assist Tomogr 1987; 11:102–107
5. Pollack HM. Long-term follow-up of the upper urinary tract for transitional cell carcinoma: how much is enough? Radiology 1988; 167:871–872

6. Ritchie JP, Ehrlich RM. Ureteral obstruction secondary to metastatic tumors. Surg Gynecol Obstet 1979; 148:355–357

7. Stefanovic V, Polenakovic MH. Balkan nephropathy: kidney disease beyond the Balkans? Am J Nephrol 1991; 11:1–11

8. Winalski CS, Lipman JC, Tumeh SS. Ureteral neoplasms. RadioGraphics 1990; 10:271–283

9. Yousem DM, Gatewood OM, Goldman SM, Marshall FF. Synchronous and metachronous transitional cell carcinoma of the urinary tract: prevalence, incidence, and radiographic detection. Radiology 1988; 167:613–618

ENDOMETRIOSIS

10. Ball TL, Platt MA. Urologic complications of endometriosis. Am J Obstet Gynecol 1962; 84:1516–1521

11. Dallemand S, Kutcher R, McPherson H, Schneider M, Farman J. Endometriosis with ureteric involvement: preoperative sonographic evaluation. NY State J Med 1979; 79:382–383

12. Jepsen JM, Hansen KB. Danazol in the treatment of ureteral endometriosis. J Urol 1988; 139:1045–1046

13. Lucero SP, Wise HA, Kirsh G, et al. Ureteric obstruction secondary to endometriosis. Report of three cases with a review of the literature. Br J Urol 1988; 61:201–204

14. Mourin-Jouret A, Squifflet JP, Cosyns JP, Pirson Y, Alexandre GP. Bilateral ureteral endometriosis with end-stage renal failure. Urology 1987; 29:302–306

15. Plous RH, Sunshine R, Goldman H, Schwartz IS. Ureteral endometriosis in post-menopausal women. Urology 1985; 26:408–411

16. Pollack HM, Wills JS. Radiographic features of ureteral endometriosis. AJR 1978; 131:627–631

SUBUROTHELIAL HEMORRHAGE

17. Antopol W, Goldman L. Subepithelial hemorrhage of renal pelvis simulating neoplasm. Urol Cutan Rev 1948; 52:189–195

18. Eisenberg RL, Clark RE. Filling defects in the renal pelvis and ureter owing to bleeding secondary to acquired circulating anticoagulants. J Urol 1976; 116:662–663

19. Kaiser JA, Jacobs RP, Korobkin M. Submucosal hemorrhage of the renal collecting system. AJR 1975; 125:311–313

20. Levitt S, Waisman J, deKernion J. Subepithelial hematoma of the renal pelvis (Antopol-Goldman lesion): a case report and review of the literature. J Urol 1984; 131:939–941

21. Miller V, Witten DM, Shin SM. Computed tomographic findings in suburothelial hemorrhage. Urol Radiol 1982; 4:11–14

22. Pollack HM, Popky GL. Roentgenographic manifestations of spontaneous renal hemorrhage. Radiology 1974; 110:1–6

23. Smith WL, Weinstein AS, Wiot JF. Defects of the renal collecting systems in patients receiving anticoagulants. Radiology 1974; 113:649–651

VASCULAR IMPRESSIONS ON THE URETER

24. Chait A, Matasar KW, Fabian CE, Mellins HZ. Vascular impressions on the ureters. AJR 1971; 111:729–749
25. Cleveland RH, Fellows KE, Lebowitz RL. Notching of the ureter and renal pelvis in children. AJR 1977; 129:837–844
26. Love L, Bush IM. Early demonstration of renal collateral arterial supply. AJR 1968; 104:296–301

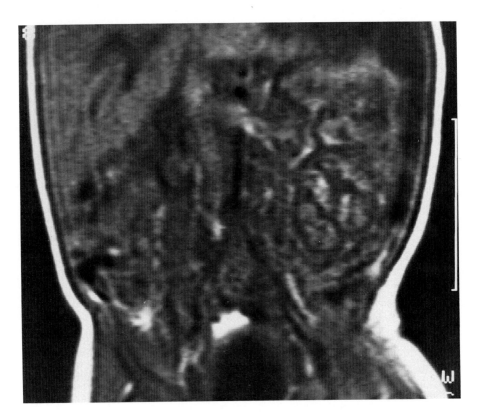

SE 500/17

Figure 21-1. You are shown a coronal MR image of the abdomen of a 2-week-old boy who became symptomatic at home following an uncomplicated birth. Additional history withheld.

Case 21: Renal Vein Thrombosis

Question 109

Which *one* of the following is the MOST likely diagnosis?

(A) Hydronephrosis
(B) Renal vein thrombosis
(C) Mesoblastic nephroma
(D) Renal infarction
(E) Multicystic dysplastic kidney

On the coronal MR image (Figure 21-1), the enlarged left kidney extends below the abdominal aortic bifurcation and displaces the descending colon laterally. There is no evidence of hydronephrosis or of any cystic structures within the kidney. The normal flow of the abdominal aorta is shown as signal void. The high signal within the left renal vein and portions of the inferior vena cava indicates thrombus or slow flow (see Figure 21-2). The evaluation of renal veins by MRI is best accomplished by coronal imaging. Renal veins have variable degrees of craniocaudal angulation, and several axial images would be required for complete visualization. Coronal images often demonstrate the renal vein in a single slice. Normal renal vessels are characterized on MRI by a lack of intraluminal signal. Renal vein thrombosis (RVT) and slow flow will show increased signal within the vessel on spin-echo imaging, as is the case in the test image **(Option (B) is correct).** On gradient-recalled-echo images, flowing blood will show high signal intensity in the plane perpendicular to flow, whereas thrombus will be intermediate in signal intensity.

Hydronephrosis (Option (A)), as demonstrated by MRI, is recognized by the low signal intensity of the dilated collecting system on T1-weighted images. There is no evidence of an enlarged collecting system in Figure 21-1; therefore, this is an unlikely diagnosis. In chronic obstruction, the cortical thickness is decreased and the corticomedullary differentiation is obscured secondary to edema.

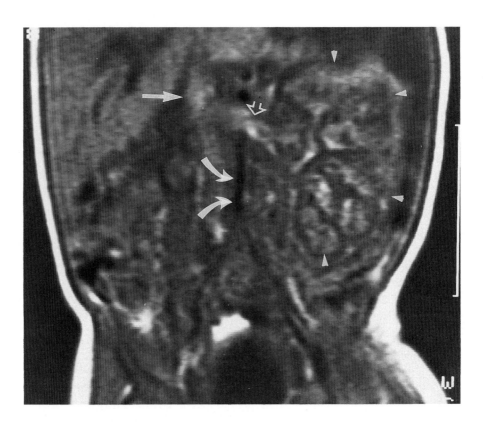

SE 500/17

Figure 21-2 (Same as Figure 21-1). Renal vein thrombosis. Coronal MR image shows enlarged left kidney (arrowheads). There is high signal intensity within the left renal vein (open arrow) and inferior vena cava (straight arrow). Aorta = curved arrows.

Mesoblastic nephroma (Option (C)) is the most common renal tumor of the neonate. It is characteristically a solid tumor that presents in the first few months of life. The typical mesoblastic nephroma is a large mass that distorts and displaces the normal renal architecture. CT and MRI show a relatively homogeneous intrarenal mass, although there may be areas of central necrosis. Figure 21-1 demonstrates an enlarged kidney, but one that is structurally intact and without cystic structures; therefore, mesoblastic nephroma is an unlikely diagnosis.

Renal infarction (Option (D)) is secondary to occlusion of the renal arterial or venous bed. Arterial thrombosis is much rarer than RVT, although many of the predisposing factors are similar. In children, arterial emboli originate from the closing ductus arteriosus or are associated with umbilical arterial catheters. Hypertension is an associated clinical finding with arterial occlusion. Arterial emboli may lodge in segmental renal arteries, resulting in focal renal changes rather than the diffuse enlargement seen in the test images. Occlusion of the main renal artery by propagation of thrombus from an umbilical arterial catheter may result in diffuse renal infarction. During the early congestive phase, renal infarction will be associated with diffuse renal enlargement similar to that in the test case. However, the infant in the test case had an uncomplicated birth and never required an umbilical arterial catheter.

Multicystic dysplastic kidney (Option (E)) is the most common renal mass in the first week of life. It is usually unilateral, and the patient has normal renal function because the contralateral kidney is functioning normally. The etiology is unknown, but it is thought most likely to represent end-stage fetal hydronephrosis. While MRI is not used for evaluating multicystic dysplastic kidneys, the expected appearance would be a group of rounded masses with cyst characteristics, i.e., long T1 and T2 relaxation times. The multicystic dysplastic kidney is characterized by multiple cysts of various sizes replacing the renal parenchyma (Figure 21-3). These cysts do not communicate with a central pelvis. The involved kidney is often enlarged and irregular. Figure 21-1 does not demonstrate multiple renal cysts, and so this is not an appropriate diagnosis.

RVT in childhood almost always occurs before the age of 2 years. One-third of the cases occur in the first week of life, and another one-third occur later in the first month. Decreased blood volume and increased blood viscosity and coagulability predispose the infant to RVT. These predisposing factors are seen in infants with hypotension, trauma, sepsis, sickle cell disease, asphyxia, or dehydration. The child may have a nonspecific clinical presentation of irritability and fever. The most helpful signs and symptoms are hematuria, an enlarged kidney on one or both sides, and thrombocytopenia.

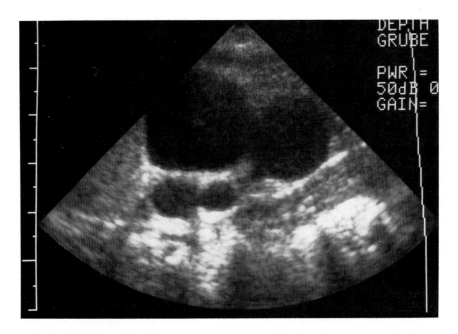

Figure 21-3. Multicystic dysplastic kidney. This longitudinal sonogram demonstrates multiple noncommunicating cysts of various sizes replacing the expected kidney.

Question 110

Concerning hydronephrosis,

(A) pelvic pressure measurements are normal after several weeks
(B) the glomerular filtration rate declines as a result of preglomerular vasoconstriction
(C) there is reduced renal blood flow in long-standing obstruction
(D) dilated ducts of Bellini are seen with chronic obstruction
(E) diuresis renography effectively separates obstruction from nonobstructive dilatation
(F) highly compliant upper tracts yield false-negative Whitaker test results

Acute ureteral obstruction can initially elevate renal pelvic pressure measurements to as high as 70 mm Hg. Ureteral peristalsis is also hyperactive following acute obstruction. The increased renal pelvic pressure gradually returns to normal over several weeks as the collecting system adapts through rupture of the fornices, dilatation of the collecting system, or pyelotubular back flow **(Option (A) is true).**

Ureteral peristalsis diminishes as the ureter fatigues and becomes dilated. The ureter then remains hypoactive until the obstruction is relieved.

Angiotensin II, thromboxane A_2, norepinephrine, and other vasoconstrictors are released because of lowered oxygen tension and are thought to be responsible for preglomerular vasoconstriction in association with obstruction. Immediately following obstruction there is increased glomerular back-pressure, resulting in a fall in the glomerular filtration rate **(Option (B) is true).** The renal blood flow increases transiently; however, it decreases after several hours. At 4 days it has dropped to levels as low as one-half of the original level, and at 4 weeks it is at 20% of the original level **(Option (C) is true).**

Ducts of Bellini are the major collecting ducts that empty directly into the renal calyces; 16 to 20 ducts of Bellini empty into each calyx at the apex of the papilla. The normal internal diameter of a duct of Bellini is 0.1 to 0.2 mm. With obstruction and hydronephrosis the calyces and collecting tubules dilate **(Option (D) is true).** Eventually, compression of the papilla by calyceal distension causes reorientation of the collecting ducts to planes parallel to the calyceal surface. Opacified distended ducts of Bellini may be seen on intravenous urograms in some cases of hydronephrosis (Figure 21-4). This gives the radiographic appearance of radiopaque linear streaks or dots immediately outside the dilated calyces.

Scintigraphic studies are used to evaluate renal perfusion, function, and, less often, morphology. Renograms are initiated with the bolus injection of the radiopharmaceutical. Images are obtained at frequent intervals through 25 to 30 minutes. Time-activity curves are constructed by flagging the renal area of interest. Normal maximum renal parenchymal activity occurs by 5 minutes. Activity progressively decreases, with one-half of normal renal activity gone by 10 minutes.

Obstructive uropathy is characterized by progressively rising time-activity curves. Diuresis or furosemide renography is utilized to assist in the differentiation of obstructive uropathy from dilated but nonobstructed renal collecting systems. Furosemide is injected intravenously 15 to 20 minutes after the injection of radiopharmaceutical. The time-activity curve following furosemide administration will demonstrate a rapid decrease with a clearance half-time of less than 10 minutes if the retained activity is contained within a dilated nonobstructed system. Mechanical obstruction will result in persistently elevated activity following furosemide administration (Figure 21-5). Published reports indicate that diuretic renography is a sensitive and reasonably specific

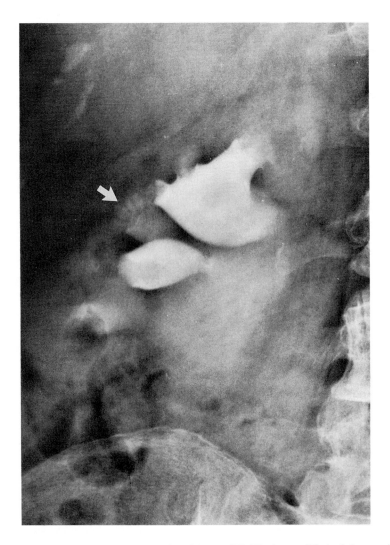

Figure 21-4. Hydronephrosis. The ducts of Bellini are dilated (arrow) in this patient with hydronephrosis due to a distal ureteral stricture. (Courtesy of Dr. Harold A. Mitty, Mount Sinai Hospital, New York.)

means to distinguish obstruction from nonobstructive dilatation (**Option (E) is true**).

Symptomatic patients who have equivocal results on a diuresis renogram need the more invasive Whitaker testing for further evaluation. While neither test is considered the "gold standard" for significant obstruction, they are complementary. When the two tests agree on the

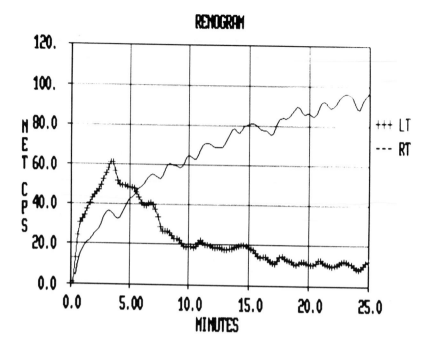

Figure 21-5. Diuresis renogram curves. There is progessively increasing activity in the right kidney, which fails to wash out after intravenous injection of furosemide at 10 minutes, a result consistent with mechanical obstruction. This same appearance may occur when there is impaired parenchymal function or if there is a grossly dilated but nonobstructed collecting system. The left kidney displays normal response of a nonobstructed collecting system.

presence or absence of obstruction, they are considered correct. Conflicting results occur, and multiple factors may be responsible for the discrepancy. Nonobstructed kidneys correctly identified by the Whitaker test but incorrectly identified as being obstructed by diuresis renography may have grossly dilated collecting systems, poor renal function, or both to explain the false-positive renogram results.

The Whitaker test is a pressure-flow study requiring placement of a nephrostomy tube in the renal pelvis and a catheter in the urinary bladder. It has been used to differentiate obstructive dilatation of the upper renal collecting systems from nonobstructive dilatation. The study is performed with the bladder empty. Following baseline pressure measurements of the renal pelvis and urinary bladder with a manometer, a saline infusion of 10 mL/minute into the renal pelvis for 1 minute is performed. The pressures are recorded for the renal pelvis and bladder to obtain a pressure gradient. In nonobstructed patients, the pressure is less than 15 cm of water. Pressures above 20 cm of water are clearly abnormal. The indeterminate zone from 15 to 20 cm of water can be clarified by continuing the infusion for 3 to 5 minutes before increasing the infusion rate incrementally to 15 mL/minute. This method of increasing the infusion rate is considered sufficient to demonstrate a pressure differential between the renal pelvis and bladder in significant ureteral obstruction. If the renal pelvis is highly compliant, a false-negative result is likely. For example, a large extrarenal pelvis may obscure pressure gradients that would be identified in smaller intrarenal and less-compliant systems **(Option (F) is true).**

Question 111

Concerning imaging of renal vein thrombosis,

(A) the characteristic finding on duplex Doppler sonography is reversed arterial diastolic flow
(B) early sonographic changes include decreased renal echogenicity
(C) a high intraluminal vascular signal on spin-echo MR images is specific for thrombosis
(D) narrow-flip-angle MR images are of little value in identifying thrombosis
(E) the intensity of contrast enhancement on CT depends on the adequacy of collateral flow

Duplex Doppler sonography has been demonstrated in multiple studies to have characteristic findings for RVT. When renal impedance exceeds diastolic pressure, blood flow is nonpropulsive and flow becomes retrograde within the arterial vasculature. This mechanism results in a dampened or reversed arterial diastolic flow (Figure 21-6) **(Option (A) is true).** While a reversed arterial diastolic wave form is a characteristic of RVT, varying degrees of a dampened wave form may be found. RVT causes increased arterial vascular resistance by transmitted back-pressure. Increased arterial vascular resistance is also seen with diffuse obliteration or compression of the renal capillary bed. Diffuse parenchymal disease such as acute tubular necrosis, transplant rejection, pyelonephritis, and extrarenal compression may also demonstrate similar duplex Doppler sonographic findings.

Ultrasonographic findings of acute RVT are an enlarged kidney and hypoechogenicity resulting from congestion **(Option (B) is true).** By 2 weeks the kidney has undergone cellular infiltration and is becoming

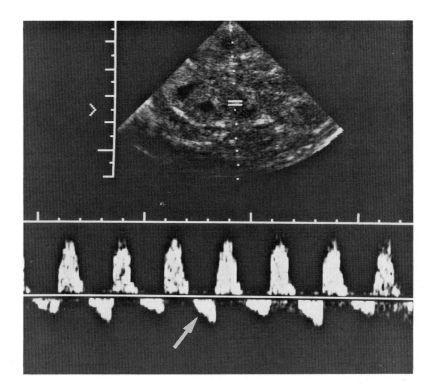

Figure 21-6. Renal vein thrombosis. Duplex Doppler sonogram of interlobar artery shows reversed diastolic flow (arrow) characteristic of RVT.

hyperechogenic. Progressive fibrosis of both the cortex and medulla
causes loss of corticomedullary differentiation.

On contrast-enhanced CT, RVT is characteristically identified as a
filling defect in the contrast-filled vein (Figure 21-7). When using rapid
bolus injections, it is necessary to obtain views of the vein after the first
transit of the contrast agent in order to avoid misinterpreting flow defects
(due to mixing of unopacified and opacified blood) as thromboses. Prior
to the contrast agent injection, the kidney will appear diffusely enlarged
with increased attenuation probably related to hemorrhagic congestion
(Figure 21-8A). Following intravenous injection of contrast agent, there
may be cortical and peripheral enhancement secondary to collateral blood
flow to the kidney (Figure 21-8B).

RVT acutely impedes blood flow through the renal venous system.
This in turn causes increased vascular back-pressure, which decreases
renal perfusion. Venous collaterals may quickly develop with renal vein
occlusion, providing improved renal perfusion. On CT, decreased renal

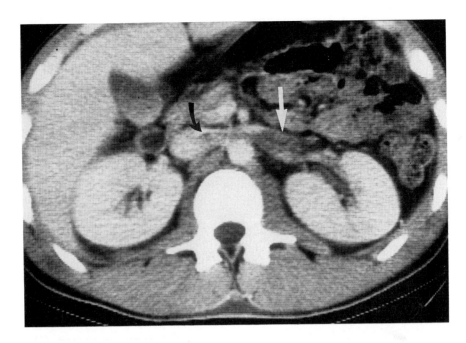

Figure 21-7. Renal vein thrombosis. Contrast-enhanced CT scan demonstrates low-attenuation filling defect in the left renal vein (straight arrow) and extending into the inferior vena cava (curved arrow).

blood flow results in diminished parenchymal enhancement and a prolonged corticomedullary-junction time (i.e., the delay before the cortex and medulla are isointense). Contrast enhancement is proportional to perfusion, which is improved by the development of extensive collateral venous drainage **(Option (E) is true).**

MRI may be used to demonstrate thromboses. Intraluminal vascular signal often signifies thrombus, but care must be taken to recognize flow artifacts that simulate disease **(Option (C) is false).** In veins, a saturation effect from slow flow may produce intraluminal signal. In addition, phase shift and flow displacement may alter the appearance of flowing blood. Presaturation of incoming blood and gradient-echo sequences help differentiate thrombus from artifact. The area of concern should be imaged with both gradient-echo and spin-echo sequences for correlation of suspected intravascular flow defects.

Narrow-flip-angle MRI utilizes a single radiofrequency pulse to produce the MR signal. The flip angle is less than 90°. As the TR is shortened, smaller flip angles provide the best signal-to-noise ratio. The narrow-flip-angle technique is known as gradient-echo imaging. These techniques

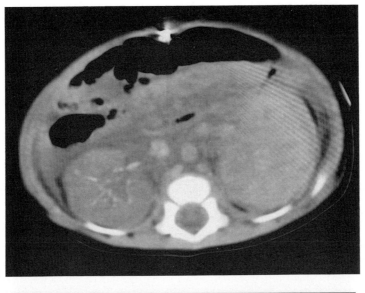

A

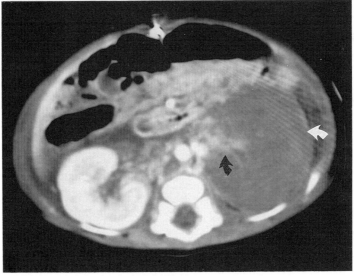

B

Figure 21-8. Renal vein thrombosis. (A) Unenhanced CT scan shows enlarged left kidney with blotchy high-attenuation areas due to hemorrhagic congestion. Note the regular linear high attenuation of the right pericalyceal and perihilar regions, thought to represent stasis of blood in dilated interlobar and segmental veins, since there is a thrombus extending into the inferior vena cava from the left renal vein. (B) Contrast-enhanced CT scan demonstrates subcapsular enhancement of the enlarged left kidney (white arrow) from collateral arterial flow, since the increased intrarenal pressure prevents normal renal arterial perfusion. Note the peripelvic linear enhancement (black arrow), possibly occurring because the urothelial microcirculation is not altered to the same extent as the parenchymal circulation.

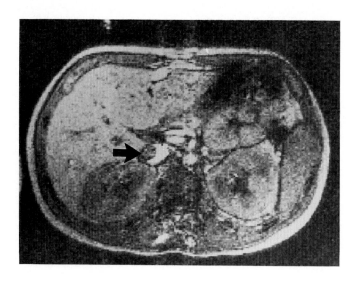

Figure 21-9. Thrombosis of inferior vena cava. This gradient-recalled-echo transverse image of the abdomen shows high signal of normally flowing unsaturated blood. The thrombus (arrow) attached to the right lateral wall is shown as a zone of intermediate signal intensity.

present moving blood as a bright signal and allow rapid imaging that is useful in MR angiography. Signal differentiation from intraluminal thrombus is improved **(Option (D) is false)** (Figure 21-9).

Peggy J. Fritzsche, M.D.
Mark McKinney, M.D.

SUGGESTED READINGS

RENAL VEIN THROMBOSIS

1. Kaveggia LP, Perrella RR, Grant EG, et al. Duplex doppler sonography in renal allografts: the significance of reversed flow in diastole. AJR 1990; 155:295–298
2. Lalmand B, Avni EF, Nasr A, Ketelbant P, Struyven J. Perinatal renal vein thrombosis: sonographic demonstration. J Ultrasound Med 1990; 9:437–442
3. Mellins HZ. Renal vein obstruction. In: Pollack HM (ed), Clinical urography. Philadelphia: WB Saunders; 1990:2119–2126
4. Parvey HR, Eisenberg RL. Image-directed Doppler sonography of the intrarenal arteries in acute renal vein thrombosis. JCU 1990; 18:512–516

5. Reuther G, Wanjura D, Bauer H. Acute renal vein thrombosis in renal allografts: detection with duplex Doppler US. Radiology 1989; 170:557–558
6. Warshauer DM, Taylor KJ, Bia MJ, et al. Unusual causes of increased vascular impedance in renal transplants: duplex Doppler evaluation. Radiology 1988; 169:367–370

HYDRONEPHROSIS

7. Griscom NT, Kroeker MA. Visualization of individual papillary ducts (ducts of Bellini) by excretory urography in childhood hydronephrosis. Radiology 1973; 106:385–389
8. Kountz PD, Siegel MJ, Shapiro E. Flank mass in a newborn. Urol Radiol 1989; 11:61–64
9. Poulsen EU, Frokjaer J, Taagehoj-Jensen F, et al. Diuresis renography and simultaneous renal pelvic pressure in hydronephrosis. J Urol 1987; 138:272–275
10. Sherwood T. Percutaneous pyeloureterodynamics (Whitaker test). In: Pollack HM (ed), Clinical urography. Philadelphia: WB Saunders; 1990:2715–2724

MR FLOW CHARACTERISTICS

11. Bradley WG Jr. Flow phenomena. In: Stark D, Bradley WG Jr (eds), Flow phenomena. In: Magnetic resonance imaging, 2nd ed. St. Louis: CV Mosby; 1992:253–298.
12. Edelman RR, Rubin JB, Buxton RB. Flow. In: Edelman RR, Hessellink JR (eds), Clinical magnetic resonance imaging. Philadelphia: WB Saunders; 1990:109–182

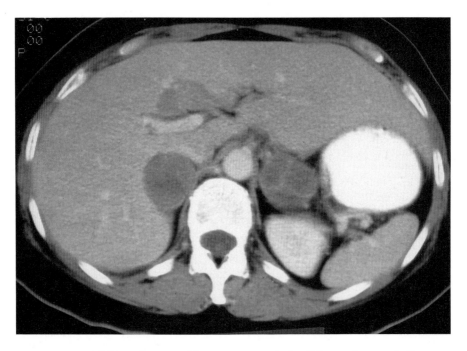

Figure 22-1. This 52-year-old man presented with weakness, lethargy, hypotension, and hyponatremia. You are shown an enhanced abdominal CT scan at the level of the adrenal glands.

Case 22: Addison's Disease

Question 112

Which *one* of the following is the LEAST likely diagnosis?

(A) Tuberculosis
(B) Adrenal hemorrhage
T (C) Autoimmune adrenal insufficiency
(D) Adrenal metastases
(E) Histoplasmosis

This enhanced abdominal CT scan (Figure 22-1) reveals bilateral adrenal masses, as well as a solitary lesion in the liver. The differential diagnosis includes metastases, granulomatous disease such as tuberculosis and histoplasmosis, and hemorrhage. Patients with autoimmune adrenal insufficiency have small atrophic glands rather than adrenal masses, and so this is an unlikely diagnosis **(Option (C) is correct).**

The clinical presentation of the test patient suggests adrenal insufficiency (Addison's disease). Additional symptoms and signs that are commonly seen in this syndrome include anorexia, nausea, vomiting, weight loss, and hyperpigmentation, which is most marked in exposed portions of the body, pressure points, and creases of the palms. The diagnosis can be confirmed by measuring the steroid secretory response, usually manifested by a rise in cortisol levels in plasma in response to a standard dose of adrenocorticotropic hormone (ACTH). Similarly, levels of 17-hydroxycorticoids in the urine are low and fail to respond to ACTH infusion. Treatment with a glucocorticoid and a mineralocorticoid results in a normal life expectancy.

Adrenal insufficiency may be caused by any process that affects the adrenal glands. However, at least 90% of functioning adrenal tissue must be destroyed before adrenal insufficiency results.

The most common cause of adrenal insufficiency in individuals in underdeveloped countries is tuberculosis (Option (A)). Acute involvement of the adrenal glands results in soft tissue masses, and low-density areas representing tissue necrosis are common. Calcification is seen in patients with chronic tuberculosis.

Adrenal insufficiency may also be caused by the soil fungus *Histoplasma capsulatum*. Histoplasmosis (Option (E)) is endemic in the Ohio and Central Mississippi River valleys, as well as in the southeastern portions of the United States, where it may infect up to 90% of the population. The usual mode of infection is by inhalation of airborne spores. Disseminated infection may be by direct extension of the pulmonary infection or by a recrudescence.

The CT manifestions of histoplasmosis are similar to those of other granulomatous diseases, such as tuberculosis. A soft tissue mass may be seen in the acute stage, whereas calcification is the hallmark of chronic infection.

The adrenal glands are a common site of metastatic disease (Option (D)); 27% of patients dying of cancer have adrenal metastases. Although adrenal metastases are common, adrenal insufficiency as a result of metastases is uncommon. Most patients, even those with bilateral adrenal metastases, do not exhibit signs or symptoms of adrenal insufficiency. The tumors most likely to cause Addison's disease are carcinoma of the lung and carcinoma of the breast. It has also been recorded as a result of other primary tumors, including primary adrenal cortical carcinoma and malignant lymphoma.

The radiographic appearance of adrenal metastases in patients with Addison's disease is the same as that in patients whose adrenal function is preserved. Bilateral involvement is essential, and most of the functioning tissue must be destroyed.

The most common cause of Addison's disease in the United States is an autoimmune disease. Adrenal antibodies are often detected in patients with autoimmune adrenal insufficiency, and their presence further supports the diagnosis. The CT appearance of autoimmune adrenal insufficiency includes small adrenal glands bilaterally. There are no soft tissue masses, and calcification is not a feature of the disease.

Adrenal hemorrhage (Option (B)) may also result in Addison's disease. Bilateral adrenal hemorrhage in the adult may occur in association with a variety of processes, including hypotension, surgery, sepsis, burns, and anticoagulation. The characteristic soft tissue masses with increased density on unenhanced scans are typically seen in the acute phase. As the acute hematoma liquefies, the density of the soft tissue masses decreases. Follow-up CT examinations often demonstrate resorption of these hematomas, as well as calcification within the gland.

The test patient had a history of pulmonary tuberculosis. Percutaneous adrenal biopsy was performed and revealed granulomas consistent with adrenal tuberculosis.

Question 113

Concerning adrenal tuberculosis,

F (A) it is the most common cause of Addison's disease
F (B) it is often due to direct spread from the kidneys
T (C) it is usually bilateral
F (D) its appearance on CT is similar to that of an adrenal adenoma
T (E) proving the tuberculous etiology of Addison's disease is often difficult

Adrenal insufficiency was first described by Addison in 1853. Six of the nine cases reported were due to tuberculous involvement of the adrenal glands. Tuberculosis remained the most common etiology until the antibiotic era. Between 1930 and 1950, tuberculosis accounted for approximately 75% of patients with Addison's disease, but by 1988 it had decreased to less than 33%. In a report from New Zealand in 1982 by Eason et al., tuberculosis was responsible for only 4% of cases of Addison's disease in Caucasians seen between 1971 and 1980 **(Option (A) is false)**.

Tuberculosis involves the adrenal glands as a secondary infection. The initial pulmonary infection occurs by inhalation of the organism. Spread to the adrenal glands is hematogenous, so patients often have involvement of other organs as well.

The kidneys are involved by tuberculosis via the same hematogenous dissemination. From the kidneys, tuberculous organisms may spread down the ureters to involve the lower genitourinary tract. A tuberculous cavity in the kidney may rupture and so involve the perinephric space and adrenal gland, but this is rare **(Option (B) is false)**.

Acute involvement of the adrenal glands results in masses of soft tissue density (Figure 22-2). Low-density areas represent tissue necrosis. Treatment at this stage may result in recovery of adrenal function. Most functioning adrenal tissue must be destroyed to produce adrenal insufficiency, and therefore involvement must be bilateral.

Adrenal glands involved with tuberculosis often maintain an adrenal configuration. Chronic tuberculous involvement of the adrenal glands is usually bilateral, and there is often dense calcification **(Option (C) is true)**. The glands are small, and no functional remnant of adrenal tissue

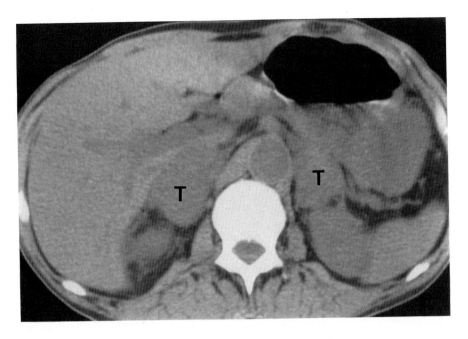

Figure 22-2. Adrenal tuberculosis. Bilateral adrenal masses (T) are seen in this unenhanced abdominal CT examination. Subsequent adrenal biopsy demonstrated noncaseating granulomas typical of tuberculosis.

is appreciated by CT. Adrenal calcification is seen in approximately 50% of patients with Addison's disease secondary to tuberculosis. However, adrenal calcification is usually idiopathic. If the adrenal glands maintain a triangular configuration, calcification seldom has clinical significance.

On CT, a benign adrenal adenoma is seen as a rounded mass, which distorts the normal adrenal contour. If the adenoma is large, it may completely replace the normal gland. Calcification is seldom seen in an adrenal adenoma unless there has been hemorrhage. Therefore, the CT appearance is not similar to that of tuberculosis **(Option (D) is false).**

The tuberculous etiology is often not apparent when the diagnosis of Addison's disease is made. The characteristic lesions of pulmonary tuberculosis may not be present on the chest radiograph, and cultures are often negative. Skin testing is frequently unrewarding in patients with adrenal failure. The CT appearance of adrenal involvement by tuberculosis is nonspecific, and the diagnosis may not be made until the adrenal gland is biopsied **(Option (E) is true).**

Question 114

Concerning adrenal hemorrhage,

T (A) it is commonly seen in newborn infants
T (B) it is unlikely to occur after trauma unless there are associated rib or spine fractures
F (C) in blunt trauma the left adrenal gland is affected more often than the right
T (D) in the absence of trauma, systemic anticoagulation is a common cause
T (E) a recent hematoma is recognized on CT as a soft tissue mass of increased density

Hemorrhage is the most common cause of an adrenal mass in infancy **(Option (A) is true).** The etiology is unknown in most cases but may be associated with a traumatic delivery, neonatal bradycardia, or asphyxia. It is more common in infants of diabetic mothers.

In most infants, adrenal hemorrhage is unilateral and Addison's disease does not develop. The most common manifestation is jaundice, which results from a breakdown of hemoglobin. If bleeding is massive, hypotension and shock can occur.

Adrenal injury is an uncommon finding after trauma, occurring in approximately 2% of patients. In severely injured patients, however, the adrenal glands are involved in as many as 25% of patients. However, the adrenal glands are unlikely to be affected unless there are associated injuries to the overlying ribs or spine **(Option (B) is true).**

In blunt trauma a hematoma of the right adrenal gland is more common than that of the left **(Option (C) is false)** (Figure 22-3A). There are two possible explanations for this. In some cases, the right adrenal gland may be crushed between the liver and the spine. This is not likely to occur on the left because the adrenal gland is near the body and tail of the pancreas, a much less rigid organ.

Another explanation involves the differences in venous drainage. The right adrenal vein is short and enters directly into the inferior vena cava (IVC). The left adrenal vein joins the left inferior phrenic vein, which enters the left renal vein before draining into the IVC. In blunt abdominal trauma, an acute rise in pressure in the IVC is more easily propagated into the right than the left adrenal vein; this may result in rupture of the small venules and hence a hematoma.

In the adult, adrenal hemorrhage may be associated with shock, burns, septicemia, severe stress, or an abnormal clotting mechanism, such as thrombocytopenia or anticoagulant therapy. Almost 33% of patients reported with nontraumatic bilateral adrenal hemorrhage have been

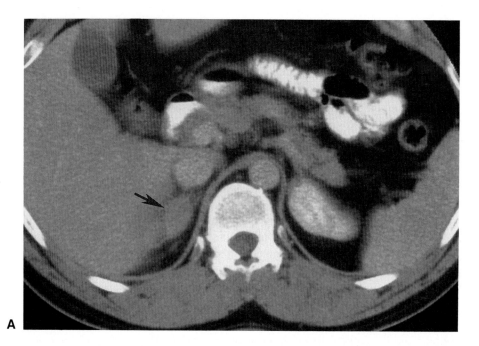

A

Figure 22-3. Hematoma of the right adrenal gland. This 42-year-old man was injured in a motor vehicle accident. (A) An enhanced abdominal CT scan reveals a right adrenal hematoma (arrow). (B) Two months later the hematoma (arrow) has been almost completely resorbed.

maintained on anticoagulant therapy **(Option (D) is true)**. Among patients being treated with anticoagulation therapy, an adrenal hematoma is usually found during the first 3 weeks of therapy. It does not seem to be due, however, to excessive anticoagulation because hematomas are not seen in other common sites, such as the rectus abdominus or psoas muscles, or in the remainder of the retroperitoneum.

In most patients an adrenal hematoma can be easily detected by CT. A rounded soft tissue mass is present and is often large enough to distort the normal contour of the gland. If the hemorrhage is recent, an increased density is present, indicating a hematoma as the etiology **(Option (E) is true)**.

With time, the density of the hematoma decreases. If the clot liquefies into a seroma, a density lower than that of soft tissue may be present. In these cases the diagnosis of adrenal hemorrhage can be supported by a normal adrenal CT scan prior to the hemorrhage or by a decrease in the size of the adrenal mass on subsequent CT examinations, as the

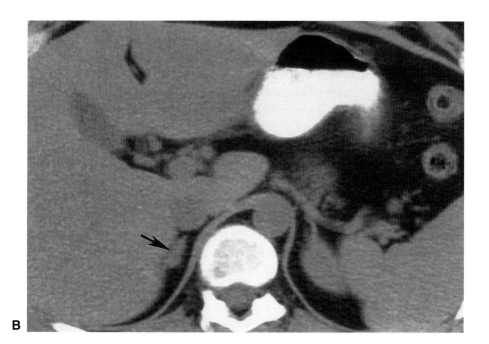

B

hematoma is resorbed (Figure 22-3B). Calcification often occurs in the later stages of adrenal hemorrhage.

Adrenal hemorrhage can also be diagnosed by MRI. With an acute hemorrhage, an adrenal mass with a high signal intensity, presumably due to the paramagnetic effects of methemoglobin, is found on both T1- and T2-weighted sequences.

Question 115

Concerning autoimmune adrenal insufficiency,

(A) it is more common among women than men
(B) patients present at an older age than those with tuberculous destruction of the adrenal glands
(C) the adrenal glands appear diffusely and symmetrically enlarged
(D) it is commonly associated with other endocrine or autoimmune diseases

Although tuberculosis was the most common cause of Addison's disease in the preantibiotic era, autoimmune disease is now a more common etiology. Eason et al. reported 48 patients for whom a cause of Addison's disease was found; 34 cases (71%) were due to an autoimmune disease, and 14 (29%) were due to tuberculosis. Among those with an autoimmune disorder, female patients outnumbered male patients 19 to 15. Of the 24 patients with idiopathic Addison's disease reported by De Rosa et al., 66% were female **(Option (A) is true).** Among patients with a tuberculous etiology for Addison's disease, the opposite is true. Only 11% of the patients with tuberculosis in the series of De Rosa et al. were women.

The clinical presentation of idiopathic Addison's disease is not significantly different from that for other etiologies. Most patients complain of weakness, anorexia, and easy fatigability. Hyperpigmentation was found in 96% of patients reported by De Rosa et al. Similarly, 96% of the patients in this series had an electrolyte imbalance. Most patients were found to have low aldosterone levels in serum and urine and a concomitant elevation of ACTH. Renin levels in plasma were more commonly elevated among patients with autoimmune disease than among those with tuberculosis. Patients with an autoimmune etiology presented at a slightly younger age than those with tuberculous destruction of the adrenal gland. However, this difference was not statistically significant **(Option (B) is false).**

The adrenal glands can be identified by CT in virtually every patient, and so this is a particularly useful examination in patients with Addison's disease. When adrenal tissue is destroyed by tuberculosis, metastases, or hemorrhage, bilateral adrenal masses are detected. However, in patients with an autoimmune disorder, both adrenal glands are small **(Option (C) is false)** (Figure 22-4). The glands are atrophic, maintain a normal adrenal configuration, and do not contain focal masses.

As many as 25% of patients with idiopathic Addison's disease have other endocrine or autoimmune disease as well **(Option (D) is true).** Two distinct syndromes are now recognized, and both have a female preponderance. Polyglandular autoimmune (PGA) syndrome type I presents during childhood. The disorder is probably inherited as an autosomal recessive trait, and it is not associated with a specific human leukocyte antigen (HLA). In addition to Addison's disease, most patients have hypoparathyroidism and chronic mucocutaneous candidiasis. Other features include chronic active hepatitis, malabsorption, pernicious anemia, alopecia, gonadal failure, and thyroid disease. PGA syndrome type II (Schmidt's syndrome) is the more common disorder and usually does not present until adulthood. Most patients also suffer from autoimmune thyroid disease (either hyperthyroidism or hypothyroidism), and type I (insulin-dependent) diabetes mellitus is common. Additional features include myasthenia gravis, celiac disease, hypogonadism, perni-

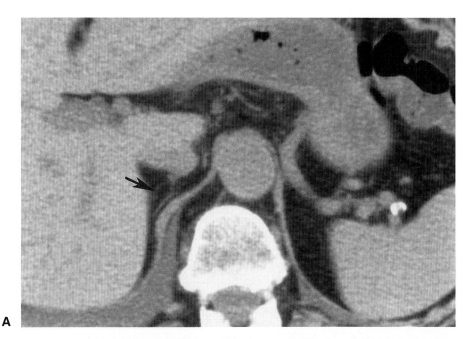

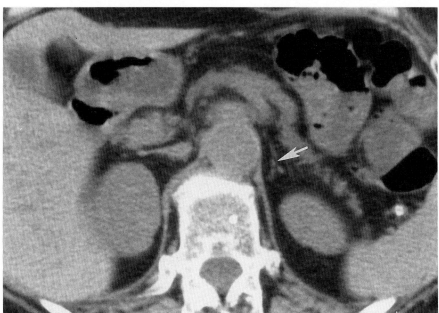

Figure 22-4. Autoimmune adrenal insufficiency. The adrenal glands are very small in patients with idiopathic Addison's disease. (A) The right adrenal gland (arrow) lies between the liver, the inferior vena cava, and diaphragmatic crus. A right pleural effusion is also present. (B) The left adrenal gland (arrow) lies between the body of the pancreas, the aorta, and the upper pole of the left kidney.

cious anemia, vitiligo, and alopecia. There is an increased incidence in persons with specific HLA types, especially in those with HLA-B8. There are specific antibodies against adrenal and thyroid microsomal antigens, gastric parietal cells, pancreatic islet cells, and Sertoli cells.

Question 116

Concerning adrenal metastases,

(A) they are common
(B) they can often be distinguished from benign adenomas by MRI
(C) they are a common cause of Addison's disease
(D) Hodgkin's disease more commonly involves the adrenal glands than does non-Hodgkin's lymphoma
(E) Addison's disease is not seen with lymphomatous infiltration of the adrenal glands

In a series of 1,000 autopsies of patients who died of cancer, Abrams et al. found adrenal metastases in 27% of patients. This was equal to the proportion of patients with bone metastases and was exceeded only by the number of patients with metastases to the lungs and liver. The adrenal glands are small and receive only about 3% of the cardiac output, but on a per-weight basis they are the most common site of metastases **(Option (A) is true).**

The most common tumors to metastasize to the adrenal glands are carcinomas of the lungs and breast. Adrenal metastases are also often secondary to renal adenocarcinoma. However, many of these are due to ipsilateral tumor spread, as the kidney and adrenal gland both lie within the perinephric space. The incidence of malignant melanoma is increasing, and this tumor often causes adrenal metastases as well. However, virtually any tumor may result in adrenal metastases. It is postulated that the high concentration of corticosteroids promotes implantation of metastases.

Adrenal metastases are best detected by CT, and they appear as soft tissue masses. Large lesions often have low-density areas, which are due to hemorrhage or necrosis. Most patients with adrenal metastases also have evidence of metastases to other sites such as the liver or retroperitoneal lymph nodes.

When other metastatic disease is present, an adrenal metastasis is not likely to be clinically significant. However, if an adrenal mass is the only site of potential metastatic tumor, it may be critical to determine whether it is a metastasis or a benign lesion, such as a nonhyperfunctioning adenoma.

MRI may be used to distinguish an adrenal metastasis from a benign adenoma. Metastases typically have a higher signal intensity on T2-weighted sequences than do benign adenomas. Despite the use of ratios of the signal intensity of the adrenal mass to a variety of nearby tissues, such as liver, muscle, or fat, there is significant overlap in the signal intensity of benign and malignant lesions. Previous studies have found 21 to 31% of patients falling in this overlap group. More recently, gadolinium enhancement has been used to improve the accuracy of this distinction. Krestin has shown that 90% of cases can be reliably classified when gadolinium enhancement is used as compared with only 72% on unenhanced studies. Adrenal metastases have greater enhancement and maintain this enhancement longer than benign adenomas (Option (B) is true).

Although adrenal metastases are common, they seldom destroy enough adrenal tissue to cause adrenal insufficiency (Option (C) is false). When Addison's disease does occur, the diagnosis may be difficult because the manifestations of Addison's disease may be attributed to the patient's neoplastic disease or other complications. Seidenwurm et al. have recommended glucocorticoid replacement therapy for patients with bilateral adrenal metastases, even if they do not have biochemical evidence of adrenal insufficiency.

Lymphoid tissue does not normally occur in the adrenal glands; however, heterotopic lymphoid elements are occasionally found and are presumably responsible for the rare cases of primary adrenal lymphoma. In most patients with adrenal lymphoma, the involvement is due to contiguous spread from adjacent retroperitoneal disease (Figure 22-5). Adrenal involvement has been detected radiographically in 4% of patients, whereas it is found histologically in 25% of patients at autopsy. Adrenal involvement is more common in patients with non-Hodgkin's lymphoma than in those with Hodgkin's disease, and with the diffuse form more commonly than with the nodular form (Option (D) is false).

Addison's disease is uncommon in patients with lymphoma, even when both adrenal glands are involved. However, just as with adrenal metastases from solid tumors, if sufficient adrenal tissue is destroyed, insufficiency will result (Option (E) is false).

N. Reed Dunnick, M.D.

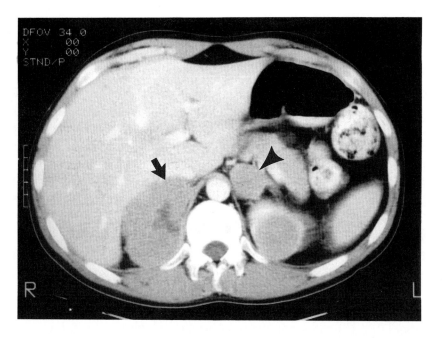

Figure 22-5. Lymphomatous involvement of both kidneys and adrenal glands. In this enhanced abdominal CT examination, a solitary mass has replaced the left adrenal gland (arrowhead), whereas the right adrenal involvement (arrow) is contiguous with renal lymphoma.

SUGGESTED READINGS

GRANULOMATOUS DISEASE

1. Doppman JL, Gill JR Jr, Nienhuis AW, Earll JM, Long JA Jr. CT findings in Addison's disease. J Comput Assist Tomogr 1982; 6:757–761
2. Osborne TM, Sage MJ. Disseminated tuberculosis causing acute adrenal failure, CT findings with post mortem correlation. Australas Radiol 1988; 32:394–397
3. Sawczuk IS, Reitelman C, Libby C, Grant D, Vita J, White RD. CT findings in Addison's disease caused by tuberculosis. Urol Radiol 1986; 8:44–45
4. Wilson DA, Muchmore HG, Tisdal RG, Fahmy A, Pitha JV. Histoplasmosis of the adrenal glands studied by CT. Radiology 1984; 160:779–783

ADRENAL HEMORRHAGE

5. Burks DW, Mirvis SE, Shanmuganathan K. Acute adrenal injury after blunt trauma: CT findings. AJR 1992; 158:503–507
6. Ling D, Korobkin M, Silverman PM, Dunnick NR. CT demonstration of bilateral adrenal hemorrhage. AJR 1983; 141:307–308

7. Wolverson MK, Kannegiesser H. CT of bilateral adrenal hemorrhage with acute adrenal insufficiency in the adult. AJR 1984; 142:311–314

8. Xarli VP, Steele AA, Davis PJ, Buescher ES, Rios CN, Garcia-Bunuel R. Adrenal hemorrhage in the adult. Medicine 1978; 57:211–221

IDIOPATHIC ADRENAL INSUFFICIENCY

9. De Rosa G, Corsello SM, Cecchini L, Della Casa S, Testa A. A clinical study of Addison's disease. Exp Clin Endocrinol 1987; 90:232–242

10. Eason RJ, Croxson MS, Perry MC, Somerfield SD. Addison's disease, adrenal autoantibodies and computerised adrenal tomography. N Z Med J 1982; 95:569–573

11. Leor J, Levartowsky D, Sharon C. Polyglandular autoimmune syndrome, type 2. South Med J 1989; 82:374–376

METASTASES

12. Baker DE, Glazer GM, Francis IR. Adrenal magnetic resonance imaging in Addison's disease. Urol Radiol 1988; 9:199–203

13. Krestin GP. Morphologic and functional MR of the kidneys and adrenal glands. New York: Field & Wood; 1991:89–106

14. Seidenwurm DJ, Elmer EB, Kaplan LM, Williams EK, Morris DG, Hoffman AR. Metastases to the adrenal glands and the development of Addison's disease. Cancer 1984; 54:552–557

15. Shea TC, Spark R, Kane B, Lange RF. Non-Hodgkin's lymphoma limited to the adrenal gland with adrenal insufficiency. Am J Med 1985; 78:711–714

16. Sheeler LR, Myers JH, Eversman JJ, Taylor HC. Adrenal insufficiency secondary to carcinoma metastatic to the adrenal gland. Cancer 1983; 52:1312–1316

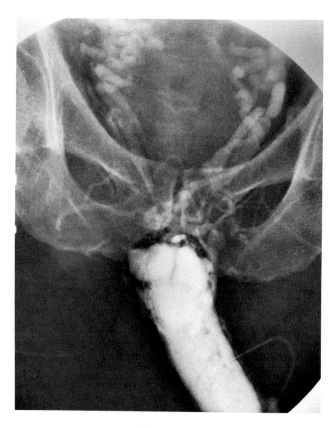

Figure 23-1. This 48-year-old man presented with impotence. Following clinical evaluation, he was referred for corpora cavernosometry and cavernosography. You are shown a corpora cavernosogram following intracorporeal administration of 60 mg of papaverine and 1 mg of phentolamine.

Case 23: Impotence

Question 117

Which *one* of the following is the MOST likely diagnosis?

(A) Veno-occlusive incompetence
(B) Peyronie's disease
(C) Psychogenic impotence
(D) Penile artery disease
(E) Multiple sclerosis

The corpora cavernosogram (Figure 23-1) demonstrates good opacification of both corpora. In addition, there is extensive venous leak with opacification of crural, periprostatic, and hypogastric veins. The normal response to intracavernosal injection of papaverine and phentolamine is smooth muscle relaxation in the trabeculae of the corpora, which leads to occlusion of the veins that exit the tunica albuginea. A normal response to these drugs is essentially no visualization of the veins, as seen in Figure 23-2. Activation of this veno-occlusive mechanism is a necessary part of the erectile process. Therefore, the test patient has veno-occlusive incompetence **(Option (A) is correct).**

On the basis of the test image, one can neither establish nor exclude the presence of associated arterial disease (Option (D)). There is no evidence of penile deformity or plaques thickening the tunica albuginea of the corpora, so the diagnosis of Peyronie's disease (Option (B)) is not correct.

Psychogenic (Option (C)) and neurogenic (Option (E)) causes of erectile dysfunction cannot be suspected on the basis of the test image. These problems may coexist with arterial insufficiency and veno-occlusive incompetence. On the other hand, it is common for patients with psychogenic and neurogenic problems to demonstrate a normal response to papaverine, phentolamine, and other vasoactive drugs such as prostaglandin E_1.

A normal male response to sexual stimulation is a rigid erection that lasts long enough for coitus and sexual satisfaction to be achieved. This

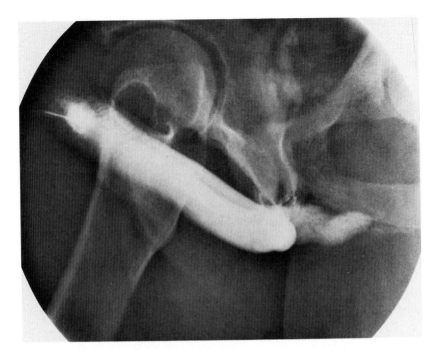

Figure 23-2. Corpora cavernosogram with normal response to papaverine. There is good tumescence of both corpora, with essentially no venous opacification.

process occurs in a normal hormonal environment with proper psychic and physical stimulation. This stimulation leads to nerve impulses from the spinal cord to the cavernous nerves, which are responsible for the innervation of the smooth muscle of the trabeculae of the corpora, as well as of the smooth muscle of the penile arteries. The neurotransmitter that is released is probably an endothelium-derived relaxing factor that is responsible for the obstruction of the venous outflow (veno-occlusive mechanism). The arterial vasodilation coupled with diminished intracorporeal resistance leads to a marked increase in blood flow into the trabecular spaces. In normal men the intracavernous pressure will reach levels ranging from 90 mm Hg up to the arterial systolic pressure. At that point the penis is rigid enough to allow coitus. Detumescence occurs when the trabeculae and arteries contract. This most probably is a response to release of norepinephrine, which is found in high concentration in erectile tissue.

Clinical and laboratory studies must be performed before the status of the arterial and venous system of the penis is evaluated. The loss of sexual desire may suggest a hormonal abnormality. This can be evaluated by determining the levels of testosterone and prolactin in plasma. In addition, alcohol abuse, adrenal tumors, and digoxin intake may lead to elevation of estradiol levels in plasma. The presence of normal neurologic function must also be established.

Many urologists screen patients with erectile dysfunction by means of nocturnal penile tumescence (NPT) studies. There is evidence that most normal men have four or five erections per night that last 10 to 15 minutes each. On the other hand, when studied in a sleep laboratory, as many as 20% of normally potent men have abnormal NPT responses. For this reason, a variety of commercial devices for use at home as well as in sleep laboratories have been developed. One of the more elaborate of these devices, Rigiscan (Dacomed, Minneapolis, Minn.), measures both tumescence and hardness. This is necessary because measuring tumescence alone does not provide information about whether adequate hardness (rigidity) has been achieved to allow coitus. Although NPT studies have limitations related to the sleep laboratory environment and the reliability of results of devices for use at home, they provide a simple way to establish whether the process of erection is to some degree physiologically intact.

Eventually, it may become necessary to establish the adequacy of penile arterial blood flow as well as veno-occlusion. The most popular noninvasive methods of evaluating these functions are duplex and color-flow Doppler sonography. The invasive arterial studies include aortography and selective pudendal arteriography. The veno-occlusive mechanism is studied by means of corpora cavernosometry and cavernosography.

Question 118

Concerning duplex and color-flow Doppler ultrasonography of the deep penile arteries after intracavernosal papaverine administration,

(A) the mean peak systolic velocity in the deep penile artery is normally 15 to 25 cm/second

(B) cavernosal arteries are constricted by the drug

(C) detectable dorsal vein flow is present during all phases of erection

(D) normally, diastolic velocity decreases below 5 cm/second as the intracavernosal pressure increases

Penile duplex and color-flow Doppler sonography have proven to be sensitive, noninvasive methods for evaluating patients with suspected vasculogenic impotence. The addition of color-flow Doppler to duplex sonography permits a more rapid examination because detection of the cavernosal artery becomes easier and correction of the Doppler angle is more accurate. Quam et al. reported on 183 patients studied by this technique. Of their patients, 61 also underwent cavernosography and cavernosometry, and 12 patients underwent selective internal pudendal arteriography. Quam et al. reported mean peak systolic velocities of less than 25 cm/second in the cavernosal arteries of patients with abnormal arteriograms. Patients with normal arteriograms had peak systolic velocities above 25 cm/second. This value has been used by other investigators as normal, although higher velocities (in the range of 45 to 55 cm/second) may be recorded **(Option (A) is false).**

Duplex sonography also provides a method of evaluating the response of the cavernosal arteries to papaverine. The smooth muscle-relaxing effects of this drug cause vasodilation **(Option (B) is false).** Thus, the normal cavernosal artery should dilate about 100% after intracorporeal administration of papaverine. Thickened arterial walls and asymmetric dilatation suggest arterial disease.

Fitzgerald et al. and Schwartz et al. (1989) described the normal Doppler spectral waveforms of the cavernosal artery during papaverine-induced erection (Figure 23-3). This drug initially causes an increase in systolic and diastolic flow. As the intracavernosal pressure increases, a dicrotic notch appears at end systole. At the same time, the diastolic flow decreases. A continuous rise in intracavernosal pressure eventually is associated with zero diastolic flow (a reflection of the activated veno-occlusive mechanism). Diastolic flow reversal also occurs with the higher intracavernosal pressures. In the final phase, the systolic envelope narrows and diastolic flow disappears completely. Clinically, this phase

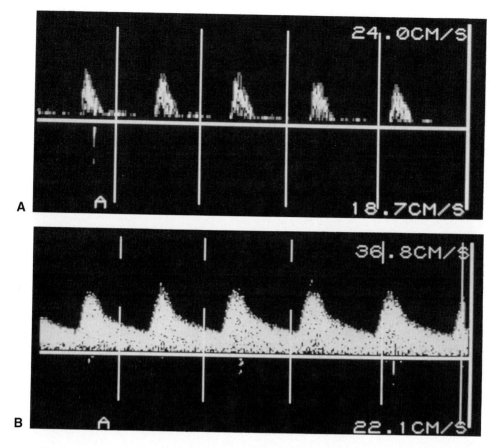

Figure 23-3. Normal progression of spectral waveforms in the cavernosal artery after papaverine injection. (A) Typical waveform before papaverine with dampened systolic envelope and minimal diastolic flow. (B) After papaverine injection, there is an abrupt increase in both systolic and diastolic flow in the cavernosal artery. Minimal tumescence usually accompanies this phase. (C) As the intracavernosal pressure rises, a transition in diastolic flow occurs. This is heralded by the development of a dicrotic notch and a decrease in diastolic flow. (D) Diastolic flow drops to zero as the intracavernosal pressure continues to rise. The systolic envelope narrows, and the systolic velocity may fluctuate. Increasing tumescence is usually present. (E) When the intracavernosal pressure exceeds the diastolic pressure within the artery, end-diastolic flow undergoes reversal. Many patients achieve maximum systolic velocity at the time of diastolic flow reversal. This may be associated with penile rigidity. (F) With maximum rigidity, intracavernosal pressure may approximate or exceed arterial systolic pressure. This results in further narrowing of the systolic envelope and usually a drop in systolic velocity. Complete obliteration of systolic flow may occur transiently. (Reprinted with permission from Fitzgerald et al. [14].)

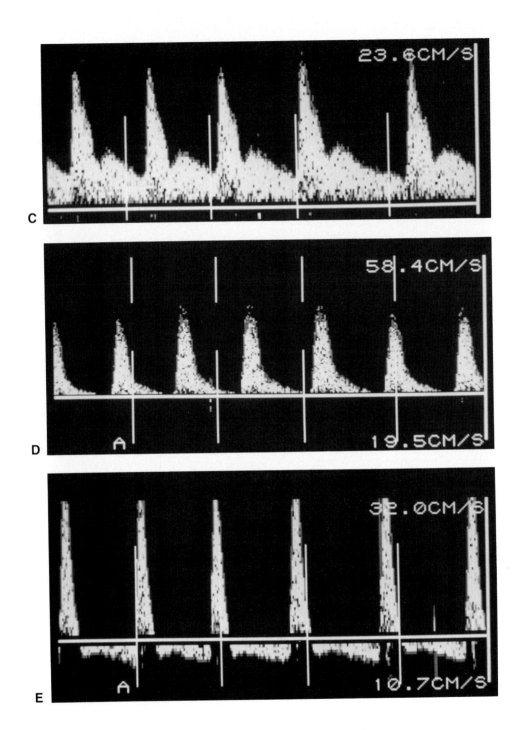

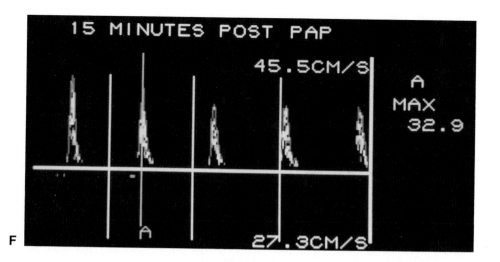

is characterized by a rigid erection. Fitzgerald et al. also emphasized the need to study these patients for an adequate length of time after the administration of papaverine. Most of their patients achieved a maximum response in the first 5 minutes, but in 10 of 75 patients significant changes in end-diastolic velocity occurred 5 to 30 minutes postinjection.

It has been established that persistent end-diastolic flow of greater than 5 cm/second indicates venous leak **(Option (D) is true)**. One may also study the dorsal vein in the assessment of suspected venous insufficiency. Transient early dorsal vein flow is normal, but with normal veno-occlusion this flow ceases **(Option (C) is false)**. Fitzgerald et al. reported that 32 patients with dorsal vein flow also had elevated end-diastolic velocities consistent with venous incompetence.

Question 119

Concerning penile arteriography,

F (A) the vessels are best studied with the penis in the flaccid state
T (B) opacification of the spongiosal artery is associated with a vascular stain
F (C) helicine branches arise from the dorsal artery
F (D) bilateral internal pudendal arteriography is sufficient for a complete evaluation of arterial disease
F (E) a single cavernosal artery indicates arteriogenic impotence

The arterial supply to the penis is from the internal pudendal arteries (Figure 23-4). The internal pudendal artery first gives rise to the scrotal branches. The spongiosal artery (artery of the penile bulb) arises next to supply the proximal corpus spongiosum. It is identified on the arteriogram by its characteristic stain (Figure 23-5) **(Option (B) is true).** The penile artery now divides into: (1) the dorsal penile artery, which supplies the glans and the skin of the penis, and (2) the cavernosal or deep penile artery, which runs in the corpus cavernosum. The deep penile artery gives rise to helicine branches **(Option (C) is false),** which are the source of blood flow to the corpora during erection.

Indications for arteriography include the following:

1. Pathologic inflow as suggested by color-flow Doppler studies.

2. Primary erectile failure. Bähren et al. emphasized that 60% of patients with primary erectile dysfunction have arterial abnormalities with or without additional causes.

3. Posttraumatic erectile dysfunction. This should be preceded by neurologic evaluation. Most of these patients have sustained pelvic trauma, usually with fracture, as a result of motor vehicle accidents. When the neurologic status is within normal limits, arterial study and revascularizing procedures can be considered.

4. Significant aortic or hypogastric artery disease. The presence of an adequate penile circulation supports the use of percutaneous transluminal angioplasty, particularly at the origin of the hypogastric arteries.

Arteriography of the internal pudendal circulation should be preceded by a study of the distal aorta and hypogastric arteries **(Option (D) is false).** This is necessary to rule out the presence of stenoses proximal to the internal pudendal branches, which might contribute to poor arterial flow. In addition, demonstration of the inferior epigastric arteries is important because these branches are used in some arterial bypass procedures to the penile circulation. It is also important to ensure that the internal pudendal artery does not have an anomalous origin.

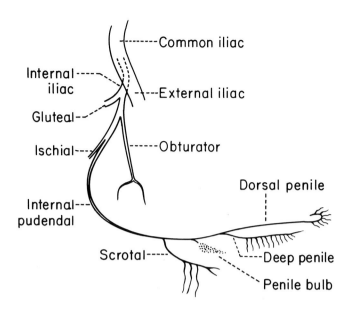

Figure 23-4. Diagram of normal blood supply to the penis.

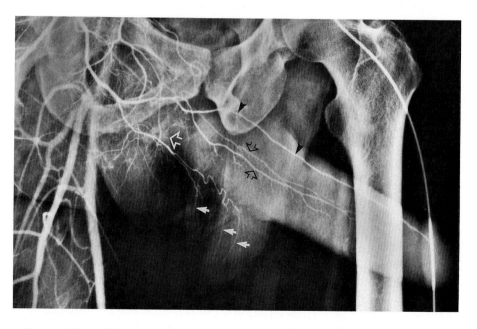

Figure 23-5. Normal selective right internal pudendal arteriogram following intracorporeal injection of 30 mg of papaverine. The dorsal penile artery (arrowheads) and scrotal arteries (white arrows) are well shown. Both cavernosal (deep penile) arteries (open black arrows) fill from the right side. The penile bulb stain (open white arrow) is shown.

Selective arteriography of the internal pudendal artery is then performed. Intracavernosal injection of 30 mg of papaverine is generally adequate to produce some tumescence so that the vessels can be studied to best advantage **(Option (A) is false)** (Figure 23-5). Some investigators increase this dose to 60 mg, and many add 1 mg of phentolamine. The penile vessels have slow flow in the flaccid state and are not maximally dilated, so it is difficult to assess their anatomy and patency adequately. On the other hand, one should not induce maximum tumescence during arteriography, because maximum penile rigidity is associated with constriction of the arteries. The patient should be positioned so that the course of the vessels is optimally demonstrated. For studying the right side, the patient is placed in a 45-degree left posterior oblique projection with the penis across the left thigh. Low-osmolar contrast agents are used so that discomfort is minimized during the injection. High-quality filming is mandatory to study these small vessels. Conventional film changers have been recommended, and Bookstein et al. have suggested twofold magnification. Digital subtraction angiography should be available because it is quite useful in selected cases.

Primary erectile dysfunction refers to the inability to have normal erections from the time of adolescence. It is important to emphasize that patients with vascular abnormalities usually have developed associated psychogenic problems. Bähren et al. reported on a group of 55 such patients with a mean age of 28.5 years. Abnormal arterial flow was shown by Doppler studies in 35 patients (64%). Twenty-four patients (44%) had venous etiologies with or without arterial abnormalities. Twenty-nine of the patients with primary erectile failure underwent arteriography. In 23 of these patients, hemodynamically significant arterial abnormalities were detected (Figure 23-6). Arteriography confirmed what other authors have stated, i.e., that cavernosal artery underdevelopment (hypoplasia or aplasia) has to be severe and bilateral to be significant **(Option (E) is false)**.

Posttraumatic erectile failure must be carefully studied. In young patients both arterial and venous abnormalities may be detected. Lurie et al. reported that 13 of 16 patients (81%) had vasculogenic impotence when studied by arteriography and by corpora cavernosometry and cavernosography. The mode of therapy depended on the findings and included venous ligation, angioplasty or bypass surgery, self-injection of papaverine, and insertion of a prosthesis. The young patient with an isolated arterial vascular lesion and no neurogenic component is said to be the best candidate for surgery or angioplasty. There are few long-term

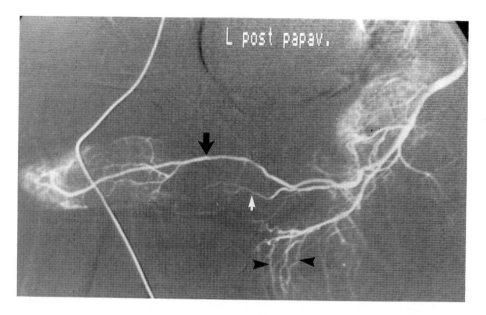

Figure 23-6. Primary erectile failure. This 26-year-old patient has never had normal erections. The dorsal penile artery (black arrow) is well opacified following papaverine administration. The deep penile vessels are hypoplastic (white arrow). Scrotal branches (arrowheads) are also shown. Injection into the contralateral side revealed no deep penile (cavernosal) or dorsal penile artery.

studies of these patients, but improvements in microsurgical techniques hold promise for improved results of revascularization.

The morphology of the pudendal and penile arteries is age related. These vessels are subject to the same risk factors for atherosclerotic disease as vessels elsewhere in the body. Arteriosclerosis reduces cavernosal arterial inflow, but collateral vessels are adequate and so ischemic damage does not occur. Nevertheless, penile arterial insufficiency is often associated with significant loss of inflow leading to erectile failure. Bähren et al. reported that in 33 of 34 patients with a mean age of 46 years, arteriographic evidence of penile arteriosclerotic lesions was associated with two or more risk factors (e.g., diabetes mellitus, hypertension, smoking, and hyperlipidemia). Patients who underwent selective angiography had a vascular etiology demonstrated up to 85% of the time.

Question 120

Concerning corpora cavernosography,

F (A) both corpora should be injected
T (B) it should be performed after cavernosometry
T (C) the saphenous vein is a potential route of penile venous drainage
F (D) opacification of the glans is abnormal

The corpora cavernosal veno-occlusive mechanism is essential for normal erectile function. Color-flow Doppler screening may indicate a venous leak, but further quantification is performed by means of cavernosometry after intracavernosal injection of papaverine and phentolamine. These studies are performed by placing one needle in each corpora cavernosum. One is used for infusion, and one is used for pressure measurements. Since there is free communication between the corpora cavernosa, only one side need be injected **(Option (A) is false).** Papaverine and phentolamine activate the veno-occlusive mechanism, thereby allowing for measurement of the amount of flow per minute necessary to maintain erection. Bookstein et al. have called this the pharmacologic maintenance erectile flow (PMEF). The normal PMEF is 2 to 12 mL/minute. Higher values are indicative of venogenic impotence. A similar approach to the study of these patients has been described by other investigators. Delcour et al. described measuring the flow rate needed to induce erection (FIE) and the flow rate needed to maintain erection (FME) with a pressure of at least 90 mm Hg during cavernosometry. They studied 10 normal volunteers who were not being given pharmacologic assistance and found that the FIE varied from 80 to 140 mL/minute while the FME ranged from 15 to 50 mL/minute.

It is important to emphasize that while cavernosometry can be performed in a variety of ways, the major goal is to establish whether an adequate erection is produced and maintained. This is usually most easily accomplished with pharmacologic assistance by the use of papaverine and phentolamine. Cavernosometry can be performed with heparinized saline. When pressure values indicate a venous leak, cavernosography is performed to demonstrate the site(s) of leakage **(Option (B) is true).**

Dilute contrast material, in the range of 10 to 15% iodine, is usually sufficient. Most recently, low-osmolar agents have been used for these studies. It is important to document the sites of venous leakage if corrective surgery or transcatheter venoablation is an option for treatment. After intracavernosal papaverine administration there is virtually complete occlusion of all venous outflow from the normal corpora

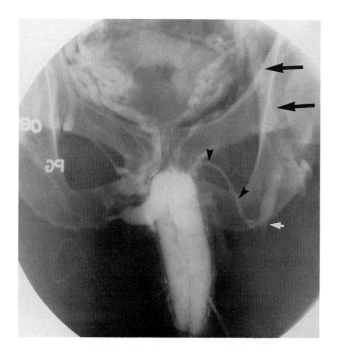

Figure 23-7. Veno-occlusive incompetence. Corpora cavernosogram demonstrating marked venous leak. There is extensive filling of periprostatic and hypogastric veins. Note also the external pudendal vein (arrowheads) draining to the left saphenous vein (white arrow), which in turn drains into the femoral and external iliac vein (black arrows).

cavernosa. Bookstein et al. reported that of 58 patients with venogenic impotence (isolated or in combination with arteriogenic disease), there was significant leakage via the deep dorsal vein in 81%, via the cavernosal perforators in 64%, via the spongiosa in 57%, and via superficial veins in 53%. Leakage of superficial penile veins to the external pudendal veins is not uncommon (Figure 23-7). It can be seen because drainage is to the saphenous and femoral veins **(Option (C) is true).** It has been suggested that another route of venous leakage is demonstrated by opacification of the glans during cavernosography. It was believed that such opacification was a sign of pathologic shunts between the corpora cavernosa and the glans. Delcour et al. demonstrated that this could be a normal finding **(Option (D) is false).** Opacification of the glans was demonstrated in five normal volunteers. In addition, among a group of 150 impotent patients, opacification of the glans was noted in 53% with venous leakage and in 36% without venous leakage.

Thus, opacification of the glans penis during cavernosography is most probably a normal variant.

Question 121

Concerning veno-occlusive incompetence,

(A) it is rarely associated with arterial disease
(B) ligation of the deep dorsal vein is a highly effective form of treatment
(C) it is due to testosterone deficiency
(D) self-administration of papaverine is beneficial

The corpora cavernosa and spongiosa are drained by three groups of veins. The superficial dorsal vein drains the cutaneous covering. The deep dorsal vein drains the glans penis and corpus spongiosum. The cavernous veins originate from the cavernous bodies. These begin as subtunical veins. The superficial and deep veins drain mainly into the periprostatic plexus, which in turn empties into the hypogastric circulation. Other connections may also be demonstrated during cavernosography, including filling of the external pudendal vein and saphenous vein.

The venous drainage of the corpora cavernosa originates from subtunical veins. Relaxation of the smooth muscle in the trabeculae allows the distending sinusoids to compress these veins, thereby severely limiting outflow from the corpora cavernosa. In patients with veno-occlusive incompetence this series of events is ineffective, so blood is not adequately contained in the penis and rigidity does not occur. Most veno-occlusive incompetence occurs in patients who have normal hormone production **(Option (C) is false).**

The idea that cavernous-venous leakage might be an important cause of erectile failure is not new. There have been reports that simple dorsal vein ligation results in transient success. This is not an effective form of treatment because it does not treat the many other sites of venous drainage **(Option (B) is false).** In fact, the surgical approaches to the venous system that include embolization or surgical ligation of the major draining veins have had mixed results, which in many cases have also proved to be transitory. This is not surprising because these interventions do not address the problem, which appears to be at the trabecular-venous level. As a result, extensive ligation or embolization of draining veins at the crural and periprostatic levels may be followed by development of new collateral routes of drainage, which lead to loss of the effectiveness of prior venous interruption.

One must be aware that arteriogenic and venogenic causes of impotence may coexist **(Option (A) is false)**. Bookstein et al. reported their results in a study of 183 patients with impotence studied by penile arterial vascular catheterization and cavernosometry and cavernosography. Of these, 29% had normal studies, 23% had pure arteriogenic impotence, 25% had pure venogenic impotence, and 23% had combined arteriogenic and venogenic impotence.

Papaverine, alone or combined with the alpha-blocker phentolamine, has been used widely in the diagnosis and treatment of impotence. Patients are identified as possible candidates for this treatment if they can be taught and accept the technique of self-injection and if they have impotence secondary to neurologic dysfunction, arterial insufficiency, or inadequate veno-occlusive mechanism. Patients with veno-occlusive incompetence report that the quality of erections improved with intracorporeal papaverine injections **(Option (D) is true)**. It is believed that residual endogenous neurotransmitters and local vasoactive substances have an additive effect when combined with intracorporeal vasoactive substances such as papaverine. Recently, prostaglandin E_1 has become increasingly popular for pharmacologically assisted erections. Priapism is a rare side effect of papaverine injections but is much less of a risk with prostaglandin E_1. In addition, intracorporeal fibrosis is thought to occur at some injection sites in patients using papaverine, whereas this does not appear to be a complication of prostaglandin E_1 injections.

Question 122

Concerning Peyronie's disease,

(A) it is a fibrous cavernositis
(B) it is associated with Dupuytren's contracture
(C) it most often begins laterally in the corpora cavernosa
(D) the corpus spongiosum is often involved
(E) calcification is common

Peyronie's disease is a disorder of the connective tissue localized to the tunica albuginea of the corpus cavernosum. It may be considered a fibrous cavernositis **(Option (A) is true)**. The corpus spongiosum is not involved **(Option (D) is false)**. Its clinical presentation ranges from a palpable

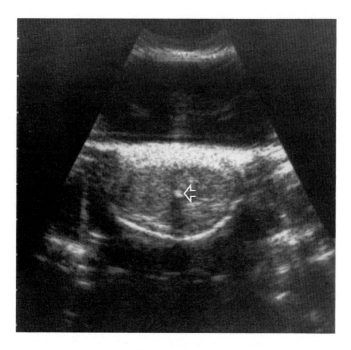

Figure 23-8. Peyronie's disease. Transverse sonogram of the corpora revealing dystrophic calcification (arrow) causing shadowing.

nodule that is asymptomatic to severe erectile pain associated with marked curvature of the penis. Dystrophic calcification is present in approximately 65% of patients **(Option (E) is true).** This may be well shown by plain radiography or by sonography (Figure 23-8). Dupuytren's contracture is associated with this condition in patients with and without associated calcification **(Option (B) is true).**

The area of the corpora most often involved is medial **(Option (C) is false).** Peyronie's disease can be grouped into two phases: early inflammation and late fibrosis. The natural history of this process is of interest. Approximately 40% of 97 patients studied by Gelbard et al. found the overall effects of pain, bending, and ability to have intercourse to be unchanged over a period of observation that ranged from 3 months to 8 years. In an additional 40% of the patients, bending and ability to have intercourse became worse during the same period of observation, whereas pain worsened in only 6% of this second group. It is of interest that 13% of these 97 patients believed that the disease gradually resolved while approximately equal numbers of the remaining patients believed that there was little or no change and 40% believed that the condition progressed during the period of observation.

Duplex Doppler ultrasonography is particularly well suited to the evaluation of patients with Peyronie's disease. It can provide information about the extent of the fibrous plaque as well as the status of the penile vasculature. This is important because patients with this condition may also develop impotence. Lopez and Jarow studied 30 impotent and 3 potent men with Peyronie's disease by means of duplex Doppler ultrasonography. They found associated arterial disease in eight (27%) of these patients. Prior to the use of ultrasonography, the extent of these fibrous plaques could be shown only by means of cavernosography. Sonography has the advantage of being a noninvasive examination and is well suited for demonstrating the extent of disease.

Harold A. Mitty, M.D.

SUGGESTED READINGS

CAVERNOSOGRAPHY, CAVERNOSOMETRY, AND VENO-OCCLUSIVE INCOMPETENCE

1. Bookstein JJ, Fellmeth B, Moreland S, Lurie AL. Pharmacoangiographic assessment of the corpora cavernosa. Cardiovasc Intervent Radiol 1988; 11:218–224
2. Bookstein JJ, Lurie AL. Selective penile venography: anatomical and hemodynamic observations. J Urol 1988; 140:55–60
3. Delcour C, Wespes E, Vandenbosch G, Schulman CC, Struyven J. Opacification of the glans penis during cavernosography. J Urol 1988; 139:732–733
4. Delcour CP, Vandenbosch GA, Struyven JL. Cavernosography and cavernosometry in the evaluation of impotence. Urol Radiol 1988; 10:144–150
5. Krane RJ, Goldstein I, Saenz de Tejada I. Impotence. N Engl J Med 1989; 321:1648–1659
6. Krysiewicz S, Mellinger BC. The role of imaging in the diagnostic evaluation of impotence. AJR 1989; 153:1133–1139
7. Melman A. The evaluation of erectile dysfunction. Urol Radiol 1988; 10:119–128

PEYRONIE'S DISEASE

8. Gelbard MK. Dystrophic penile calcification in Peyronie's disease. J Urol 1988; 139:738–740
9. Gelbard MK, Dorey F, James K. The natural history of Peyronie's disease. J Urol 1990; 144:1376–1379
10. Lopez JA, Jarow JP. Duplex ultrasound findings in men with Peyronie's disease. Urol Radiol 1991; 12:199–202

11. Metz P, Ebbehöj J, Uhrenholdt A, Wagner G. Peyronie's disease and erectile failure. J Urol 1983; 130:1103–1104

COLOR-FLOW AND DUPLEX DOPPLER SONOGRAPHY

12. Benson CB, Vickers MA. Sexual impotence caused by vascular disease: diagnosis with duplex sonography. AJR 1989; 153:1149–1153
13. Fitzgerald SW, Erickson SG, Foley WD, Lipchik EO, Lawson TL. Color Doppler sonography in the evaluation of erectile dysfunction: patterns of temporal response to papaverine. AJR 1991; 157:331–336
14. Fitzgerald SW, Erickson SJ, Foley WD, Lipchik EO, Lawson TL. Color Doppler sonography in the evaluation of erectile dysfunction. RadioGraphics 1992; 12:3–17
15. Gerstenberg TC, Nordling J, Hald T, Wagner G. Standardized evaluation of erectile dysfunction in 95 consecutive patients. J Urol 1989; 141:857–862
16. Mueller SC, von Wallenberg-Pachaly H, Voges GE, Schild HH. Comparison of selective internal iliac pharmaco-angiography, penile brachial index and duplex sonography with pulsed Doppler analyses for the evaluation of vasculogenic (arteriogenic) impotence. J Urol 1990; 143:928–932
17. Quam JP, King BF, James EM, et al. Duplex and color Doppler sonographic evaluation of vasculogenic impotence. AJR 1989; 153:1141–1147
18. Schwartz AN, Lowe M, Berger RE, Wang KY, Mack LA, Richardson ML. Assessment of normal and abnormal erectile function: color Doppler flow sonography versus conventional techniques. Radiology 1991; 180:105–109
19. Schwartz AN, Wang KY, Mack LA, et al. Evaluation of normal erectile function with color flow Doppler sonography. AJR 1989; 153:1155–1160
20. Shabsigh R, Fishman IJ, Shotland Y, Karacan I, Dunn JK. Comparison of penile duplex ultrasonography with nocturnal penile tumescence monitoring for the evaluation of erectile impotence. J Urol 1990; 143:924–927

ARTERIOGENIC IMPOTENCE

21. Bähren W, Gall H, Scherb W, Stief C, Thon W. Arterial anatomy and arteriographic diagnosis of arteriogenic impotence. Cardiovasc Intervent Radiol 1988; 11:195–210
22. Bookstein JJ, Valji K. The arteriolar component in impotence: a possible paradigm shift. AJR 1991; 157:932–934
23. Kirschenbaum A, Mitty HA. Penile prostheses. Urol Radiol 1988; 10:160–165
24. Lurie AL, Bookstein JJ, Kessler WO. Angiography of posttraumatic impotence. Cardiovasc Intervent Radiol 1988; 11:232–236
25. Rosen MP, Schwartz AN, Levine FJ, Greenfield AJ. Radiologic assessment of impotence: angiography, sonography, cavernosography, and scintigraphy. AJR 1991; 157:923–931
26. Rosen MP, Walker TG, Greenfield AJ. Arteriography and radiology of impotence. Urol Radiol 1988; 10:136–143
27. Zorgniotti AW, Lizza E. Nonprosthetic surgical strategies for impotence. Urol Radiol 1988; 10:151–155

Notes

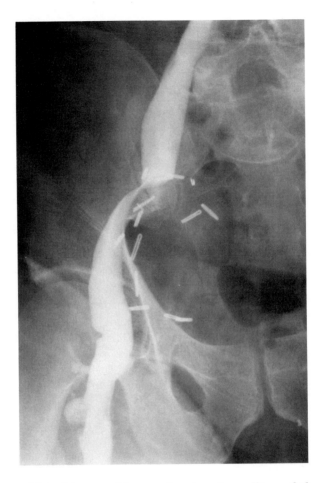

Figure 24-1. This 64-year-old man developed swelling of the right leg 2 weeks after a prostatectomy for adenocarcinoma. You are shown a venogram of the right leg.

Case 24: Pelvic Lymphocele

Question 123

Likely diagnoses include:

   (A) thrombosis of the iliac vein
   (B) extrinsic compression of the iliac vein by metastatic prostatic carcinoma
   (C) lymphocele
   (D) pelvic lipomatosis
   (E) pelvic hematoma

    The venogram (Figure 24-1) shows surgical clips in the pelvis from the recent lymphadenectomy performed before prostatectomy. The right femoral vein and common iliac vein are well opacified with contrast material and appear normal. There is extrinsic compression of the external iliac vein by a pelvic mass just medial to the vein.
    Iliac venous thrombosis is a reasonable consideration in this patient given the history of leg swelling and recent pelvic surgery. However, thrombosis is an intrinsic process and thus would produce a filling defect within the vein (Figure 24-2).The thrombus may cause complete occlusion of the vein. The abnormality in the test patient is an extrinsic process, and no filling defects are present **(Option (A) is false).**
    The extrinsic compression of the right iliac vein may be caused by any focal mass including pelvic lymphadenopathy. However, lymph node metastases from adenocarcinoma of the prostate usually produce only modest lymph node enlargement. Furthermore, the prostatectomy was performed only 2 weeks before the venogram, and the pelvic clips indicate that lymphadenectomy was also performed; it is unlikely that a tumor of this size would have been missed, and a small tumor could not have reached this size in only 2 weeks **(Option (B) is false).**
    Patients whose tumors are confined within the prostatic capsule are the most suitable candidates for prostatectomy. A prostatectomy with regional lymphadenectomy is preferred when there is involvement of the seminal vesicles or limited pelvic lymph node metastases. Pelvic surgery, especially with lymphadenectomy, predisposes patients to both venous

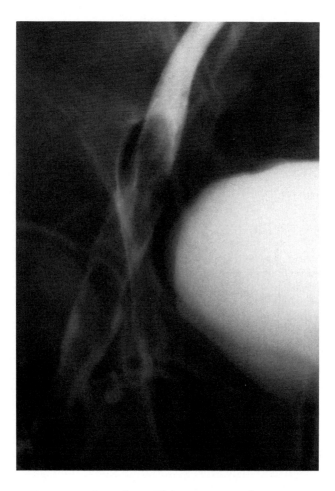

Figure 24-2. Iliac vein thrombus. This venogram demonstrates contrast material surrounding a filling defect, indicating an intraluminal process such as thrombosis.

thrombosis and lymphocele formation. When heparin is used as prophylaxis for venous thrombosis, the incidence of lymphocele increases. In general, lymphatics tend to follow the course of the veins. Thus, this location, adjacent to the iliac vein, is a common site of lymphocele. A lymphocele in this region would typically cause extrinsic compression of the adjacent iliac vein **(Option (C) is true).**

Pelvic lipomatosis is an abnormal accumulation of fat within the pelvis. It causes extrinsic compression of both sides of the bladder, resulting in a vertical bladder orientation. The process is generally asymmetric and seldom causes complications. Ureteral obstruction occurs occasionally, but vascular compromise is rare **(Option (D) is false).**

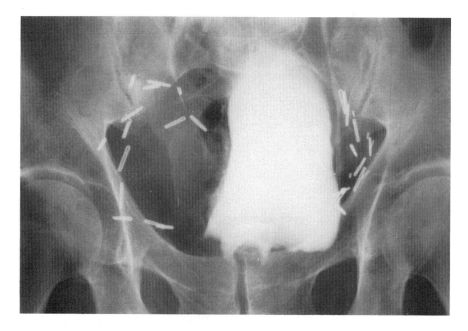

Figure 24-3. Same patient as in Figure 24-1. The contrast material used for the venogram is excreted by the kidneys. Opacification of the bladder demonstrates leftward deviation caused by the right pelvic mass.

The pelvis is a vascular area, and a hematoma could easily develop during surgery. It would not be surprising to find a large hematoma exerting extrinsic compression on the iliac vein 2 weeks after a prostatectomy **(Option (E) is true).**

A pelvic radiograph (Figure 24-3) obtained after the venogram demonstrates opacification of the bladder by excreted contrast material. The bladder is displaced to the left and is deformed by an extrinsic mass. These findings corroborate those seen on the venogram.

Question 124

Which *one* of the following is the MOST appropriate examination for this patient after the venogram?

(A) Retrograde pyelography
(B) Ultrasonography
(C) CT
(D) MRI
(E) Arteriography

The most likely etiologies for the right pelvic mass in this patient are a pelvic hematoma and a lymphocele. Although both are benign and self-limited, the patient is symptomatic and intervention is indicated. Therefore, further delineation is needed.

Retrograde pyelography (Option (A)) opacifies the intrarenal collecting system and the ureter. It is possible that the ureter was injured during surgery and that the mass is a urinoma. If this were the case, a retrograde pyelogram would be diagnostic. However, a urinoma is not as likely as a hematoma or lymphocele. Opacification of the right ureter would also demonstrate any extrinsic compression on the ureter and further define the extent of the mass. However, this indirect information would be less specific than information gained from one of the cross-sectional imaging techniques.

Ultrasonography is an excellent modality for imaging the pelvis. In most patients, the iliac vessels are clearly visualized and an adjacent mass can be defined. Sonography is often used to distinguish a cystic from a solid mass. Cystic lesions transmit sound easily and demonstrate a strong posterior echo, indicating increased through transmission. Simple cysts have no internal echoes. If the cyst has been complicated by hemorrhage or infection, internal echoes will be present but will move within the fluid-filled mass. Lymphoceles are cystic lesions; they are usually hypoechoic on sonography due to fine septations and scattered debris, but they may be anechoic. There is increased through transmission (Figure 24-4).

A hematoma can often be distinguished from a lymphocele by ultrasonography. The dense echoes from clotted blood in a hematoma would not be expected in a lymphocele unless there has also been bleeding into the lymphocele. For these reasons, ultrasonography would be the most appropriate examination in the test patient **(Option (B) is correct).**

Pelvic masses are also well defined by CT (Option (C)). Solid lesions can often be distinguished from cystic lesions on the basis of the tissue

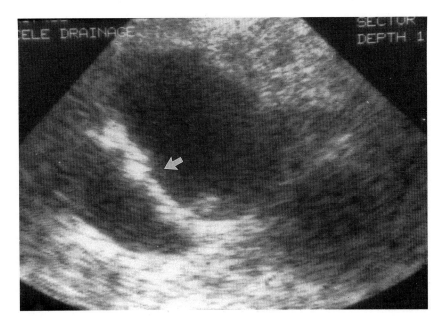

Figure 24-4. Lymphocele. This sonogram shows a cystic mass in the right pelvis. The internal septation (arrow) and scattered internal echoes are typical of a lymphocele.

density. Cystic masses are usually at or slightly greater than water density (0 to 10 Hounsfield units [HU]) (Figure 24-5), whereas solid masses have soft tissue density (25 to 40 HU). Acute hemorrhage can be recognized by an increased density (50 to 90 HU) of the blood clot. However, CT depends upon opacification of the entire bowel within the pelvis so that masses can be distinguished from fluid-filled loops of bowel. Although this can be accomplished in most patients, it may require several hours for the oral contrast material to reach the pelvis. Intravascular contrast may be needed to define the iliac vessels on CT. This is particularly true in patients with a paucity of pelvic fat. If intravascular contrast material must be used, the expense of CT is further increased. The time and expense make CT less appropriate than ultrasonography.

MRI (Option (D)) has been particularly useful in imaging the pelvis. The multiple planes in which images can be acquired often help define relationships that are more difficult to appreciate on CT, which is limited largely to the axial projection. Furthermore, blood can often be recognized by its specific signal characteristics. However, MRI is the most expensive and least readily available of the cross-sectional imaging techniques. Furthermore, many patients are too claustrophobic to undergo MRI, and

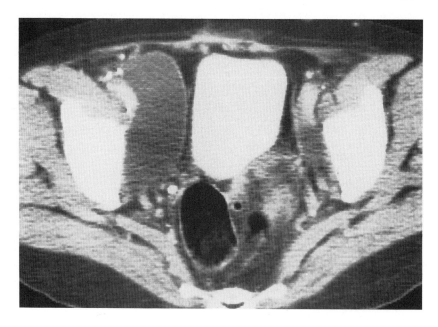

Figure 24-5. Lymphocele. On this pelvic CT examination a water-density mass is seen in the right pelvis, displacing the bladder to the left.

acutely ill patients cannot be monitored or attended during the examination. MRI is therefore less appropriate than ultrasonography.

Arteriography (Option (E)) is an invasive procedure and is not likely to provide additional information. The size of the mass certainly could be surmised from the draping of vessels supplying the adjacent structures, but the mass is better defined by cross-sectional imaging techniques. Since the mass is most probably a lymphocele or hematoma, it will not demonstrate neovascularity. Although an arterial injury may be the etiology, it is not likely to be demonstrated on an arteriogram in a patient who is hemodynamically stable.

Question 125

Concerning lymphoceles,

T (A) they occur after disruption of the lymphatic system
T (B) septations are commonly seen on ultrasonography
F (C) the diagnosis is confirmed by visual inspection of the aspirated fluid
F (D) the lymphatic etiology of the cyst can be predicted by MRI
F (E) they are readily cured by percutaneous aspiration

Lymphoceles are collections of extravasated lymph. They usually occur after surgery or other trauma in which the efferent lymphatic channels have been disrupted **(Option (A) is true).** Lymphoceles occur most commonly after pelvic lymphadenectomy combined with radical hysterectomy, where they may arise in 13 to 50% of cases. The incidence of lymphocele seems to be lower in patients undergoing pelvic lymphadenectomy for urologic cancer.

Most lymphoceles are seen within the first few weeks after surgery. The symptoms arising from lymphoceles are usually due to compression or displacement of adjacent structures. Small lymphoceles are asymptomatic.

Lymphoceles must be differentiated from other abnormal fluid collections, including urinomas, hematomas, bilomas, and abscesses. Whereas a hematoma or urinoma arises very quickly after injury, the development of a lymphocele may take several weeks.

Sonography is an excellent method of detecting lymphoceles. The cystic nature of these lesions distinguishes them from fibrosis and solid tumors, and they often occur in areas such as the pelvis or retroperitoneum, which are usually easily amenable to ultrasonographic evaluation.

The typical sonographic appearance of a lymphocele is that of a hypoechoic or anechoic mass with increased through transmission, consistent with the lesion's cystic nature (Figure 24-4). Internal echoes from scattered debris may be present. Thin septations are characteristic although not pathognomonic **(Option (B) is true).** The presence of a large amount of internal debris suggests infection.

Percutaneous aspiration is very helpful in confirming the diagnosis of a lymphocele. However, visual inspection of aspirated lymph is not sufficient for diagnosis **(Option (C) is false).** Lymphoceles range from almost clear to yellow or tan, and a small amount of cellular debris is often present. Measurement of the fluid creatine level of the aspirated fluid is needed to distinguish a lymphocele from a urinoma, while an elevated bilirubin level indicates a biloma or mature hematoma (seroma). Gram stain and culture may be used to exclude infection. Although fat globules are seldom demonstrated, their presence is virtually pathognomonic of a lymphocele.

MRI is often used in evaluating patients with prostate carcinoma. Unlike CT, no artifact is generated by surgical clips. Lymphoceles are recognized by their fluid content, which results in long T1 and T2 relaxation times. However, these features are found in other fluid collections and do not allow a specific diagnosis of lymphocele **(Option (D) is false).**

Small lymphoceles are often asymptomatic and seldom require treatment. Furthermore, they often resolve spontaneously. Large or symptomatic lymphoceles may be treated by surgical marsupialization into the peritoneal cavity. However, percutaneous treatments are often successful and surgery can be avoided. Simple needle aspiration is not adequate, because the lymphocele will usually recur **(Option (E) is false).** Long-term catheter drainage may be effective because there may be sufficient reactive inflammation to seal the leaking lymphatics. In most patients, however, it is necessary to use a sclerosing agent.

Reported series of percutaneous lymphocele drainage are too small to be statistically significant. However, Cohan et al. reported the percutaneous drainage of 13 pelvic lymphoceles; only three of six lymphoceles (50%) treated with catheter drainage were cured, whereas six of seven lymphoceles (86%) treated with povidone-iodine sclerosis were cured.

Question 126

Concerning pelvic lipomatosis,

T (A) it is most commonly seen in black men
F (B) it is associated with chronic urinary tract infection
T (C) large amounts of benign adipose tissue compress the bladder and rectum
F (D) ureteral obstruction is a common problem among older men
F (E) it is associated with transitional cell carcinoma

Pelvic lipomatosis is a benign proliferation of fibrofatty tissue within the pelvis. Most patients are asymptomatic, and the diagnosis is based on characteristic radiographic features. Therefore, the diagnosis is usually an incidental finding in patients who are being evaluated for other problems.

The age at presentation ranges from 9 to 80 years, but the majority of patients are between 30 and 70 years of age. Approximately two-thirds of reported patients are black, and very few women have been reported to be affected **(Option (A) is true)**.

No specific etiology has been found. Obesity has been suggested as the cause, but the correlation of lipomatosis with weight is poor. Patients with lipomatosis who have undergone cystoscopy reportedly have a high incidence of inflammatory changes in the bladder, including cystitis cystica and cystitis glandularis. However, an increased incidence of urinary tract infection has not been demonstrated in patients with pelvic lipomatosis **(Option (B) is false)**.

The diagnosis of pelvic lipomatosis is usually made on the basis of characteristic radiographic findings. Excessive pelvic fat compresses the bladder and rectum **(Option (C) is true)**. The bladder is elevated and has a vertical orientation, often resulting in a teardrop- or pear-shaped configuration (Figure 24-6). The posterior urethra is elongated due to the cephalic displacement of the bladder. Both distal ureters are medially deviated. The rectosigmoid colon is effaced and pushed out of the true pelvis.

The differential diagnosis of this constellation of findings includes pelvic hematoma, pelvic tumor, bilateral iliac artery aneurysms, occlusion of the inferior vena cava with extensive collateral vessels, retroperitoneal fibrosis, and iliopsoas muscle hypertrophy. The excess fat associated with pelvic lipomatosis produces a lucency on both sides of the bladder, whereas the other entities in the differential diagnosis have soft tissue density (Figure 24-6). Although this difference can often be appreciated on an abdominal radiograph, it is difficult to establish the diagnosis of lipomatosis with confidence based on conventional radiographs alone. Therefore, before CT became available, many patients underwent surgery to confirm the diagnosis of pelvic lipomatosis. The density differentiation afforded by CT is sufficiently accurate so that the presence of fat and the diagnosis of pelvic lipomatosis can be determined with a high degree of confidence.

The fatty nature of the excess tissue in the pelvis can also be determined by MRI. Since fat has short T1 and long T2 times, it has a strong signal intensity on both T1- and T2-weighted images.

The most common complications of pelvic lipomatosis are ureteral obstruction and iliac vein compression with secondary thrombosis. Crane and Smith found ureteral obstruction in 14 of more than 65 reported patients with pelvic lipomatosis. However, many asymptomatic patients go undiagnosed, so this complication is probably much less common than the reported frequency would suggest.

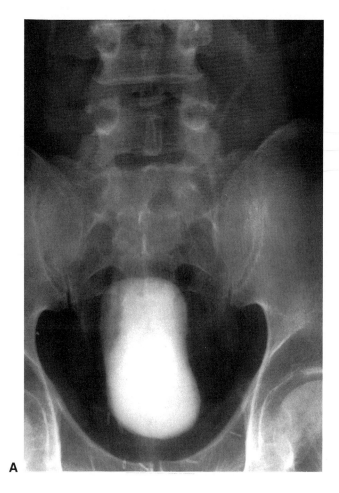

A

Figure 24-6. Pelvic lipomatosis. (A) On excretory urography, the bladder
has a vertical orientation and both distal ureters are medially deviated.
Increased lucency within the pelvis on both sides of the bladder indicates
fat. (B) This CT examination shows no pelvic mass and confirms the
presence of fat on both sides of the bladder.

Patients with pelvic lipomatosis may be divided into two groups. In
elderly men pelvic lipomatosis is usually diagnosed as an incidental
finding and rarely progresses **(Option (D) is false).** Younger men are
more prone to developing ureteral obstruction, and therefore follow-up
may be indicated.

Cystitis glandularis, cystica, or follicularis is found in 75% of patients
with pelvic lipomatosis. It has been postulated that these changes may
be related to venous or lymphatic stasis caused by the abundant pelvic
fat, leading to submucosal edema.

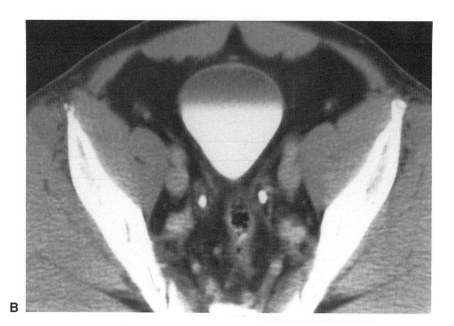

B

Cystitis glandularis is considered a premalignant lesion leading to adenocarcinoma. Despite the strong association of cystitis glandularis with pelvic lipomatosis, only two patients with both pelvic lipomatosis and adenocarcinoma of the bladder have been reported. There is no association of pelvic lipomatosis with transitional cell carcinoma **(Option (E) is false),** and the relationship with adenocarcinoma is based only on the two patients described above.

Question 127

Concerning pelvic hematoma,

T (A) it is uncommon in the absence of pelvic trauma
T (B) an acute hemorrhage can be diagnosed on CT by its high density
T (C) ultrasonography may reveal either an anechoic or an echogenic mass
F (D) the MR appearance is a function of the iron content
T (E) it rarely causes venous obstruction

The pelvic organs have a rich vascular supply. Injury or damage to either arteries or veins may create a large pelvic hematoma. Trauma, including iatrogenic injury such as vascular catheterization, biopsy, or surgery, is the most common cause of a pelvic hematoma. There are other

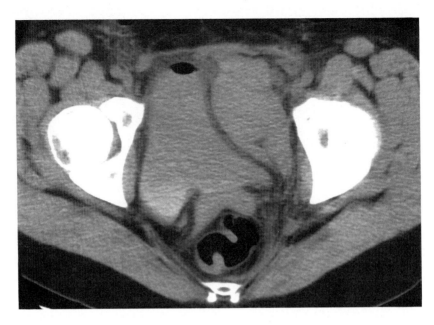

Figure 24-7. Hematoma. This CT scan shows a mass in the left pelvis deviating the bladder to the right. The density of this mass is higher than would be expected for a lymphocele or urinoma. In this patient, the occurrence of the mass after arteriography is most consistent with a hematoma.

causes, such as spontaneous bleeding from a malignant or benign pelvic tumor, ectopic pregnancy, aneurysm, or arteriovenous malformation, but these are rare **(Option (A) is true)**.

An acute hemorrhage into the pelvis is easily diagnosed by CT (Figure 24-7). Fluid-filled loops of bowel, which are occasionally confused with a pelvic hematoma, can be clearly defined by opacification with orally administered contrast material. An acute hemorrhage is distinguished by the higher attenuation coefficient of clotted blood **(Option (B) is true)**. Later, as the blood clot liquefies, the density decreases and may approach that of water.

The sonographic appearance of a pelvic hematoma depends on its age. A collection of clotted blood is seen as an echogenic mass. With time the clot may retract and be resorbed or may liquefy and become a serous fluid collection. This is seen as an anechoic mass **(Option (C) is true)**.

The appearance of blood on MRI is complex but is only partially due to the presence of iron **(Option (D) is false)**. The change of hemoglobin to deoxyhemoglobin and, finally, in chronic stages, to methemoglobin is the primary determinant of the MR signal characteristics. In the acute phase, hematoma has a medium signal intensity on T1-weighted images, making it difficult to distinguish from soft tissue. However, it has a high signal intensity on T2-weighted images. Sometimes a "hematocrit" phenomenon due to sedimentation of blood cell elements may be found. In the subacute phase, the hematoma has a high signal intensity on both T1- and T2-weighted sequences.

Occasionally, hematomas will demonstrate concentric rings of different signal intensity on T1-weighted images. The outer ring of low signal intensity reflects hemosiderin within macrophages around the hematoma. The inner ring has a higher signal intensity due to the hemoglobin degradation product methemoglobin.

A pelvic hematoma may displace the pelvic viscera. The bladder is easily compressed so that a pelvic hematoma extending to both sides of the bladder may mimic pelvic lipomatosis. The prostate gland and ureters are more firmly anchored in position, but adnexal structures, bowel loops, and renal allografts are easily moved by large pelvic hematomas. Despite this potential compressive effect, it is seldom sufficient to cause venous obstruction **(Option (E) is true)**.

N. Reed Dunnick, M.D.

SUGGESTED READINGS

LYMPHOCELES

1. Cohan RH, Saeed M, Schwab SJ, Perlmutt LM, Dunnick NR. Povidone-iodine sclerosis of pelvic lymphoceles: a prospective study. Urol Radiol 1988; 10:203–206
2. Gittes RF. Carcinoma of the prostate. N Engl J Med 1991; 324:236–245
3. Jensen SR, Voegeli DR, McDermott JC, Crummy AB. Percutaneous management of lymphatic fluid collections. Cardiovasc Intervent Radiol 1986; 9:202–204
4. Sogani PC, Watson RC, Whitmore WF Jr. Lymphocele after pelvic lymphadenectomy for urologic cancer. Urology 1981; 17:39–43
5. van Sonnenberg E, Wittich GR, Casola G, et al. Lymphoceles: imaging characteristics and percutaneous management. Radiology 1986; 161:593–596

PELVIC LIPOMATOSIS

6. Allen FJ, de Kock MLS. Pelvic lipomatosis: the nuclear magnetic resonance appearance and associated vesicoureteral reflux. J Urol 1987; 138:1228–1230

7. Crane DB, Smith MJ. Pelvic lipomatosis: 5-year followup. J Urol 1977; 118:547–550
8. Hatten HP Jr, Chuang VP, Rosenbaum HD. When is biopsy necessary in pelvic lipomatosis? Urology 1977; 9:333–336
9. Heyns CF. Pelvic lipomatosis: a review of its diagnosis and management. J Urol 1991; 146:267–273
10. Heyns CF, De Kock ML, Kirsten PH, van Velden DJ. Pelvic lipomatosis associated with cystitis glandularis and adenocarcinoma of the bladder. J Urol 1991; 145:364–366
11. Werboff LH, Korobkin M, Klein RS. Pelvic lipomatosis: diagnosis using computed tomography. J Urol 1979; 122:257–259

Notes

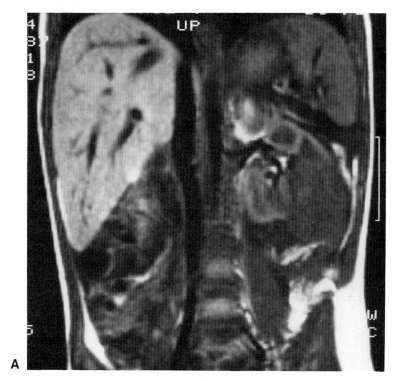

SE 500/17

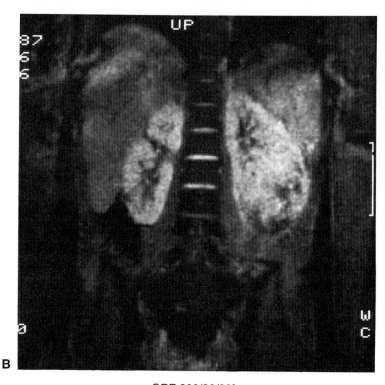

GRE 300/30/20°

Figure 25-1. This 4-year-old girl has left flank pain and fever. You are shown coronal T1-weighted (A) and gradient-recalled-echo (B) MR images.

Case 25: Wilms' Tumor with Perinephric Hemorrhage

Question 128

Which *one* of the following is the MOST likely diagnosis?

- (A) Traumatic subcapsular hematoma
- (B) Mesoblastic nephroma
- (C) Burkitt's lymphoma
- (D) Wilms' tumor
- (E) Renal abscess

The coronal T1-weighted abdominal MR image (Figure 25-1A) shows an area of low to intermediate slightly heterogeneous signal intensity attributable to a mass arising from the left kidney with more heterogeneous perinephric extension (see Figure 25-2) . The gradient-recalled-echo (GRE) image (Figure 25-1B) demonstrates intermediate to high signal intensity of the lower-pole renal mass and mixed signal intensity in the perinephric space. The areas of decreased signal intensity in the perinephric space are characteristic of hemorrhage. On GRE imaging, hemorrhage, regardless of its age, has a low signal intensity because of the magnetic susceptibility of blood products. These hemorrhagic areas are visible as areas of both T1 lengthening and T1 shortening on the T1-weighted image, presumably because of the various ages of the hemorrhages. The right kidney is normal. The MR findings in the test patient are most consistent with Wilms' tumor with an associated perinephric hemorrhage **(Option (D) is correct).** The patient's age and clinical presentation are also typical for this tumor.

Imaging modalities such as ultrasonography, CT, and MRI help to differentiate Wilms' tumor from the other possible causes of pediatric abdominal masses such as multicystic dysplastic kidney, hydronephrosis, neuroblastoma, polycystic renal disease, mesoblastic nephroma, renal abscess, subcapsular hematoma, and Burkitt's lymphoma. It is important to assess whether the mass is solid or cystic and whether it is intrarenal or extrarenal. The superior spatial resolution of sonography and CT

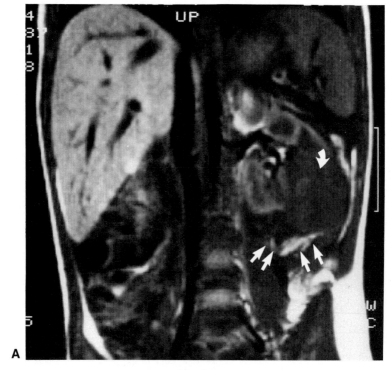

SE 500/17

Figure 25-2 (Same as Figure 25-1). Wilms' tumor with perinephric hemorrhage. (A) Coronal MR image demonstrating a left-lower-pole slightly heterogeneous mass (curved arrow). There is mixed low and high signal intensity in the perinephric space inferiorly (arrowheads). (B) Coronal GRE MR image at 1.0 T showing patchy areas of low signal intensity consistent with hemorrhage (straight arrows). These areas of hemorrhage were of variable signal intensity on the SE image (panel A).

provides for accurate depiction of the opposite kidney, whereas MRI and intravenous urography (IVU) are limited in this regard.

The typical Wilms' tumor is a bulky intrarenal mass that replaces most of the normal renal parenchyma and distorts the renal collecting structures. In many cases, the tumor contains areas of central hemorrhage and necrosis and is delineated sharply by a fibrous pseudocapsule on sonography and CT. On occasion, as in the test case, Wilms' tumor disrupts the renal borders and extends into the perirenal space. Midline extension occurs in only 20% of cases. Metastases occur either by direct extension into adjacent organs or by invasion of the intrarenal vessels with propagation into the renal vein and inferior vena cava (Figure 25-3).

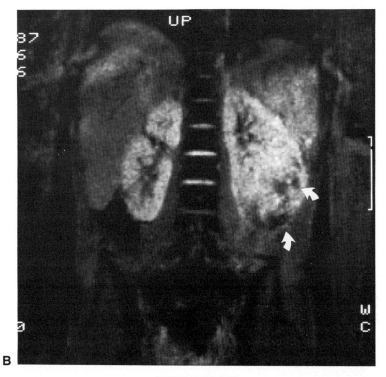

GRE 300/30/20°

B

Venous invasion explains the preponderance of pulmonary and hepatic metastases, which are present at the time of diagnosis in 12 to 20% and 8 to 10% of cases, respectively. Intra-abdominal extension takes the form of retroperitoneal lymphadenopathy in 20 to 40% of cases.

Another pediatric intrarenal mass is mesoblastic nephroma (Option (B)), but the age of the test patient and the perinephric extension argue against this diagnosis. Mesoblastic nephroma is the most common renal tumor during the first few months of life and should be suspected when a newborn or infant under 6 months of age has an intrarenal mass simulating a Wilms' tumor. It is a benign tumor composed mostly of fibrous and mesenchymal stroma that grows between intact nephrons, almost entirely replacing normal renal parenchyma. Mesoblastic nephromas characteristically are unencapsulated and infiltrating. Hemorrhage and necrosis, so common in Wilms' tumor, are generally absent. Prenatally, mesoblastic nephroma is detected as an intrarenal mass by ultrasonography, which is also the preferred postnatal method of diagnosis. On ultrasonography, the mass demonstrates low-intensity echoes that tend to be more uniform than in children with Wilms' tumor.

Case 25 / 425

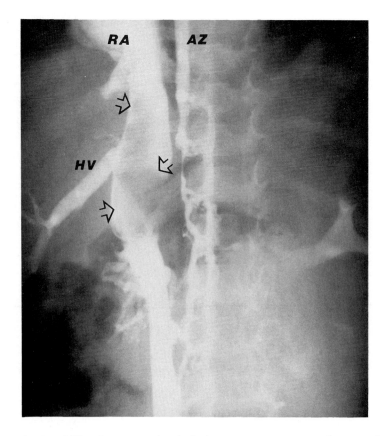

Figure 25-3. Wilms' tumor. An inferior venacavagram shows a large, left-sided tumor that has extended into the vena cava, producing a lobulated filling defect (arrows). RA = right atrium; HV = hepatic vein; AZ = azygous vein. (Courtesy of Harold A. Mitty, M.D., Mount Sinai Hospital, New York, N.Y.)

Burkitt's lymphoma (Option (C)) is the most common type of lymphoma in childhood. The age distribution of this tumor shows a peak at 4 to 7 years of life and again in adult life. Boys are affected two or three times more frequently than girls. An affected patient usually presents with an abdominal mass, which may originate in the bowel, kidneys, or gonads and may be accompanied by massive ascites. Patterns of renal involvement include multiple nodules, solitary nodules, invasion from perirenal disease, and diffuse perirenal retroperitoneal adenopathy (Figure 25-4). The perinephric hemorrhagic extension and lack of concomitant retroperitoneal or bowel disease make Burkitt's lymphoma an unlikely diagnosis in the test case.

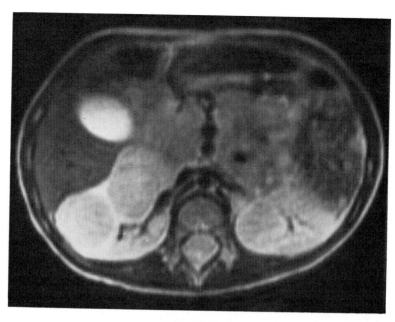

SE 2,000/84

Figure 25-4. Burkitt's lymphoma. Transverse MR image showing multiple bilateral renal nodules, one of the characteristic appearances of intrarenal Burkitt's lymphoma. (Courtesy of Rosalind Dietrich, M.D., University of California, Irvine.)

Patients with traumatic subcapsular hematoma (Option (A)) present with a palpable mass and tenderness in the flank and upper abdomen. There is usually associated gross hematuria. On cross-sectional imaging, a subcapsular hematoma appears as a lenticular fluid collection limited to the renal periphery and separated from Gerota's fascia by fat. It occupies the space between the renal parenchyma and the capsule. Limited by the relatively inelastic renal capsule, it flattens the underlying renal parenchyma but does not displace the kidney. The abdominal MR image in the test case shows a rounded intrarenal mass lacking the elliptical or lenticular configuration typical of a subcapsular hematoma.

Renal abscess (Option (E)) occurs at any age, and the patient commonly presents with spiking fever and leukocytosis. The clinical presentation of the patient in the test case is compatible with abscess. A renal abscess certainly could cause an intrarenal mass and could also give rise to a perinephric extension. Perinephric extension of an abscess would likely show similar MR signal intensity to the intrarenal component. In the test case, there is a striking difference of signal intensity present within the renal mass compared to the signal intensity of the hemorrhage in the perinephric space. The presence of perinephric hemorrhage mitigates against abscess.

Question 129

Concerning the MR appearance of hemorrhage,

T (A) it is determined partially by the pulse sequences
T (B) the age of the hemorrhage influences the signal intensity
T (C) narrow-flip-angle images are more sensitive for detection of hemorrhage than are standard spin-echo images
F (D) a bright signal on short-TR/short-TE images is specific for hemorrhage
T (E) hemorrhage can be differentiated from proteinaceous fluid on narrow-flip-angle GRE images

The appearance of hemorrhage on MRI is related to the specific type of hemoglobin present and the integrity of the erythrocytes. Initially, extravascular hemoglobin is in the form of oxyhemoglobin with no unpaired electrons available, so T1 and T2 relaxation times are intermediate. As the oxyhemoglobin becomes deoxygenated to deoxyhemoglobin, the resulting unpaired electrons cause a nonuniform magnetic field between the intact erythrocytes and the plasma, leading to T2 shortening. As the blood clot contracts it dehydrates, resulting in an increasing hematocrit; this also contributes to T2 shortening. This T2 shortening effect is more noticeable at higher field strengths, although it is also noted at intermediate field strengths, particularly on GRE images. Later the deoxyhemoglobin is oxidized to methemoglobin, which has five unpaired electrons and is paramagnetic, resulting in T1 shortening (Figure 25-5).

The pulse sequence selected will determine the appearance of hemorrhage on an MR image **(Option (A) is true)**. Acute hemorrhage has a signal intensity similar to that of muscle on T1-weighted (short-TR/short-TE) images and a lower signal intensity on T2-weighted (long-TR/long-TE) images, representing intracellular deoxyhemoglobin. Later, with the development of methemoglobin, the hemorrhage shows increasing signal intensity on T1-weighted images. As the erythrocytes lyse, the signal of the extracellular methemoglobin becomes bright on both T1- and T2-weighted images **(Option (B) is true)**.

Subacute hemorrhage is readily identified on spin-echo MR images by its high signal intensity on T1-weighted images, whereas acute hemorrhage lacks T1 shortening. Therefore, acute hemorrhage is seen as low

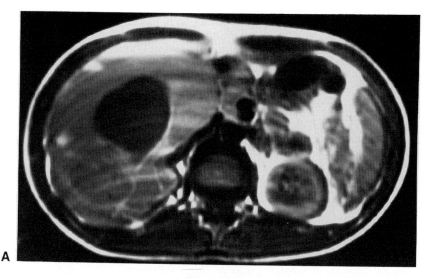

SE 2,000/20

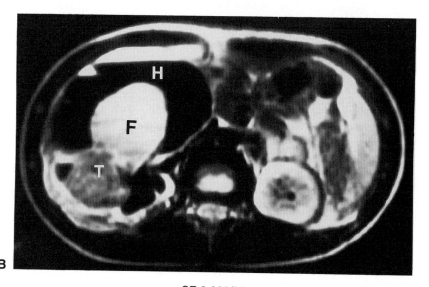

SE 2,000/80

Figure 25-5. Right renal sarcoma. (A) A transverse proton-density MR image shows an enlarged right kidney. There is a central rounded area of low signal intensity that is high in signal intensity on the T2-weighted image (see panel B), a finding that is characteristic of fluid. (B) This transverse T2-weighted MR image demonstrates heterogeneous signal intensity of tumor (T) located posteriorly. The fluid collection (F) is now high in signal intensity. Note the surrounding zone of very low signal intensity (H) with a fluid level anteriorly; this was found at surgery to represent relatively acute hemorrhage. (C) A coronal gradient-echo-recalled MR image shows intermediate signal intensity of tumor in the middle of the right kidney. The surrounding low signal intensity represents the hemorrhage. (Courtesy of George Bisset, III, M.D., Children's Hospital Medical Center, Cincinnati, Ohio.)

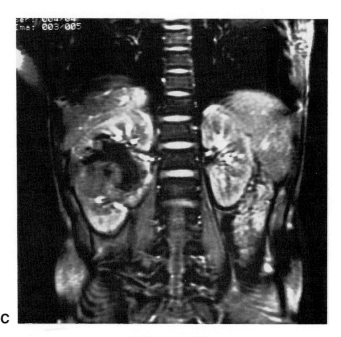

C

GRE 25/13/20°

signal intensity on T1-weighted images, particularly with high-field-strength magnets.

Spin-echo imaging uses the 90° pulse and then a 180° pulse to refocus the protons and correct for local field inhomogeneities. In GRE imaging, the initial pulse is less than 90° and the refocusing is accomplished through gradient reversal. Lacking the traditional 180° refocusing pulse, GRE images are more sensitive to local field inhomogeneities. With spin-echo techniques the contrast is dependent largely upon the T2 time, whereas the contrast created by GRE sequences is dependent on both T2 and the flip angle.

Narrow-flip-angle GRE images are more sensitive to methemoglobin concentration than are T1-weighted spin-echo images. On GRE images, hemorrhage, regardless of age, shows decreased signal intensity because of the magnetic susceptibility of blood products **(Option (C) is true).** On T1-weighted (short-TR/short-TE spin-echo) sequences, fresh hemorrhage appears as low to intermediate signal intensity and subacute hemorrhage appears as high signal intensity (Figure 25-6). Certain concentrations of protein and paramagnetic substances will also demonstrate high signal intensity on T1-weighted sequences **(Option (D) is false).** Narrow-flip-angle GRE imaging can be used to verify the presence of hemorrhage,

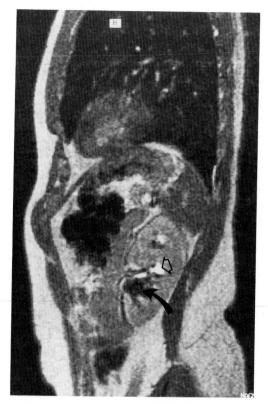

GRE 70/6/80°

Figure 25-6. Hemorrhagic multiloculated renal cyst. Sagittal gradient-echo-recalled MR image at 1.0 T demonstrating the low signal intensity of the cystic mass (solid arrow), verified to be a hemorrhagic cyst. The pure fluid of the adjacent normal collecting system (open arrow) has high signal intensity.

thereby differentiating protein-containing structures from those that contain blood products **(Option (E) is true).**

Question 130

Concerning mesoblastic nephroma,

(A) it is the most common intrarenal tumor in neonates
(B) it is occasionally associated with nephroblastomatosis
(C) calcification is common
(D) it is considered premalignant

The major clinical feature of mesoblastic nephroma is its onset early in infancy. The tumor is usually discovered as an abdominal mass in an infant younger than 6 months of age and is the most common intrarenal tumor in neonates **(Option (A) is true).** The congenital nature of the onset is further supported by prenatal detection. There is a reported association with polyhydramnios, but the relationship remains unclear. Male preponderance has been noted, as well as hypertension caused by hyperreninemia.

Grossly, congenital mesoblastic nephroma is a massive, firm, infiltrative, solitary renal mass. The histologic appearance of this lesion is distinctive, and it is considered an entity independent of Wilms' tumor: i.e., a hamartoma (fetal renal hamartoma) rather than a neoplasm. Calcification is uncommon **(Option (C) is false).** The infiltrative margins are difficult to delineate histologically from normal or dysplastic renal stroma, and there may be cartilaginous areas at this margin, a finding considered a hallmark of dysplasia.

The occasional "cellular" congenital mesoblastic nephroma may appear more ominous, and the distinction between this disorder and clear cell sarcoma may be arbitrary. The distinction is critical because congenital mesoblastic nephroma is virtually always benign **(Option (D) is false).** Local recurrence is unusual and results from incomplete excision. Mesoblastic nephroma is cured if it is completely resected; however, some pediatric oncologists treat it as a stage I Wilms' tumor. Nephrectomy is accompanied by tumor precautions including ligation of the vascular pedicle prior to tumor mobilization and minimal handling of the tumor to prevent rupture.

Nephroblastomatosis is a condition in which the renal cortex is diffusely infiltrated by undifferentiated cells of the renal blastema. These represent precursors of Wilms' tumor, but they undergo spontaneous regression in the majority of cases. Nephroblastomatosis is not associated with congenital mesoblastic nephroma **(Option (B) is false).**

Question 131

Concerning Wilms' tumor,

T (A) about 80% are diagnosed in patients less than 6 years old
T (B) it is composed of tubular, epithelial, and stromal tissue
T (C) aniridia is an associated feature
T (D) cell type is a better predictor of long-term prognosis than is the stage at presentation
F (E) nonfunction of the affected kidney is typical

In children more than 1 year old, Wilms' tumor (nephroblastoma) is the most common malignant intrarenal tumor and accounts for about one-fifth of all abdominal masses. It is responsible for 95% of malignant urinary tract neoplasms in children under age 16. Wilms' tumor is bilateral in about 10% of children.

The annual incidence of Wilms' tumor is 7.8 cases per million children, and there are over 500 new cases per year in the United States. The diagnosis is usually made between the ages of 1 and 5 years (78% of all cases), with a peak incidence at 3 years of age **(Option (A) is true).** This tumor is rarely found at birth or during the neonatal period. There have been occasional cases of Wilms' tumor in adolescence and adulthood. There is no sex or race predominance.

Affected children present with a palpable flank mass (about 80%) and less frequently with abdominal pain (30%), hematuria (25%), or fever (20%). Mild hypertension may be present in as many as 75 to 95% of patients with Wilms' tumor, along with increased plasma renin levels. The elevated levels of renin presumably are due either to renin production by neoplastic cells or to ischemia of the normal renal parenchyma caused by compression by the intrarenal neoplasm. Hypertension usually resolves after tumor resection.

Rare familial cases of Wilms' tumor have been observed. The heritable form is usually bilateral and is inherited as an autosomal dominant trait with incomplete penetrance. An individual with either a parent or a sibling with bilateral Wilms' tumor has a risk of up to 30% for developing a similar tumor. Approximately 15% of patients with Wilms' tumor have associated congenital abnormalities. Genitourinary abnormalities such as renal hamartomas or renal enlargement are most commonly associated. Other associated conditions include congenital hemihypertrophy, sporadic nonfamilial aniridia, Beckwith-Wiedemann syndrome, cerebral gigantism (Soto's syndrome), pseudohermaphroditism (Drash's syndrome), and neurofibromatosis. Wilms' tumor has been reported with chromosomal abnormalities, e.g., deletion of the short arm of chromosome 11 in patients with sporadic nonfamilial aniridia. Wilms' tumor will develop in approximately 30% of individuals with aniridia **(Option (C) is true)**. Etiologic factors for the more common nonhereditary Wilms' tumor have not been evaluated.

The main differential diagnostic consideration of Wilms' tumor in the young child is neuroblastoma. The vanillylmandelic acid (VMA) spot test is often performed to differentiate the two tumors. This test should be negative in Wilms' tumor patients and positive in at least 70% of patients with neuroblastoma. Another differentiating feature is that Wilms' tumor extends across the midline and displaces the major vessels in only 20% of cases, whereas neuroblastoma commonly extends across the midline, encircling the major vessels. Stippled calcification in an abdominal mass in children is more likely to indicate a neuroblastoma since these tumors calcify 60% of the time compared with 10% of Wilms' tumors.

Wilms' tumor may be central or polar and displaces normal renal tissue. In only 10% of patients will the affected kidney fail to function, attributable to infiltration of tumor throughout the kidney, tumor compressing the renal pelvis, or tumor invasion of the renal vein (Figure 25-7) **(Option (E) is false)**. Grossly, the tumor is usually pale and lobulated and is surrounded by a pseudocapsule of compressed renal tissue. Cut sections of Wilms' tumor usually demonstrate a mucinoid, gray-white lobular appearance secondary to multiple fibrous septa. It is composed of tubular, epithelial, and stromal tissue **(Option (B) is true)**. Microscopic classification of Wilms' tumor is made according to the degree of differentiation. Two major histologic types have been identified: favorable (no anaplasia, nonsarcomatous) and unfavorable (anaplasia, sarcomatous), with prevalences of 90 and 10%, respectively, and survival rates of 90% and 20 to 30%. Sarcomatous and anaplastic cell type tumors occur in older children and are associated with a poor prognosis even when discovered at an early stage **(Option (D) is true)**.

The clinicopathologic system of staging was designed by the National Wilms' Tumor Study (NWTS):

I. Tumor limited to kidney and completely excised
II. Tumor extending beyond the kidney but completely excised
III. Residual nonhematogenous tumor confined to the abdomen
IV. Hematogenous metastases
V. Bilateral renal involvement at diagnosis

Effective therapeutic modalities include surgery, radiation therapy, and chemotherapy. The multimodal treatment used depends on the clin-

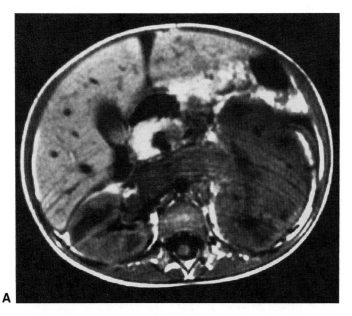

SE 600/12

Figure 25-7. Wilms' tumor with venous thrombus. (A) A transverse T1-weighted MR image shows a left renal mass with enlargement of the left renal vein and inferior vena cava as a result of tumor extension. (B) A sagittal T1-weighted MR image demonstrates the intermediate signal intensity of the tumor thrombus expanding the inferior vena cava. Note that the superior aspect of the thrombus (T) extends past the hepatic veins into the right atrium. (Courtesy of George Bisset III, M.D.)

icopathologic staging and histologic type of the tumor and the clinical condition of the individual patient. Wilms' tumor is the first human cancer to be successfully treated with adjuvant therapy (defined as chemotherapy given after all measurable tumor has been removed). Adjuvant therapy is used to eradicate micrometastases or microscopic residual disease.

Surgical resection remains the cornerstone of therapy for all children with Wilms' tumor. Nephrectomy is usually performed through a generous transperitoneal incision with early ligation of the renal pedicle. Careful inspection and palpation of the peritoneal contents are mandatory, with particular attention directed toward the periaortic lymph nodes, liver, spleen, and contralateral kidney. The 5 to 10% incidence of bilateral Wilms' tumor means that the opposite kidney must be thor-

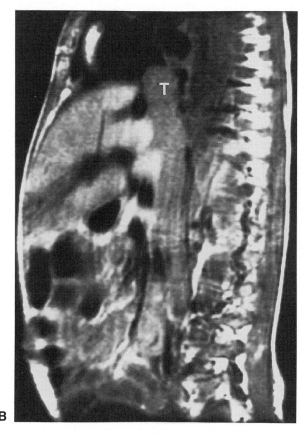

SE 600/12

oughly inspected. Extreme care must be taken to avoid spillage of tumor, because this has resulted in a higher rate of abdominal recurrence and higher mortality. Spillage of tumor necessitates more extensive radiation therapy with significant risk of side effects and complications.

Peggy J. Fritzsche, M.D.

SUGGESTED READINGS

PRIMARY RENAL NEOPLASMS

1. Beckwith JB, Palmer NF. Histopathology and prognosis of Wilms tumor: results from the First National Wilms' Tumor Study. Cancer 1978; 41:1937–1948

2. Beckwith JB, Weeks DA. Congenital mesoblastic nephroma: when should we worry? Arch Pathol Lab Med 1986; 110:98–99

3. Chan HS, Cheng MY, Mancer K, et al. Congenital mesoblastic nephroma: a clinicoradiologic study of 17 cases representing the pathologic spectrum of the disease. J Pediatr 1987; 111:64–70

4. Fernbach SK, Schlesinger AE, Gonzalez-Crussi F. Calcification and ossification in a congenital mesoblastic nephroma. Urol Radiol 1985; 7:165–167

5. Franken EA Jr, Yiu-Chiu V, Smith WL, Chiu C. Nephroblastomatosis: clinicopathologic significance and imaging characteristics. AJR 1982; 138:950–952

6. Hartman DS, Lesar MS, Madewell JE, Lichtenstein JE, Davis CJ Jr. Mesoblastic nephroma: radiologic-pathologic correction of 20 cases. AJR 1981; 135:69–74

7. Kirks DR, Kaufman RA, Babcock DS. Renal neoplasms in infants and children. Semin Roentgenol 1987; 22:292–302

8. Montgomery P, Kuhn JP, Berger PE, Fisher J. Multifocal nephroblastomatosis: clinical significance and imaging. Pediatr Radiol 1984; 14:392–395

9. Reiman TA, Siegel MJ, Shackelford GD. Wilms tumor in children: abdominal CT and US evaluation. Radiology 1986; 160:501–505

10. Rosenfield NS, Shimkin P, Berdon W, Barwick K, Glassman M, Siegel NJ. Wilms tumor arising from spontaneously regressing nephroblastomatosis. AJR 1980; 135:381–384

11. Sleight G, Lock MM. Clear cell sarcoma of the kidney: a renal tumor of childhood that metastasizes to bone. AJR 1986; 146:65–66

TRAUMATIC SUBCAPSULAR HEMATOMA

12. Belville JS, Morgentaler A, Loughlin KR, Tumeh SS. Spontaneous perinephric and subcapsular renal hemorrhage: evaluation with CT, US, and angiography. Radiology 1989; 172:733–738

13. Pollack HM, Wein AJ. Imaging of renal trauma. Radiology 1989; 172:297–308

LYMPHOMA

14. Negendank WG, al-Katib AM, Karanes C, Smith MR. Lymphomas: MR imaging contrast characteristics with clinical–pathologic correlations. Radiology 1990; 177:209–216

15. Weinberger E, Rosenbaum DM, Pendergrass TW. Renal involvement in children with lymphoma: comparison of CT with sonography. AJR 1990; 155:347–349

RENAL ABSCESS

16. Soulen MC, Fishman EK, Goldman SM, Gatewood OM. Bacterial renal infection: role of CT. Radiology 1989; 171:703–707

MRI OF HEMORRHAGE

17. McRitchie HA, Ridgway JP, Turbull LW, Kean DM. An observation of increased contrast due to both T1 and T2 weighting in a synthetic image. Magn Reson Imaging 1990; 8:261–266
18. Paajanen H, Schmiedl U, Aho HJ, Revel D, Terrier F, Brasch RC. Magnetic resonance imaging of experimental renal hemorrhage. Invest Radiol 1987; 22:792–798
19. Unger EC, Cohen MS, Brown TR. Gradient-echo imaging of hemorrhage at 1.5 Tesla. Magn Reson Imaging 1989; 7:163–172

KIDNEY MRI

20. Baumgartner BR, Chezmar JL. Magnetic resonance imaging of the kidneys and adrenal glands. Semin US CT MR 1989; 10:43–62
21. Belt TG, Cohen MD, Smith JA, Cory DA, McKenna S, Weetman R. MRI of Wilms' tumor: promise as the primary imaging method. AJR 1986; 146:955–961
22. Eilenberg SS, Lee JK, Brown J, Mirowitz SA, Tartar VM. Renal masses: evaluation with gradient-echo Gd-DTPA-enhanced dynamic MR imaging. Radiology 1990; 176:333–338
23. Fritzsche PJ. Current state of MRI in renal mass diagnosis and staging of RCC. Urol Radiol 1989; 11:210–214
24. Hricak H, Thoeni RF, Carroll PR, Demas BE, Marotti M, Tanagho EA. Detection and staging of renal neoplasms: a reassessment of MR imaging. Radiology 1988; 166:643–649
25. Kangarloo H, Dietrich RB, Ehrlich RM, Boechat MI, Feig SA. Magnetic resonance imaging of Wilms' tumor. Urology 1986; 28:203–207

Notes

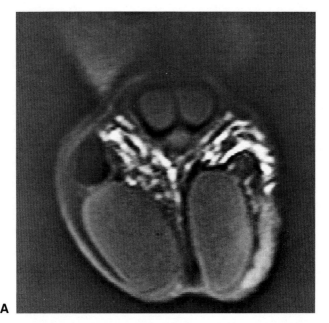

SE 500/26

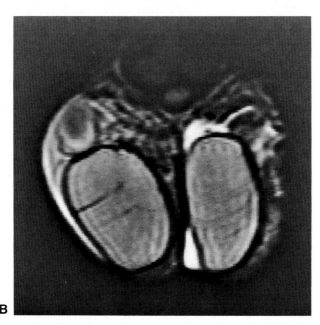

SE 2,500/80

Figure 26-1. This 46-year-old man presented with a palpable mass
the scrotum. You are shown coronal T1-weighted (A) and T2-weight
(B) MR images.

Case 26: Spermatocele

Question 132

Which *one* of the following is the MOST likely diagnosis?

(A) Varicocele
(B) Spermatocele
(C) Epididymal cyst
(D) Epididymitis
(E) Embryonal cell carcinoma

The testes can be seen in the test MR images as ovoid structures of intermediate signal intensity, each sharply defined by its dense fibrous capsule, the tunica albuginea (Figure 26-1). The epididymis lies along the posterior aspect of the testes and is subdivided into three regions: the head (globus major, located superiorly), the body, and the tail (globus minor, located inferiorly). A tortuous tubular structure located above the epididymal head represents the pampiniform plexus.

The lesion in the test MR images is a complex cyst (arrows, Figure 26-2) with low signal intensity centrally and intermediate signal intensity of the rim inferiorly. It is located outside the testicle in the head of the right epididymis. A spermatocele (Option (B)) and an epididymal cyst (Option (C)) are both cystic lesions and must be considered in the differential diagnosis in this patient. These lesions are indistinguishable by sonography because they have identical characteristics, i.e., well-marginated and anechoic epididymal lesions with good posterior sound transmission. Epididymal cysts contain serous fluid and appear on MRI as round, well-demarcated lesions with homogeneous T1 and T2 lengthening characteristic of simple fluid. Spermatoceles are also well demarcated but contain thick creamy fluid with spermatozoa and cellular debris; therefore, the MR signal is heterogeneous. The variable MR signal intensity of the extratesticular mass on the test images is characteristic of a spermatocele rather than an epididymal cyst **(Option (B) is correct).** A spermatocele is always located in the head of the epididymis.

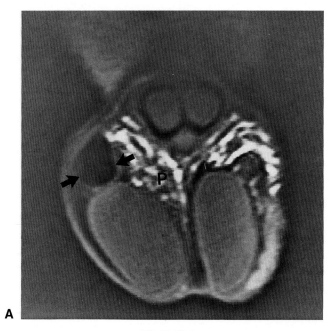

SE 500/26

Figure 26-2 (Same as Figure 26-1). Spermatocele. (A) Coronal T1-weighted MR image showing a unilocular mass with T1 lengthening characteristic of fluid but also an inferior thick rim of intermediate signal intensity (arrows) more consistent with the mixed fluid and debris of a spermatocele than with the simple fluid of an epididymal cyst. The serpiginous structures are consistent with the pampiniform plexus (P). (B) Coronal T2-weighted MR image confirms the heterogeneous signal intensity consistent with spermatocele and again shows the thicker rim inferiorly (straight arrows). The lesion was later confirmed to contain fluid, spermatozoa, and cellular debris. A small amount of high-signal-intensity fluid surrounds the testes and is within normal limits. The tunica albuginea is seen as a low-intensity structure surrounding the testis (curved arrows). The low-signal-intensity horizontal band in the mid right testis is an artifact.

While an epididymal cyst is more commonly found in the head of the epididymis, it may be located in the body or tail of the epididymis as well.

A varicocele (Option (A)) consists of an abnormal dilatation of the veins of the pampiniform plexus and the spermatic vein of the spermatic cord. A primary varicocele is idiopathic, possibly a result of incompetent valves in the internal spermatic vein leading to dilatation of the pampiniform plexus. A primary varicocele will decompress when the patient is supine.

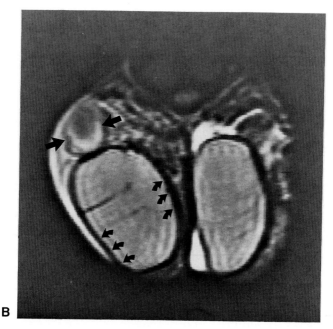

SE 2,500/80

A secondary varicocele results from chronic stasis caused by increased pressure on the spermatic vein by abdominal tumors, massive hydronephrosis, enlarged liver, aberrant renal artery, or compression of the renal vein. These secondary spermatoceles do not decompress in the supine position. A left-sided varicocele is more common than a right-sided varicocele, occurring in up to 15% of the male population. This is due to the longer and more tortuous anatomic pathway for venous drainage on the left; the internal spermatic vein first flows into the left renal vein before reaching the inferior vena cava. On the right side, drainage of the internal spermatic vein goes directly into the inferior vena cava. Unilateral right-sided varicoceles are rare, being noted in only 2% of normal men, and should suggest the possibility of a venous anatomic anomaly such as a left-sided inferior vena cava or obstruction (tumor or thrombus) of the internal spermatic vein or the inferior vena cava.

The diagnosis of a varicocele is usually made by physical examination, on which the lesion characteristically feels like a "bag of worms." The dilated veins are best palpated with the patient standing and performing the Valsalva maneuver. The majority of varicoceles are asymptomatic; they are usually incidentally detected during the investigation for male infertility. Up to 40% of infertile males may have a varicocele. The

40%

fertility problems are felt to be due to venostasis, increased scrotal heat, and abnormal anastomosis of draining veins resulting in retrograde blood flow. The subfertility that results is apparently responsible for the stress-pattern seminal fluid containing abnormally formed sperm. Small subclinical varicoceles have been shown to have the same effect of decreased sperm motility as large lesions. Varicoceles are visible on MRI as numerous extratesticular structures of high signal intensity on T2-weighted images. They can be differentiated from other extratesticular masses since they will extend into the inguinal region and will demonstrate a pronounced flow artifact.

Epididymitis (Option (D)) is a common extratesticular scrotal infection. It presents in any age group as sudden onset of scrotal pain and swelling. Hence, the finding of only a scrotal mass in the test patient argues against epididymitis. Fever and chills may develop, and patients usually have pyuria and bacteriuria. In sexually active men under 35 years old, *Chlamydia trachomatis* and *Neisseria gonorrhoeae* are the most common etiologic agents. In children and in men over 35 years old, *Escherichia coli* is the most common pathogen. The signal intensity of the infected portions of the epididymis in epididymitis is intermediate or high on T2-weighted images.

Embryonal cell carcinoma (Option (E)) represents about 25% of testicular tumors and occurs in the age range from 26 to 33 years and in infants. These testicular tumors present as fullness or heaviness in the affected testicle. Testicular pain also occurs and is thought to be secondary to hemorrhage into the tumor mass. Patients can also have scrotal swelling; however, in the majority of cases the mass is asymptomatic. Physical examination and ultrasonography differentiate intratesticular from extratesticular processes. Transillumination differentiates solid from fluid-filled masses. Of the options listed, embryonal cell carcinoma is the least likely, both because it would be an intra- rather than an extratesticular lesion and because it should appear as a solid rather than as a fluid-filled mass.

On MRI, intratesticular tumors show heterogeneous signal intensity lower than the intensity of the normal testis on T2-weighted images. Embryonal cell carcinoma is characteristically the most heterogeneous intratesticular neoplasm on MRI, with multiple areas of high and low signal intensity on the proton-density and T2-weighted images. Heterogeneity results from the presence of various stages of hemorrhage. This tumor is the most aggressive of intratesticular tumors and frequently invades the tunica albuginea. The size, margination, and location of testicular tumor are demonstrated on sonograms and MR images (Figure

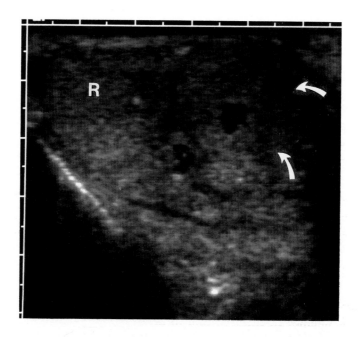

Figure 26-3. Intratesticular neoplasm. Transverse sonogram of both testes showing a left intratesticular mixed malignant tumor with indistinct margination (arrows) and central necrosis. The right testis (R) is homogeneous.

26-3). The superior contrast resolution of MRI provides better tissue demarcation than sonography and excellent depiction of the extent of the tumor. With extratesticular extension, the tunica albuginea becomes discontinuous, losing its characteristic low signal intensity, and the epididymis becomes heterogeneous in signal intensity.

Question 133

Concerning spermatoceles,

(A) they are located in the head of the epididymis
(B) typical components include lymphocytes and fat
(C) they are often confused with sperm granulomas
(D) they are incorporated within the tunica albuginea

Spermatoceles are either solitary or multiloculated extratesticular masses (Figure 26-4) that arise from obstructed ductules in the head of the epididymis **(Option (A) is true)** and lie just above and posterior to the testis outside the tunica albuginea **(Option (D) is false)**. Typical components of a spermatocele are spermatozoa, probably dead; a cloudy fluid; and a sediment made of lymphocytes, fat globules, and cellular debris **(Option (B) is true)**.

On MR images, spermatoceles are identified as extratesticular lesions in the head of the epididymis. They have a long T2 time because of their water content, and they demonstrate high signal intensity on T2-weighted images. Heterogeneous signal intensities appear as a result of the sensitivity of MRI to fluid and debris composition (Figure 26-5). Spermatoceles occur in older men and are often bilateral. Most spermatoceles are less than 1 cm in diameter, although they are occasionally quite large. Spermatoceles are usually discovered by the physician during routine examination of the genitalia; at times they are large enough to come to the attention of the patient, but they are always painless. They may be firm, simulating solid tumor. Examination reveals a freely movable transilluminating cystic mass lying above the testicle.

Cystic degeneration secondary to vasectomy rarely occurs, causing cystic distension of the tubules. If there is rupture of the cyst and leakage of sperm, a sperm granuloma may form. A sperm granuloma is a solid nodule of reactive granulomatous tissue located along the body of epididymis. Therefore a sperm granuloma should not be confused with a spermatocele **(Option (C) is false)**.

Sonographically, a multiloculated spermatocele may be difficult to distinguish from a varicocele; however, the physical findings of the two lesions are vastly different and are quite specific.

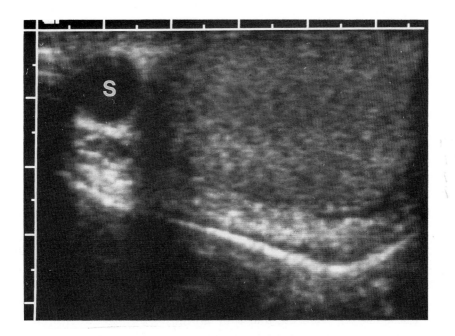

Figure 26-4. Spermatocele. Longitudinal sonogram showing the extra-testicular unilocular cystic lesion (S). The back wall enhancement indicates the fluid content of the lesion. This particular lesion cannot be distinguished sonographically from an epididymal cyst in the head of the epididymis because it is unilocular and because both lesions would be anechoic with back wall enhancement.

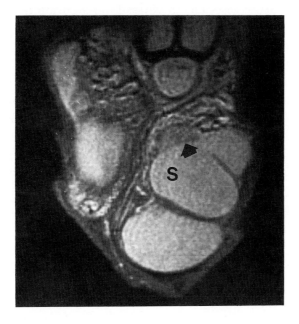

Figure 26-5. Spermatocele. A coronal T2-weighted MR image demonstrates a multiloculated extratesticular mass (S). There is T2 lengthening in most of the lesion, but variable T2 characteristics in a small, apparently loculated portion (arrow). (Courtesy of Robert Mattrey, M.D., University of California, San Diego.)

Question 134

Concerning epididymal cysts,

(A) they occur anywhere along the course of the epididymis
(B) the MR characteristics are those of a simple cyst
(C) they are often confused with varicoceles on MR imaging
(D) they are usually secondary to infection
(E) they are associated with adenomatoid extratesticular tumors

[handwritten annotations in left margin: T, T, F, F, F next to options; "Congenital but uncommon in children"]

Epididymal cysts are secondary to cystic dilatation of epididymal tubules and are considered a congenital abnormality of the epididymis. They most commonly occur in the head of the epididymis but are found anywhere along the course of the epididymis **(Option (A) is true)**. They are uncommon in children, and they are not associated with prior infection **(Option (D) is false)**. These cysts occur in normal men, but their incidence is increased in men who were exposed *in utero* to diethylstilbestrol.

Epididymal cysts usually present as painless swelling of the scrotum in young men. They rarely rupture spontaneously resulting in a hydrocele. They may rupture secondary to trauma with bleeding and then present as an acute scrotum. In general, an accurate diagnosis can be made by palpation, transillumination, and sonography; surgical exploration is not necessary unless the cyst grows. The effect of epididymal cysts on fertility is uncertain.

The MR characteristics of epididymal cysts are similar to those of other simple cysts containing serous fluid (i.e., long T1/long T2) **(Option (B) is true)**. Epididymal cysts are unilocular and therefore should not be confused with varicoceles **(Option (C) is false)**. As noted previously, they may be located in the head of the epididymis like spermatoceles, but, unlike spermatoceles, they are filled with simple fluid (Figure 26-6).

Adenomatoid tumors are the most common neoplasm of the epididymis and usually arise in the head or tail region (Figure 26-7). Rarely, they are found in the spermatic cord. These benign tumors have epithelial and fibrous elements. They are not associated with epididymal cysts **(Option (E) is false)**. They have the characteristics of a solid lesion on sonography.

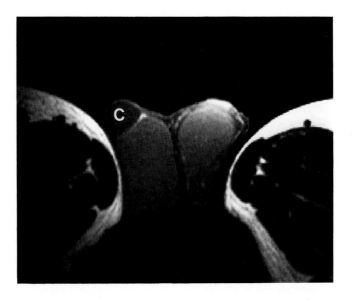

Figure 26-6. Epididymal cyst. A transverse T1-weighted image of the scrotum shows the well-demarcated low signal intensity of an epididymal cyst (C).

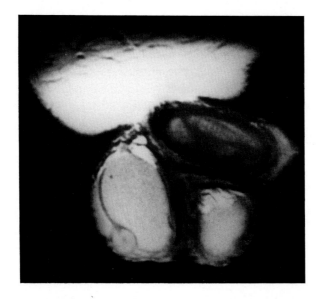

Figure 26-7. Adenomatoid tumor. A coronal proton-density MR image shows a well-demarcated extratesticular mass in the epididymal tail. Note the displacement of the tunica albuginea. (Courtesy of Robert Mattrey, M.D.)

Question 135

Concerning imaging of the scrotum,

(A) on T2-weighted MR images, the normal epididymis has low signal intensity
(B) ultrasonography is the modality of choice for differentiating intratesticular from extratesticular masses
(C) diffuse bilateral testicular involvement by leukemia is better detected by MRI than by ultrasonography
(D) MRI is the best method for diagnosing a varicocele
(E) tumor and abscess are reliably differentiated by signal characteristics on T2-weighted MR images

MRI of the scrotum is best accomplished with a surface coil because the coil can be easily applied near the structure of interest. A small distance between the suspended coil and the testes is preferable, since symptomatic patients may not be able to tolerate the discomfort of direct contact. The scrotum can be elevated by a towel draped over the thighs for easier positioning of the testes.

Short-TR/short-TE sequences show good testis-fat contrast, with the testis being lower in signal intensity than fat. On long-TR/long-TE sequences, the intensity of the testis becomes equal to or greater than that of fat. The tunica albuginea is composed of fibrous tissue, which has a short T2 relaxation time and shows a low signal intensity on both T1-and T2-weighted sequences. The epididymis varies in signal intensity, depending on the amount of fat between the tubules. Epididymal cysts, spermatoceles, and hydroceles have a long T2 time owing to their fluid content and demonstrate high signal intensity on T2-weighted images. The signal intensity of epididymitis may be normal or increased on T2-weighted images. Intratesticular neoplasms and inflammatory processes both show inhomogeneous areas of decreased signal intensity on T2-weighted images.

Transverse or coronal planes are preferred for detecting intratesticular tumor or inflammation since comparison of signal intensity between the two testes is thus more easily performed. The sagittal plane is the most effective plane for evaluation of the anteroposterior margins of the scrotum, since use of the coronal plane causes partial volume artifacts at the extreme anterior and posterior margins. The presence or absence of a spermatic cord is most reliably evaluated in the transverse and coronal planes but may also be identified in the sagittal plane.

MRI allows visualization of the scrotum and its contents in excellent anatomic detail (Figure 26-8). The differences in signal intensity between

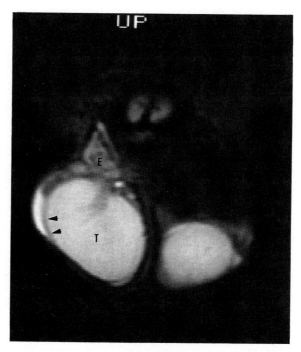

SE 2,500/80

Figure 26-8. Normal scrotum. Coronal T2-weighted MR image of the scrotum showing the intermediate to high intensity of the testis and the distinct low intensity of the circumferential tunica albuginea (arrowheads). The epididymis (E) is lower in signal intensity than the testis (T).

the epididymis, testis, tunica albuginea, fluid, fat, and spermatic cord allow clear delineation of these structures. On sonography, the tunica albuginea is seen as an echogenic circumferential line (Figure 26-9). It is more consistently visualized by MRI than by sonography. Both sonography and MRI will accurately distinguish between intratesticular and extratesticular disease. They will also be able to identify focal intratesticular lesions. Thurnher et al. demonstrated 4 false-negative evaluations in 20 patients evaluated for intratesticular disease when there was a diffuse infiltrating malignant tumor, including 2 with leukemic involvement, 1 with lymphomatous involvement, and 1 with a large Leydig cell tumor. Lymphomatous lesions are the most common testicular lesions in men over 50 years of age and account for nearly 5% of all testicular neoplasms. These lesions are usually infiltrative and may be a late manifestation of disseminated disease. Children with leukemia are often followed for leukemic infiltration of the testes since these are a

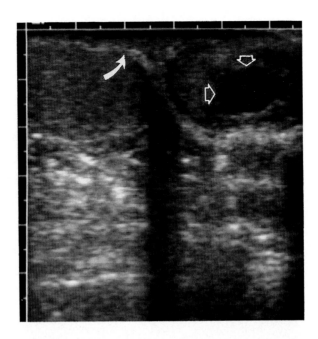

Figure 26-9. Testicular tumor. Transverse sonogram of both testes showing a well-demarcated Sertoli-Leydig cell tumor (open arrows). Note the hyperechoic circumferential tunica albuginea outlining the testes (curved arrow).

well-known site for recurrence. In these cases with leukemic or lymphomatous infiltration, the entire testis can be affected diffusely with decreased signal intensity (Figure 26-10). MRI is considered superior to sonography for evaluating bilateral testicular lymphomatous or leukemic infiltration since the signal intensity may be altered diffusely in both testes **(Option (C) is true).**

On MRI, the normal testis appears as a sharply defined oval structure. It has homogeneous intermediate signal intensity on T1-weighted and proton-density images and high signal intensity on T2-weighted images in comparison with the appearance of subcutaneous fat. Its intensity on T2-weighted images is similar to or slightly lower than that of the fluid frequently present between the layers of the tunica vaginalis. The testes are surrounded by a thin layer (less than 1 mm) of low signal intensity called the tunica albuginea. It has lower signal intensity than the testis on T2-weighted images and is the border separating intratesticular and extratesticular processes.

The outer parietal and inner visceral layers of the tunica vaginalis are frequently separated by a small layer of fluid (up to 2 mm thick). In-

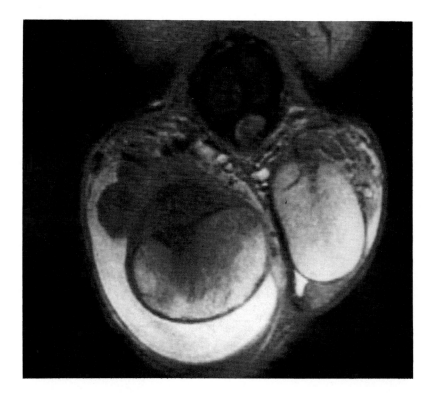

Figure 26-10. Lymphoma. A coronal T2-weighted MR image demonstrates diffuse lymphomatous infiltration of the right testis. The normal high signal intensity of the testis has been replaced by the low signal intensity of the lymphoma. The tumor also involves the head of the epididymis. (Courtesy of Robert Mattrey, M.D.)

creased amounts of fluid are consistent with the diagnosis of a hydrocele (Figure 26-11). The fluid may completely surround the testes, except for the posteromedial "bare area" where the testis is attached to the scrotal wall.

The head, body, and tail of the epididymis are easily delineated. Furthermore, the epididymis is clearly demarcated from the high signal intensity of the testis and the low signal intensity of the tunica albuginea. On balanced images, the epididymis is seen as an area of heterogeneous intermediate signal intensity lower than or equal to that of normal testicular tissue. On T2-weighted images, it is markedly less intense than the testis (see Figure 26-8) **(Option (A) is true).**

The key question to be answered in scrotal imaging is whether a lesion is intratesticular or extratesticular. The multiplanar imaging capabilities of both sonography and MRI make these modalities ideal for performing

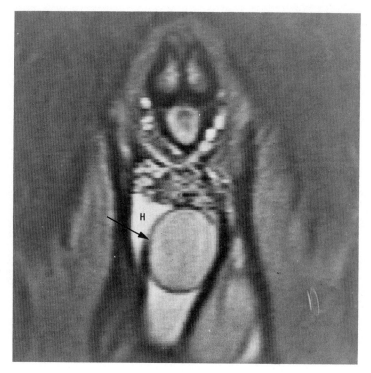

SE 2,500/70

Figure 26-11. Hydrocele. Coronal T2-weighted MR image of the scrotum showing a hydrocele (H) surrounding the right testis. The tunica albuginea (arrow) separates the hydrocele from the testes.

this differentiation. MRI has the advantages of a larger field of view, which permits simultaneous assessment and comparison of the right and left hemiscrotal contents, and outstanding contrast resolution, which permits detailed visualization of scrotal anatomy. However, since the most important question is simply whether the lesion is intratesticular or extratesticular, sonography, as the more accessible and less costly method, remains the modality of choice for scrotal imaging **(Option (B) is true).**

The spermatic cord contains the vas deferens and testicular vessels. Tortuous tubular structures of low signal intensity located at the posterosuperior aspect of the testes represent the pampiniform plexus, which can be followed into the inguinal canal. Serpiginous areas of high signal intensity within the cord on proton-density and T2-weighted images are presumed to represent phase-shift artifact as a result of slow

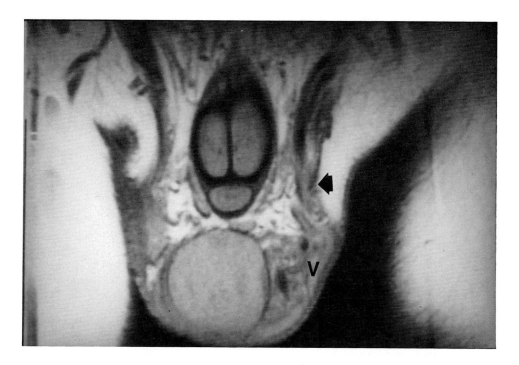

Figure 26-12. Varicocele. A coronal proton-density MR image shows serpiginous extratesticular structures (V) following the spermatic cord (arrow) into the inguinal region. (Courtesy of Robert Mattrey, M.D.)

flow in the venous plexus. The vas deferens is more likely to be identified separately from the vessels on a transverse image.

Varicoceles have characteristics that allow them to be differentiated from other scrotal processes. Their presence produces enlargement of the spermatic cord, which can be followed from the inguinal ring to the mediastinum testis (Figure 26-12). The cord has characteristically greater numbers of high-intensity, serpiginous structures on both proton-density and T2-weighted images owing to the phase shift artifact produced by slow flow. Since this artifact may interfere with the evaluation of a varicocele by MRI, sonography remains the procedure of choice for diagnosis **(Option (D) is false).**

Tumors are of heterogeneous signal intensity that is equal to or lower than the intensity of the normal testis on proton-density images and markedly lower on T2-weighted images. The low signal intensity of intratesticular lesions is nonspecific, occurring with neoplasm, infarction, infection, and scarring. Therefore, one cannot rely on signal intensity for differentiation of testicular infection and tumor **(Option (E) is false).**

Tumors are usually well-defined masses, whereas infection is patchy and less well defined. Associated epididymal infection and clinical presentation would be helpful in the diagnosis of orchitis.

Peggy J. Fritzsche, M.D.
May Kinaly, M.D.

SUGGESTED READINGS

TESTIS AND EPIDIDYMIS

1. Gooding GA, Leonhardt W, Stein R. Testicular cysts: US findings. Radiology 1987; 163:537–538
2. Hamm B, Fobbe F, Loy V. Testicular cysts: differentiation with US and clinical findings. Radiology 1988; 168:19–23
3. Johnson JO, Mattrey RF, Phillipson J. Differentiation of seminomatous from nonseminomatous testicular tumors with MR imaging. AJR 1990; 154:539–543
4. Nemcek AA Jr, Fisher MR, Leschorn E, et al. Mixed sex-cord stromal tumor of the testis: evaluation by ultrasonography and magnetic resonance imaging. Urol Radiol 1989; 11:186–189

IMAGING OF THE SCROTUM

5. Baker LL, Hajek PC, Burkhard TK, et al. MR imaging of the scrotum: pathologic conditions. Radiology 1987; 163:93–98
6. Baker LL, Hajek PC, Burkhard TK, et al. MR imaging of the scrotum: normal anatomy. Radiology 1987; 163:89–92
7. Fritzsche PJ. MRI of the scrotum. Urol Radiol 1988; 10:52–57
8. Fritzsche PJ, Wilbur MJ. The male pelvis. Semin US CT MR 1989; 10:11–28
9. Rholl KS, Lee JK, Ling D, Heiken JP, Glazer HS. MR imaging of the scrotum with a high-resolution surface coil. Radiology 1987; 163:99–103
10. Seidenwurm D, Smathers RL, Lo RK, Carrol CL, Bassett J, Hoffman AR. Testes and scrotum: MR imaging at 1.5 T. Radiology 1987; 164:393–398
11. Thurnher S, Hricak H, Carroll PR, Pobiel R, Filly RA. Imaging the testis: comparison between MR imaging and US. Radiology 1988; 167:631–636

Notes

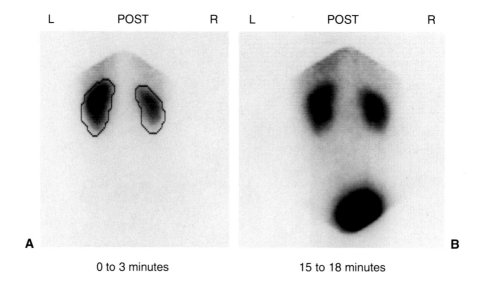

L POST R L POST R

A
0 to 3 minutes

B
15 to 18 minutes

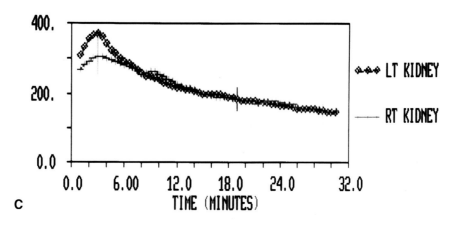

◆◆◆ LT KIDNEY

— RT KIDNEY

C

Figure 27-1

Figures 27-1 and 27-2. This 33-year-old hypertensive woman with normal renal function underwent Tc-99m DTPA renal scintigraphy before (Figure 27-1) and after (Figure 27-2) the oral administration of captopril.

Case 27: Renovascular Hypertension

Question 136

Concerning the test patient,

(A) left renal artery stenosis is likely to be present
(B) a greater discrepancy in relative tracer accumulation after captopril administration would have been present if I-131 *o*-iodohippurate had been used instead of Tc-99m DTPA
(C) the changes seen after captopril administration are secondary to efferent arteriolar vasodilatation
(D) a satisfactory blood pressure response to renal revascularization is likely

Figures 27-1A and B are images obtained during Tc-99m DTPA renal scintigraphy prior to administration of captopril. Figure 27-1A, obtained during the first 3 minutes after injection of the tracer, shows prompt, relatively symmetric accumulation of the radiopharmaceutical by the kidneys. The right kidney is slightly smaller than the left and has slightly less uptake of Tc-99m DTPA. Figure 27-1B, a 15–18 minute image, demonstrates normal symmetric clearance of the Tc-99m DTPA. The renogram curves (Figure 27-1C) confirm these findings of mildly reduced right-sided uptake and essentially symmetric excretion of Tc-99m DTPA by the kidneys.

Figure 27-2 consists of corresponding renal images and renogram curves in the same patient following reinjection of Tc-99m DTPA 1 hour after oral administration of captopril. The 0–3 minute image (Figure 27-2A) shows a dramatic change from the baseline study, with markedly decreased tracer accumulation by the right kidney, a finding that is still apparent on the 15–18 minute image (Figure 27-2B). The postcaptopril renogram curves (Figure 27-2C) also show the marked decrease in right renal accumulation of Tc-99m DTPA. In this patient the postcaptopril change is obvious from inspection of the scintigraphic images; the renogram curves are merely confirmatory.

Renal scintigraphy in conjunction with administration of an angiotensin-converting enzyme (ACE) inhibitor, such as captopril, is performed

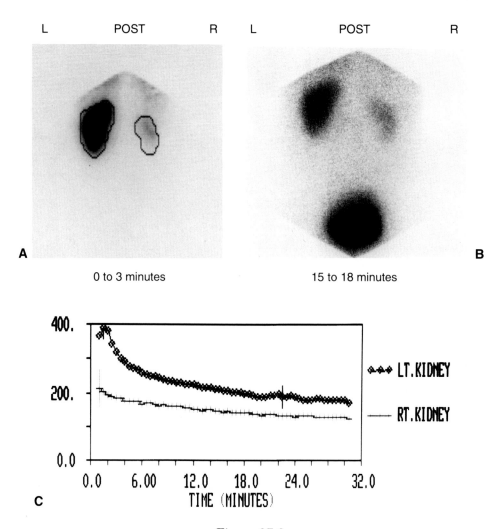

A

B

0 to 3 minutes

15 to 18 minutes

C

Figure 27-2

in patients with hypertension suspected to be caused by renal artery stenosis (RAS). The study is relatively noninvasive and can easily be performed in outpatients without special preparation, except that use of ACE inhibitors should be discontinued before the study. Therapy with other antihypertensive drugs need not be discontinued, although for safety reasons the patients should not be severely sodium or fluid depleted. Some investigators therefore recommend that diuretics should be discontinued for at least 5 days before the study. Specific protocols vary, but the general approach is similar. Some investigators favor imaging with and without captopril on two separate days, whereas others recommend a 1-day protocol. Still other investigators have recommended performing the initial study with captopril and performing a baseline study without captopril only if the first examination gives equivocal results.

A sample 1-day protocol is as follows. Initially, the patient's blood pressure is checked. If fluid loading is not contraindicated, the patient is hydrated intravenously to ensure good urine flow during the study. The patient is injected with a first dose of radiopharmaceutical (the test patient received Tc-99m DTPA). A standard renal scintigraphic study is performed, with acquisition of both analog and digital images, so that differential renal function can be determined by standard methods and renogram curves can be generated. The second portion of the study is begun approximately 90 to 120 minutes after injection of the first dose of radiopharmaceutical; this delay is necessary to allow for the clearance of the tracer used for the first scintigraphic study. The patient's blood pressure is again recorded. The patient is then given 50 mg of captopril by mouth. (Administering the captopril on an empty stomach will facilitate oral absorption, as will crushing the captopril tablet.) The blood pressure should be monitored every 15 minutes, and the patient should continue to receive intravenous fluids. Sixty minutes after captopril administration, a second dose of radiopharmaceutical is injected and standard images are acquired again.

Pre- and postcaptopril images and time-activity curves are then analyzed for evidence of captopril-induced deterioration of renal function. Captopril does not affect the glomerular filtration rate (GFR) in normal patients or in those with essential hypertension, but it does cause decreased renal function in kidneys affected with hemodynamically significant RAS. As is illustrated in Figure 27-3 and discussed further in Question 138, the reason that captopril causes decreased renal function in a kidney with RAS is that it acts to produce efferent arteriolar vasodilatation by blocking the conversion of angiotensin I to angiotensin II **(Option (C) is true).** In a kidney with RAS, increased production of angiotensin II causes preferential efferent arteriolar vasoconstriction. This increases pressure in the glomerulus, and thus filtration continues. With ACE inhibition and the resultant decline in the angiotensin II level, efferent arteriolar vasodilation occurs. Even though overall renal blood flow may actually increase, the drop in perfusion pressure at the glomerulus leads to a net drop in filtration, resulting in both decreased Tc-99m DTPA uptake and decreased urine flow. In the test patient, the postcaptopril study (Figure 27-2) shows markedly decreased right renal uptake of Tc-99m DTPA by comparison with the baseline study (Figure 27-1). Therefore, this is the kidney that is likely to have RAS. The left

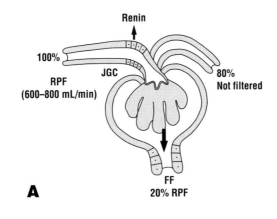

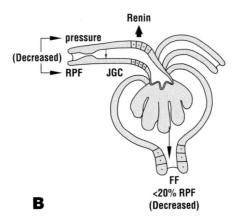

Figure 27-3. Physiologic effects of renal artery stenosis and angiotensin-converting enzyme inhibition on the kidney. (A) In the normal kidney, renal plasma flow (RPF) is 600 to 800 mL/minute and the filtration fraction (FF) is 20%. Renin is produced in normal quantities in response to variations in afferent arteriolar pressure detected by the juxtaglomerular complex (JGC). (B) In the kidney with significant renal artery stenosis, the renal plasma flow is decreased, the glomerular filtration rate is also decreased, and the filtration fraction is usually decreased. The decreased afferent arteriolar blood pressure is detected by the juxtaglomerular apparatus, resulting in increased renin secretion. (C) Compensated renal artery stenosis. The increased renin secretion leads to increased production of angiotensin II, which causes efferent arteriolar vasoconstriction. This raises the glomerular pressure, which helps to preserve the glomerular filtration rate and to restore the filtration fraction. (D) In the kidney with renal artery stenosis, angiotensin-converting enzyme inhibition produces efferent arteriolar vasodilatation, which leads to a decrease in the glomerular filtration rate and the filtration fraction. (Adapted with permission from Sfakianakis et al. [17].)

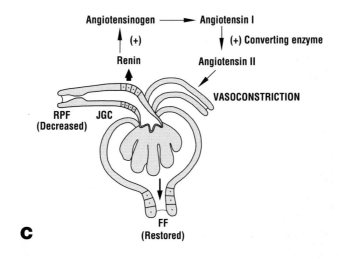

C

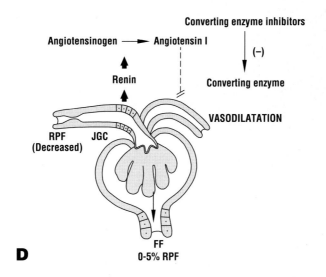

D

kidney does not show an obvious change in its uptake or excretion of Tc-99m DTPA following captopril administration, and thus left RAS is unlikely to be present **(Option (A) is false).** Figure 27-4 is an angiogram of the test patient, confirming right RAS. No significant left RAS is identified.

Captopril renal scintigraphy can be performed with Tc-99m DTPA, with either I-131 or I-123 *o*-iodohippurate (OIH), or with Tc-99m mercaptoacetylglycylglycylglycine (Tc-99m MAG3) (see below). When captopril renal scintigraphy is performed with Tc-99m DTPA, the accumulation

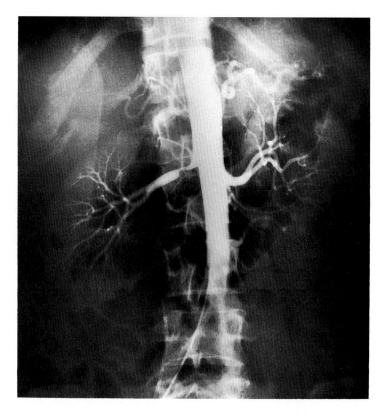

Figure 27-4. Same patient as in Figures 27-1 and 27-2. Renal arteriography demonstrates a high-grade stenosis of the proximal right renal artery. The left renal artery is normal.

and the rate of excretion of the tracer by the kidney with RAS decrease, as seen in the test patient. This is because Tc-99m DTPA is excreted by glomerular filtration. The efferent arteriolar vasodilatation produced by captopril causes a decrease in GFR and urine flow in the kidney with RAS (and, consequently, causes a decrease in renal uptake and excretion of Tc-99m DTPA) (Figure 27-5).

When I-131 OIH is used for captopril renal scintigraphy, the chief effect of captopril on the kidney with RAS is prolongation of the transit of the radiopharmaceutical in the kidney (Figure 27-5). OIH is excreted by the kidney predominantly through tubular secretion; glomerular filtration is only a minor component of total excretion because about 70% of the drug in plasma is bound to proteins. When captopril renal scintigraphy is performed with I-131 OIH, there is continued accumulation of tracer (reflecting maintained tubular uptake and secretion) in the kidney with

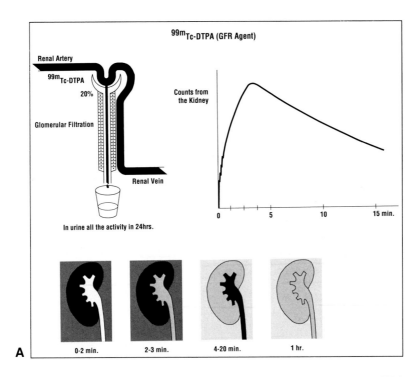

Figure 27-5. Illustration of the renal handling of Tc-99m DTPA and I-131 OIH. (A) Tc-99m DTPA handling by the normal kidney and by one with compensated renal artery stenosis (RAS). Tc-99m DTPA is eliminated by glomerular filtration. There is no tubular secretion or reabsorption. The normal renogram curve and sequential images reflect prompt uptake and excretion of the radiopharmaceutical. (B) In the kidney with renal artery stenosis, captopril-induced decompensation causes a dramatic decrease in glomerular filtration. There is flattening of the time-activity curve, reflecting the decreased uptake and delayed excretion of Tc-99m DTPA by the kidney. With bilateral renal artery stenosis, both kidneys will show changes as a result of the decrease in glomerular filtration. (C) I-131 OIH handling by the normal kidney and by one with compensated renal artery stenosis. I-131 OIH is eliminated by both filtration (ca. 20%) and tubular secretion (ca. 80%). Again, the normal renogram curve and sequential images reflect prompt uptake and excretion of this radiopharmaceutical. (D) In the kidney affected by RAS, captopril-induced decompensation causes a dramatic decrease in glomerular filtration. Renal uptake of I-131 OIH is little changed, but, because of the decrease in the rate of urine flow, there is marked prolongation of the cortical transit time of the radiopharmaceutical in the affected kidney. (Adapted with permission from Sfakianakis et al. [17].)

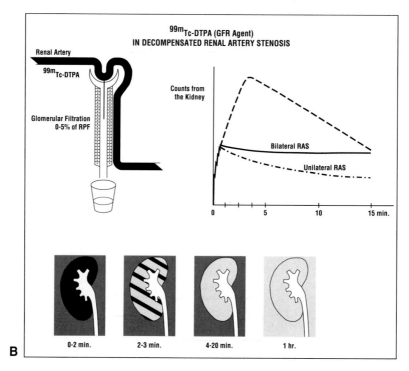

**99mTc-DTPA (GFR Agent)
IN DECOMPENSATED RENAL ARTERY STENOSIS**

Renal Artery

99mTc-DTPA

Glomerular Filtration
0-5% of RPF

Counts from
the Kidney

Bilateral RAS

Unilateral RAS

0   5   10   15 min.

0-2 min.   2-3 min.   4-20 min.   1 hr.

B

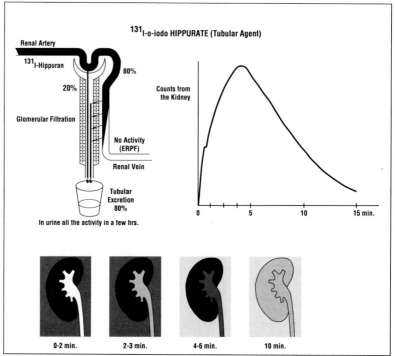

131I-o-iodo HIPPURATE (Tubular Agent)

Renal Artery

131I-Hippuran

20%

80%

Glomerular Filtration

No Activity
(ERPF)

Renal Vein

Tubular
Excretion
80%

In urine all the activity in a few hrs.

Counts from
the Kidney

0   5   10   15 min.

0-2 min.   2-3 min.   4-6 min.   10 min.

C

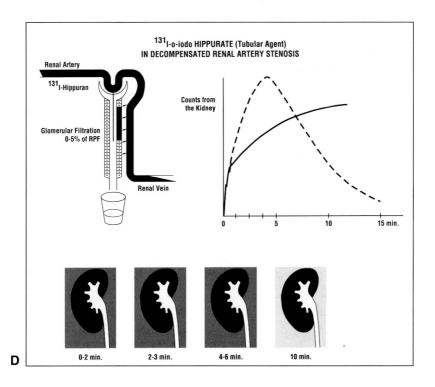

131I-o-iodo HIPPURATE (Tubular Agent)
IN DECOMPENSATED RENAL ARTERY STENOSIS

Renal Artery

131I-Hippuran

Counts from
the Kidney

Glomerular Filtration
0-5% of RPF

Renal Vein

0   5   10   15 min.

0-2 min.   2-3 min.   4-6 min.   10 min.

D

RAS. However, the captopril-induced decline in glomerular filtration results in a decrease in the rate of urine flow, and cortical activity thus persists for longer than normal (reflecting the delayed intrarenal transit time). Serial monitoring for a long enough period shows that the I-131 OIH is eventually cleared from the kidney. The discrepancy in relative tracer accumulation in the affected kidney between the pre- and postcaptopril images is therefore much smaller with I-131 OIH than with Tc-99m DTPA, the agent used in the test case **(Option (B) is false).**

In 1990, a new radiopharmaceutical for renal imaging, Tc-99m MAG3, was approved for use in the United States. Tc-99m MAG3 provides images of superb quality, even in patients with poor renal function, and will probably replace Tc-99m DTPA and I-131 OIH for renal imaging for most clinical indications, including captopril renal scintigraphy. Tc-99m MAG3 is secreted predominantly by the renal tubules, with only a small amount filtered (the plasma protein binding of this drug is approximately 90%). Consequently, scintigraphic images obtained with this agent are similar in appearance to those obtained with I-131 OIH; i.e., during captopril renal scintigraphy, a kidney with RAS will exhibit delayed radiopharmaceutical transit and persistent cortical activity. However, the images obtained with Tc-99m MAG3 are of substantially better quality than those obtained with I-131 OIH.

Captopril renal scintigraphy has been shown to be accurate in predicting which patients are likely to respond well to revascularization. For example, Geyskes et al. studied 34 patients suspected to have renovascular hypertension (RVH). Arteriography demonstrated unilateral RAS in 21 of these 34 patients, and all underwent angioplasty or nephrectomy. Fifteen patients had improved blood pressure control or cure of hypertension postrevascularization (or postnephrectomy); these patients were considered to have RVH. Captopril scintigraphy was abnormal unilaterally in 12 of these 15 patients. Six patients did not respond to angioplasty and were defined as having nonfunctional RAS (i.e., RAS not causally related to the hypertension), and 13 patients had normal renal arteries. Captopril scintigraphy gave negative results not only in the 13 patients with normal renal arteries, but also in all 6 patients with nonfunctional RAS. Overall, these investigators obtained a sensitivity of 80% and a specificity of 100% for captopril scintigraphy in detection of RVH. In the test patient, a satisfactory blood pressure response to revascularization of the right kidney is likely **(Option (D) is true).** Captopril renal scintigraphy also has an advantage over other radiologic imaging techniques in that it may easily be performed for follow-up assessment of patients who have undergone surgery or angioplasty. A small study by Fommei et al. obtained results similar to those of Geyskes et al. They also studied, at various intervals postintervention, patients who had undergone repair of RAS by surgical revascularization or angioplasty. They found a good correspondence of captopril scintigraphy with therapeutic outcome of revascularization. Some investigators suggest that captopril scintigraphy may be a more physiologic test than arteriography. Captopril scintigraphy detects lesions of hemodynamic significance, whereas an arteriogram may detect RAS that is not causing the patient's hypertension.

Bilateral false-positive captopril studies, simulating the findings of bilateral RAS, have been reported in association with an excessive drop in diastolic blood pressure after captopril administration. Thus, some investigators recommend repeating bilaterally positive studies in patients who have had a marked decline in diastolic blood pressure. Ensuring that patients are adequately hydrated and not excessively salt depleted may avoid these dangerous and potentially misleading blood pressure changes. Available data suggest that the accuracy of captopril scintigraphy is otherwise similar in patients with bilateral and those with unilateral RAS.

A false-positive result may also be due to an interpretation error. For example, changes in the renogram curve due to pelvicalyceal retention of radiopharmaceutical may be confused with a true-positive test showing cortical retention. Sfakianakis et al. have proposed giving furosemide 3 minutes after radiopharmaceutical administration to better delineate true cortical activity and avoid these false interpretations. Additionally, both quantitative analysis of the renogram curves and subjective assessment of the scintigraphic images will help to avoid such errors in interpretation.

Poorly functioning kidneys are a potential cause of false-negative examinations, since changes induced by captopril may not be detectable. However, a patient with hypertension and poor visualization of one kidney by scintigraphy should undergo angiography to exclude RAS. A captopril study under these circumstances should not be interpreted as negative, even though no changes are noted between the pre- and postcaptopril portions of the study. As Sfakianakis et al. have noted, with very advanced or complete renal artery obstruction, there may not be enough renal function to ensure scintigraphic changes after ACE inhibition. Currently available data suggest that the sensitivity and specificity of captopril renal scintigraphy are equivalent in patients with mild renal failure and those with normal renal function.

Question 137

Regarding renovascular hypertension,

(A) if there is no lateralization of renal vein renin activity, revascularization is unlikely to be beneficial
(B) intravenous digital subtraction angiography has poor sensitivity for detecting fibromuscular dysplasia
(C) the results of intravenous digital subtraction angiography correlate well with those of conventional arteriography for detecting atheromatous disease in the renal artery
(D) peripheral plasma renin measurements are unreliable for its exclusion

Approximately 60 million Americans are affected with hypertension, a disorder of considerable clinical importance because it is a major risk factor for morbidity and mortality from cardiovascular disease. Primary (or essential) hypertension, without known cause, accounts for at least 95% of cases of hypertension. Between 1 and 5% of cases of hypertension have known causes (secondary hypertension). RVH caused by obstruction of the renal artery is the most common cause of secondary hypertension. Identifying RVH is important, since it can be treated successfully with balloon angioplasty or surgery. In fact, RVH is defined as the presence of RAS and improvement or cure of hypertension following angioplasty, surgical repair, or nephrectomy of the involved kidney. The requirement that an appropriate blood pressure response to therapy occur is an important component of the definition of RVH, since hemodynamically insignificant RAS is frequently identified in normotensive individuals who are undergoing arteriography for unrelated reasons. In fact, in the review of 500 angiograms by Eyler et al., almost as many normotensive patients as hypertensive patients had RAS. Similarly, an autopsy study performed by Holley et al. found that 49% of normotensive patients had moderate to severe RAS.

Pathologically, the two most common etiologies for RAS and RVH are atherosclerosis and fibromuscular dysplasia. Other causes of RVH include traumatic injury to the renal artery, renal arterial embolism, middle aortic syndrome (a syndrome that narrows the abdominal aorta and other abdominal arteries, including the renal arteries), Takayasu's arteritis, irradiation, neurofibromatosis type 1, and congenital narrowing of the renal artery, all of which are rare.

Hypertension is a common disease, and patients undergoing screening for RVH should be carefully selected, since the predictive value of a positive test varies with the prevalence of the disease. For a test with both sensitivity and specificity of 95% (better than any current screening examination for RVH) and another with more realistic values of 80%, Table 27-1 shows how the predictive value of a positive test falls when it is applied to populations with low disease prevalence.

The exact prevalence of RVH is unknown, but it is probably present in about 1% of all hypertensive patients. From Table 27-1, it therefore follows that if all patients with hypertension were screened for RVH by using a test that had 95% sensitivity and specificity, the predictive value of a positive test would be only 16%. For a test with only 80% sensitivity and specificity, the corresponding positive predictive value would be only 4%. Therefore, it is important to use clinical history and physical findings to select a subset of hypertensive patients with a higher than average probability of having RVH. Although no clinical features are entirely specific for RVH, assessment of both clinical history and physical examination findings permits identification of patients most likely to have RAS due to atherosclerosis or fibromuscular dysplasia. As reported by Saddler and Black, the clinical findings that suggest atherosclerotic RAS include (1) resistant, severe, or accelerated hypertension; (2)

Table 27-1. Predictive value of a screening test in relation to the prevalence of disease

Disease prevalence (%)	Predictive value for:			
	Sensitivity and specificity of 95%		Sensitivity and specificity of 80%	
	Positive (%)	Negative (%)	Positive (%)	Negative (%)
1	16.1	99.9	3.9	99.7
2	27.9	99.9	7.5	99.5
5	50.0	99.7	17.4	98.7
10	67.9	99.4	30.7	97.3
20	82.6	98.7	50.0	94.1

hypertension initially presenting in a patient over 60 years of age; (3) previously well-controlled hypertension that has become difficult to control; (4) evidence of vascular disease elsewhere (coronary artery disease, cerebrovascular disease, peripheral vascular disease); (5) presence of abdominal bruits, especially if systolic and diastolic; (6) history of heavy cigarette smoking (more than 25 pack-years); (7) Caucasian race; and (8) unexplained renal dysfunction in a patient with recent onset of hypertension. The clinical findings that suggest RAS caused by fibromuscular dysplasia include (1) resistant, severe, or accelerated hypertension in a white woman (under 30 years of age) and (2) the presence of abdominal bruits, especially if diastolic and systolic, in a patient with significant hypertension.

Once it has been determined that a patient belongs to a subset that should undergo screening for RVH, the clinician must decide which of the many available laboratory or radiographic tests to use. This is a difficult task because the literature dealing with hypertension is replete with studies in which RAS is incorrectly equated with RVH. There is no laboratory or radiologic "gold standard" for RVH; definitive diagnosis depends on retrospective evaluation of blood pressure response to surgery or angioplasty. Even standard renal arteriography is an imperfect test for RVH; it is well documented that not all hypertensive patients with RAS improve despite technically successful angioplasty or surgical revascularization.

The radiologic screening tools for RVH available to the clinician include conventional renal arteriography, intravenous and intra-arterial digital subtraction angiography (DSA), and captopril renal scintigraphy. In the past, rapid-sequence excretory urography, radionuclide renography, and renal scintigraphy (without ACE inhibitors) were used, but these are now generally believed to have insufficient sensitivity, specificity, or both to be useful as screening tools and have been largely abandoned. Intravenous DSA shares with urography the advantage of being relatively noninvasive, requiring only catheterization of a vein. More importantly, it allows the main renal artery to be assessed directly and so is more specific than urography, which must rely on comparisons of the two nephrograms for detection of RAS. In addition, if intravenous DSA is performed with a catheter placed in the inferior vena cava through a femoral approach, blood samples for renal vein renin determinations may be obtained concurrently. When intravenous DSA is technically well performed, its results correlate well with those of conventional renal arteriography for detecting atherosclerotic disease in the renal artery **(Option (C) is true);** this was demonstrated in the 1989 study by Dunnick et al., who evaluated 94 patients judged to be at high risk for RVH. Each of these patients underwent both intravenous DSA and arteriography. Relative to arteriography, intravenous DSA had a sensitivity of 100% and a specificity of 93%, with positive and negative predictive values of 83% and 100%, respectively, in this subset of patients with a 27% prevalence of RAS. Patients must be selected carefully for intravenous DSA, since uncooperative patients or those with decreased cardiac function are more likely to have technically inadequate studies and so require examination by intra-arterial DSA or arteriography. Intravenous DSA is relatively insensitive for detecting RAS due to fibromuscular dysplasia **(Option (B) is true).** This is not surprising because even with conventional arteriography it may be difficult to identify the subtle abnormalities associated with this disease.

Captopril renal scintigraphy provides quantitative information on differential renal function that is not afforded by angiography, provides more information on the physiologic significance of RAS, and provides a safe method to assess angioplasty or surgical repair of RAS. In addition to these advantages, it is relatively noninvasive and is the least expensive of the radiologic screening tools. The best criteria for defining a positive study are still being refined; various investigators have proposed the use of quantifiable changes in GFR, time to peak activity, renal transit time, residual cortical activity, and relative delay in excretion to determine the presence of hemodynamically significant RAS. As noted above, subjective evaluation of the scintigraphic images is also important.

A variety of blood tests have also been proposed as screening tools to detect patients likely to have RVH. All involve measurements of plasma renin levels. Available tests include peripheral plasma renin assay, sampling of renal vein renins, and the captopril test. The last of these should not be confused with captopril renography or scintigraphy. In the captopril test, peripheral plasma renin activity is determined just before and then 60 minutes after ingestion of captopril. The physiologic rationale for performing the test is that captopril produces a greater rise in renin production in patients with RVH than in patients with essential hypertension. Despite the apparent simplicity of this test, there are many potential sources of error, including those caused by concomitant use of a variety of medications and by coexisting renal parenchymal disease or extrarenal disease affecting renin secretion. A number of different criteria for a positive test have been proposed. The utility of the captopril test as a screening tool for RVH is extremely controversial. Two recent groups of investigators came to entirely different conclusions; one group (Fredrickson et al.) recommended it, and another (Postma et al.) did not. An editorial by McCarthy and Weder accompanying these two papers concluded that the captopril test could not be simplified enough to recommend its use in the routine clinical evaluation of hypertensive patients.

Peripheral plasma renin measurements have also been used in attempts to diagnose RVH. Unfortunately, the majority of patients with elevated peripheral renin levels do not have RVH, and, conversely, only approximately 50 to 60% of patients with RVH have elevated peripheral plasma renin levels. Therefore, the high false-positive and false-negative rates of this examination make it of limited clinical utility **(Option (D) is true)**.

Selective renal vein renin sampling has been perhaps the most widely used method to attempt to predict which patients will respond favorably to renal revascularization. Although a variety of complicated formulas have been advocated to diagnose RVH from renal vein renin assays, the simplest and most widely used approach is to determine a simple ratio of the relative renin activity between each renal vein. An arbitrary value of 1.5:1 is considered positive or "lateralizing." A positive renal vein renin ratio predicts a satisfactory clinical outcome in approximately 90% of cases; however, the converse is not true, since the false-negative rate ranges from 30 to 70%. Therefore, failure of lateralization does not imply that a particular patient will not respond favorably to a revascularization procedure **(Option (A) is false)**.

A variety of differential strategies have been used in an attempt to increase the specificity of selective renal vein renin sampling, including altering the patient's position, restricting dietary sodium, and using various pharmacologic agents (most commonly furosemide). Recently the addition of captopril stimulation to the selective sampling technique has been proposed, but in a prospective study Roubidoux et al. reported that the stimulated renal vein renin ratio still demonstrated a low sensitivity (65%) and specificity (52%) when cure or improvement of hypertension following renal revascularization was used as the end point. In this study, 48% of the patients with proven essential hypertension had falsely elevated renal vein renin ratios. The authors concluded that captopril-stimulated renal vein renin sampling is not sufficiently sensitive to predict which patients will benefit from renal revascularization and therefore offers little benefit over conventional sampling techniques.

The poor predictive value of renal vein renin sampling has led many authorities to conclude that renal revascularization can be undertaken without waiting for the results of sampling in patients who have severe hypertension and RAS and in whom the procedure can be undertaken with a relatively low complication rate. This implies that a diagnostic arteriogram and a renal angioplasty can be performed together in patients for whom the risk-benefit ratio suggests that the procedure should be attempted.

Question 138

Regarding captopril,

T   (A) it is an angiotensin-converting enzyme inhibitor
F   (B) it is the antihypertensive agent of choice in patients with bilateral renal artery stenosis
F   (C) in a kidney with renal artery stenosis, its primary effect is to increase glomerular filtration
T   (D) it occasionally produces a profound hypotensive response
F   (E) captopril scintigraphy with Tc-99m DTPA is effective in assessing for renovascular hypertension in patients with poor renal function

Captopril is a member of the class of antihypertensive drugs that competitively inhibit ACE **(Option (A) is true).** The other commercially available drugs in this class are enalapril and lisinopril (Table 27-2). The use of enalapril in its intravenous form (enalaprilat) can shorten the total examination time for renal scintigraphy, since it is necessary to wait for 1 hour after oral administration of captopril but only 15 minutes after intravenous administration of enalaprilat before imaging. In addition, the use of enalaprilat ensures that an effective blood level is achieved.

Table 27-2. Properties of ACE inhibitors

Drug	Usual dose, frequency, and route of administration	Dose for scintigraphy	T_{Biol}* (h)	Minimum time (days) to withhold drug prior to scintigraphy
Captopril	Up to 50 mg 2 or 3 times/day, oral	50 mg orally (patient should fast 1–4 h before dose)	<2	1
Enalapril	10–40 mg once a day, oral	–	11	2.25
Enalaprilat	1.25 mg over 5 min every 6 h, intravenous	0.04 mg/kg (max. 2.5 mg) intravenous over 5 min	11	2.25
Lisinopril	20–40 mg once a day, oral	–	12	2.5

*Biologic half-time (T_{Biol}) may be prolonged if renal failure is present.

The mechanism of action of this class of drugs is inhibition of the renin-angiotensin-aldosterone system. Normally, renin is secreted by the cells of the juxtaglomerular apparatus in the kidneys in response to decreased tension in the afferent arteriolar wall or a decreased rate of delivery of sodium to the distal tubule. Renin is a proteolytic enzyme that acts on angiotensinogen, a circulating α_2-globulin produced in the liver, to form angiotensin I. ACE cleaves two C-terminal amino acids from angiotensin I to produce angiotensin II. This conversion takes place both peripherally and locally in the kidney. Angiotensin II is a potent pressor and also stimulates the release of aldosterone, which in turn causes salt and water retention.

In patients with RAS, angiotensin II is crucial in preserving the GFR. When RAS develops, the decreased renal perfusion pressure and filtration of sodium are detected and the juxtaglomerular apparatus increases renin production. By the pathway discussed above, angiotensin II is ultimately produced. Angiotensin II causes preferential postglomerular (efferent arteriolar) vasoconstriction in the affected kidney, and this leads to increased vascular resistance, which in turn restores glomerular pressure and allows the GFR to be maintained. When ACE inhibitors are administered to patients with RAS, conversion of angiotensin I to angiotensin II is blocked. The decrease in angiotensin II levels leads to efferent arterial vasodilatation, and the net effect is a decrease in the GFR **(Option (C) is false).**

The resultant decreased glomerular perfusion pressures and the fall in GFR can be quite marked in patients with RAS who depend on angiotensin II-induced vasoconstriction to maintain the GFR. Thus, ACE inhibitors are not the antihypertensive agents of choice for patients with bilateral RAS but are in fact contraindicated in these patients and in patients with stenosis of an artery to a transplanted kidney or other solitary functioning kidney **(Option (B) is false).** When treated with ACE inhibitors, these patients can rapidly develop oliguric renal failure that is unrelated to drug hypersensitivity or nephrotoxicity but is instead directly related to the decreased GFR. When the ACE inhibitors are withdrawn, renal function recovers. This prompt reversibility of renal failure is expected, since the mechanism of renal failure is hemodynamic and not true nephrotoxicity. However, as Wenting et al. have pointed out, the potential long-term consequences of a captopril-mediated reduction in GFR are not necessarily so benign, since captopril-induced renal artery thrombosis has been reported to occur in a patient with preexisting RAS.

Profound hypotension is a potential complication of captopril administration, and this may occur with the initial dose **(Option (D) is true).** A precipitous blood pressure drop is most likely in salt- or volume-depleted patients, such as those who are severely salt restricted, taking diuretics, or being treated by dialysis. Patients who are referred for captopril renal scintigraphy are often salt or volume depleted, and extreme care should be taken to hydrate these patients before administering captopril. Even with hydration, some degree of blood pressure decline occurs in virtually all patients following the first administration of captopril, and this is a useful indicator that the captopril has been adequately absorbed. Because of the risk of hypotension, careful blood pressure monitoring is suggested when performing captopril renal scintigraphy. Some investigators recommend both oral and intravenous hydration. Hypotension, should it occur, usually responds to saline infusion. In addition to the usual medical reasons for avoiding severe hypotension, there is an important theoretical reason as well, since Dondi et al. documented false-positive captopril scintigraphic studies in several patients whose postcaptopril diastolic blood pressures fell below 60 mm Hg. The results simulated the findings of bilateral RAS.

< 60 mm Hg

Angioedema is also a reported complication of ACE inhibitor therapy. This may be fatal as a result of airway obstruction if the tongue, glottis, or larynx is involved. Angioedema is reported to occur in approximately 1 in 1,000 patients. Physicians performing captopril renal scintigraphy should be prepared to treat possible allergic reactions to the drug.

Captopril renal scintigraphy performed with Tc-99m DTPA is not effective in detecting RAS in patients with poor renal function (**Option (E) is false**). In the 1987 study by Sfakianakis et al., patients with decreased renal function had abnormal baseline studies with both I-131 OIH and Tc-99m DTPA. However, only the I-131 OIH studies were able to help differentiate between the contribution of RAS and intrinsic renal disease to the decrease in renal function. Kidneys with intrinsic renal disease had flat I-131 OIH renogram curves, whereas kidneys with decreased renal function as a result of severe RAS had slowly rising I-131 OIH renogram curves.

Janice W. Semenkovich, M.D.
Carl M. Sandler, M.D.

SUGGESTED READINGS

CAPTOPRIL SCINTIGRAPHY

1. Blaufox MD. Cost effectiveness of nuclear medicine procedures in renovascular hypertension. Semin Nucl Med 1989; 19:116–121
2. Blaufox MD. Procedures of choice in renal nuclear medicine. J Nucl Med 1991; 32:1301–1309
3. Chen CC, Hoffer PB, Vahjen G, et al. Patients at high risk for renal artery stenosis: a simple method of renal scintigraphic analysis with Tc-99m DTPA and captopril. Radiology 1990; 176:365–370
4. Dondi M, Franchi R, Levorato M, et al. Evaluation of hypertensive patients by means of captopril enhanced renal scintigraphy with technetium-99m DTPA. J Nucl Med 1989; 30:615–621
5. Dondi M, Monetti N, Fanti S, et al. Use of technetium-99m-MAG3 for renal scintigraphy after angiotensin-converting enzyme inhibition. J Nucl Med 1991; 32:424–428
6. Dubovsky EV, Russell CD. 99mTc-MAG3: the multipurpose renal radiopharmaceutical. In: Freeman LM (ed), Nuclear medicine annual 1991. New York: Raven Press; 1991:1–35
7. Erbslöh-Möller B, Dumas A, Roth D, Sfakianakis GN, Bourgoignie JJ. Furosemide-131I-hippuran renography after angiotensin-converting enzyme inhibition for the diagnosis of renovascular hypertension. Am J Med 1991; 90:23–29

8. Fine EJ, Sarkar S. Differential diagnosis and management of renovascular hypertension through nuclear medicine techniques. Semin Nucl Med 1989; 19:101–115

9. Fommei E, Ghione S, Palla L, et al. Renal scintigraphic captopril test in the diagnosis of renovascular hypertension. Hypertension 1987; 10:212–220

10. Geyskes GG, Oei HY, Puylaert CB, Mees EJ. Renovascular hypertension identified by captopril-induced changes in the renogram. Hypertension 1987; 9:451–458

11. Maher ER, Othman S, Frankel AH, Sweny P, Moorhead JF, Hilson AJ. Captopril-enhanced ^{99m}Tc DTPA scintigraphy in the detection of renal artery stenosis. Nephrol Dial Transplant 1988; 3:608–611

12. Nally JV Jr, Black HR. State-of-the-art review: captopril renography—pathophysiological considerations and clinical observations. Semin Nucl Med 1992; 22:85–97

13. Nally JV Jr, Chen C, Fine E, et al. Diagnostic criteria of renovascular hypertension with captopril renography. A consensus statement. Am J Hypertens 1991; 4:749S–752S

14. Pedersen EB, Jensen FT, Eiskjaer H, et al. Differentiation between renovascular and essential hypertension by means of changes in single kidney ^{99m}Tc-DTPA clearance induced by angiotensin-converting enzyme inhibition. Am J Hypertens 1989; 2:323–334

15. Saddler MC, Black HR. Captopril renal scintigraphy: a clinician's perspective. In: Hoffer PB (ed), Yearbook of nuclear medicine. Chicago: Mosby-Year Book; 1990:xiii–xxxiv

16. Sfakianakis GN, Bourgoignie JJ, Jaffe D, Kyriakides G, Perez-Stable E, Duncan RC. Single-dose captopril scintigraphy in the diagnosis of renovascular hypertension. J Nucl Med 1987; 28:1383–1392

17. Sfakianakis GN, Sfakianakis E, Bourgoignie J. Renal scintigraphy following angiotensin-converting enzyme inhibition in the diagnosis of renovascular hypertension (captopril scintigraphy). In: Freeman LM (ed), Nuclear medicine annual 1988. New York: Raven Press; 1988:125–170

18. Taylor A Jr, Halkar R. Radionuclide renal studies. Curr Opin Radiol 1989; 1:460–467

19. Wilcox CS, Smith TB, Fredrickson ED, Wingo CD, Phillips MI, Williams CM. The captopril glomerular filtration rate renogram in renovascular hypertension. Clin Nucl Med 1989; 14:1–7

RENOVASCULAR HYPERTENSION

20. Baert AL, Wilms G, Amery A, Vermylen J, Suy R. Percutaneous transluminal renal angioplasty: initial results and long-term follow-up in 202 patients. Cardiovasc Intervent Radiol 1990; 13:22–28

21. Dunnick NR, McCallum RW, Sandler CM. Textbook of uroradiology. Baltimore: Williams & Wilkins; 1991:172–188

22. Dunnick NR, Sfakianakis GN. Screening for renovascular hypertension. Radiol Clin North Am 1991; 29:497–510

23. Dunnick NR, Svetkey LP, Cohan RH, et al. Intravenous digital subtraction renal angiography: use in screening for renovascular hypertension. Radiology 1989; 171:219–222

24. Eyler WR, Clark MD, Garman JE, Rian RL, Meininger PE. Angiography of the renal areas including a study of renal artery stenosis in patients with or without hypertension. Radiology 1962; 78:879–892

25. Fredrickson ED, Wilcox CS, Bucci M, et al. A prospective evaluation of a simplified captopril test for detection of renovascular hypertension. Arch Intern Med 1990; 150:569–572

26. Gaul MK, Linn WD, Mulrow CD. Captopril-stimulated renin secretion in the diagnosis of renovascular hypertension. Am J Hypertens 1989; 2:335–340

27. Hillman BJ. Imaging advances in the diagnosis of renovascular hypertension. AJR 1989; 153:5–14

28. Holley KE, Hunt JC, Brown AL Jr, Kincaid OW, Sheps SG. Renal artery stenosis: a clinicopathologic study in normotensive and hypertensive patients. Am J Med 1964; 37:14–22

29. Illescas FF, Braun SD, Cohan RH, Sussman SK, Saeed M, Dunnick NR. Fibromuscular dysplasia of renal arteries: comparison of intravenous digital subtraction angiography with conventional angiography. Can Assoc Radiol J 1988; 39:167–171

30. Klinge J, Mali WP, Puijlaert CB, Geyskes GG, Becking WB, Feldberg MA. Percutaneous transluminal renal angioplasty: initial and long-term results. Radiology 1989; 171:501–506

31. Marks LS, Maxwell MH. Renal vein renin: value and limitations in the prediction of operative results. Urol Clin North Am 1975; 2:311–325

32. Martin LG, Casarella WJ, Alspaugh JP, Chuang VP. Renal artery angioplasty: increased technical success and decreased complications in the second 100 patients. Radiology 1986; 159:631–634

33. Martin LG, Price RB, Casarella WJ, et al. Percutaneous angioplasty in clinical management of renovascular hypertension: initial and long-term results. Radiology 1985; 155:629–633

34. Maxwell MH, Marks LS, Lupo AN, Cahill PJ, Franklin SS, Kaufman JJ. Predictive value of renin determinations in renal artery stenosis. JAMA 1977; 238:2617–2620

35. McCarthy JE, Weder AB. The captopril test and renovascular hypertension. A cautionary tale. Arch Intern Med 1990; 150:493–495

36. Peters AM. Renal artery stenosis, reno-vascular hypertension and predicting the blood pressure response to renal revascularization. Nucl Med Commun 1990; 11:1–5

37. Pickering TG. Renovascular hypertension: etiology and pathophysiology. Semin Nucl Med 1989; 19:79–88

38. Pickering TG. Diagnosis and evaluation of renovascular hypertension. Indications for therapy. Circulation 1991; 83(suppl 2):I147–I154

39. Postma CT, van der Steen PH, Hoefnagels WH, de Boo T, Thien T. The captopril test in the detection of renovascular disease in hypertensive patients. Arch Intern Med 1990; 150:625–628

40. Roubidoux MA, Dunnick NR, Klotman PE, et al. Renal vein renins: inability to predict response to revascularization in patients with hypertension. Radiology 1991; 178:819–822

41. Rudnick MR, Maxwell MH. Limitations of renin assays. In: Narins RG (ed), Controversies in nephrology and hypertension. New York: Churchill Livingstone; 1984:123–160

42. Sos TA, Crystal S, Pickering TG. Percutaneous transluminal angioplasty of the renal arteries. In Dondelinger RF, Rossi P, Kurdziel JC, Wallace S (eds), Interventional radiology. New York: Thieme; 1990:596–609

43. Sos TA, Pickering TG, Sniderman K, et al. Percutaneous transluminal renal angioplasty in renovascular hypertension due to atheroma or fibromuscular dysplasia. N Engl J Med 1983; 309:274–279

44. Tack C, Sos TA. Radiologic diagnosis of renovascular hypertension and percutaneous transluminal renal angioplasty. Semin Nucl Med 1989; 19:89–100

45. Tegtmeyer CJ, Kellum CD, Ayers C. Percutaneous transluminal angioplasty of the renal artery. Results and long-term follow-up. Radiology 1984; 153:77–84

46. Tegtmeyer CJ, Selby JB. Percutaneous transluminal angioplasty of the renal arteries. In: Castañeda-Zúñiga WR, Tadavarthy SM (eds), Interventional radiology, 2nd ed. Baltimore: Williams & Wilkins; 1992:77–84

47. Vaughan ED Jr, Case DB, Pickering TG, Sosa RE, Sos TA, Laragh JH. Clinical evaluation of renovascular hypertension and therapeutic decisions. Urol Clin North Am 1984; 11:393–407

48. Vidt DG. The diagnostic dilemma: a clinician's viewpoint. Semin Nucl Med 1989; 19:75–78

49. Wise KL, McCann RL, Dunnick NR, Paulson DF. Renovascular hypertension. J Urol 1988; 140:911–924

50. Working Group on Renovascular Hypertension. Detection, evaluation, and treatment of renovascular hypertension. Final report. Arch Intern Med 1987; 147:820–829

ACE INHIBITORS

51. Johnston CI, Jackson B. Overview: angiotensin converting enzyme inhibition in renovascular hypertension. Kidney Int 1987; 31(suppl):S154–S156

52. Levenson DJ, Dzau VJ. Effects of angiotensin-converting enzyme inhibition on renal hemodynamics in renal artery stenosis. Kidney Int 1987; 31(suppl):S173–S179

53. Tunny TJ, Klemm SA, Hamlet SM, Gordon RD. Diagnosis of unilateral renovascular hypertension: comparative effect of intravenous enalaprilat and oral captopril. J Urol 1988; 140:713–715

54. Wenting GJ, Derkx FH, Tan-Tjiong LH, van Seyen AJ, Man in't Veld AJ, Schalekamp MA. Risks of angiotensin converting enzyme inhibition in renal artery stenosis. Kidney Int 1987; 31(suppl):S180–S183

Notes

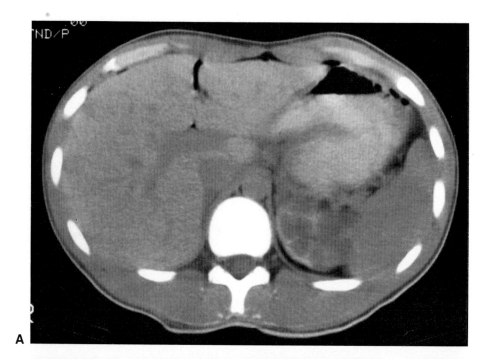

A

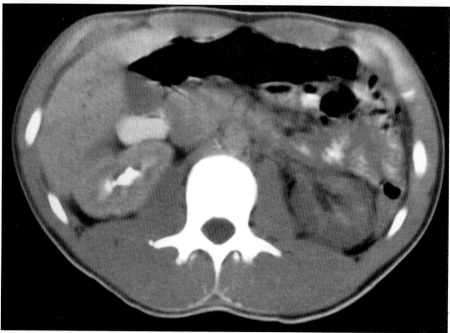

B

Figure 28-1. History withheld. You are shown CT scans made at the level of the upper pole of the left kidney (A) and through the midportion of both kidneys (B) following an excretory urogram.

Case 28: Traumatic Renal Artery Occlusion with Renal Infarction

Question 139

Which *one* of the following is the MOST likely diagnosis?

(A) Acute ureteral obstruction
(B) Renal vein thrombosis
(C) Acute cortical necrosis
(D) Acute pyelonephritis
(E) Acute renal infarction

Both images from the CT scan (Figure 28-1) were performed after an initial excretory urogram (Figure 28-2), which demonstrated absence of contrast material excretion from the left kidney. The upper CT image (Figure 28-1A) demonstrates a thin rim of enhancing renal cortex in the left kidney. This pattern of enhancement extends into the septal cortex. In the image performed at the level of the renal hilum (Figure 28-1B), there is a marked discrepancy in the amount of contrast material excretion between the right and left kidneys with absence of both the nephrogram and pyelogram on the left side. A minimal amount of patchy increased density in the renal parenchyma is present in Figure 28-1B. The combination of a rim of cortical enhancement (the "cortical rim sign") and markedly diminished excretion is most suggestive of acute renal infarction **(Option (E) is correct).** The test patient is a 17-year-old boy who had been involved in a motor vehicle accident. In the setting of acute trauma, renal infarction is most likely a manifestation of an acute renal artery thrombosis secondary to an intimal tear of the main renal artery. This diagnosis was confirmed on a digital subtraction arteriogram (Figure 28-3) performed a few minutes after the CT scan.

The cortical rim sign was originally described as a urographic sign of acute renal infarction and was demonstrated on high-dose nephroto-

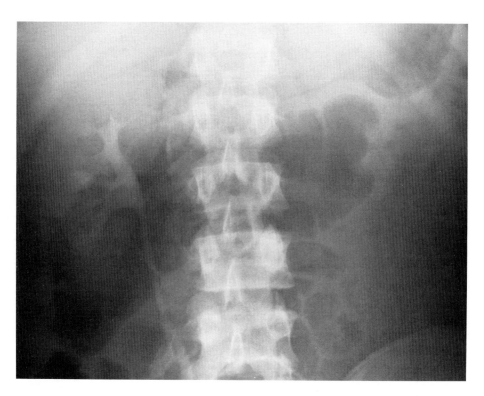

Figure 28-2. Same patient as in Figure 28-1. Close-up view of the kidneys from the excretory urogram that preceded the CT images shown in Figure 28-1. The patient is a 17-year-old boy who had been involved in a motor vehicle accident approximately 2 hours prior to the study. No excretion of contrast material is present from the left kidney. The right kidney appears normal.

mography. The rim of enhancement is thought to be secondary to collateral circulation to the kidney via capsular, adrenal, pelvic, and ureteral vessels. The rim sign is much more readily demonstrated on CT than on nephrotomography because of the superior contrast resolution of CT, and it is said to be present in approximately 50% of the cases of both global and segmental infarction described by Wong et al. Lupetin et al., however, found the cortical rim sign in only 3 of 10 patients with renal artery occlusion who underwent CT following blunt abdominal trauma. Although the cortical rim sign has also been described in acute renal vein thrombosis, acute tubular necrosis, and acute cortical necrosis, it is much more commonly associated with acute renal infarction; even when associated with these other conditions, it is nonetheless a manifes-

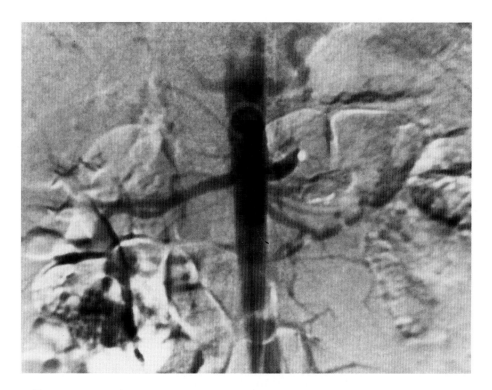

Figure 28-3. Same patient as in Figures 28-1 and 28-2. Intra-arterial digital subtraction arteriogram demonstrates a sharp cut-off in the left renal artery diagnostic of traumatic renal artery thrombosis. A rounded artifact, related to the digital technique, is also present adjacent to the abnormal vessel.

tation of the diminished renal blood flow that can occur with these disorders. In addition, since both acute tubular necrosis and acute cortical necrosis are usually bilateral conditions and acute renal vein thrombosis is generally associated with a swollen but nonetheless functioning kidney, these diagnoses are less likely than acute renal infarction as the cause of the CT findings in the test case.

The finding of minimal patchy areas of contrast enhancement has been previously reported in patients with renal artery occlusion. The cause of this phenomenon is poorly understood, but it may be a manifestation of contrast medium reaching the kidney via a partially occluded vessel prior to complete thrombosis.

Acute ureteral obstruction (Option (A)) is generally associated with a dense rather than a diminished or absent nephrogram (Figure 28-4). Acute cortical necrosis (Option (C)) is generally bilateral, as described

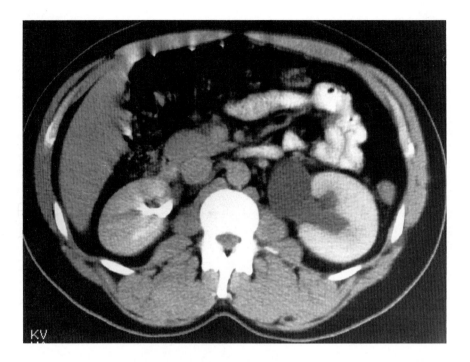

Figure 28-4. Acute ureteral obstruction. CT image at the level of the midportion of the kidneys shows increased density in the left renal cortex ("obstructive nephrogram") and no excretion of the contrast material into a dilated left collecting system.

above, and is associated with acute renal failure. Therefore, it is unlikely that an excretory urogram would have been performed in a patient with acute cortical necrosis. The CT findings in patients with acute renal vein thrombosis (Option (B)) have been described by Gatewood et al.; they include renal enlargement; persistent, inhomogeneous parenchymal opacification following contrast medium administration and parenchymal retention of the contrast agent; the presence of dilated perirenal collateral veins ("perirenal cobwebs"); and visualization of the thrombus within the renal vein (Figure 28-5). None of these findings were present in the test patient. Additional findings in patients with renal vein thrombosis include compression of the collecting system secondary to renal edema, absent or delayed pyelocalyceal visualization, and demonstration of perirenal collateral vessels. Acute pyelonephritis (Option (D)) is generally characterized by narrow striate zones of diminished excretion of contrast material throughout the involved segment of renal parenchyma on CT (Figure 28-6). With more-severe forms of renal inflammatory disease,

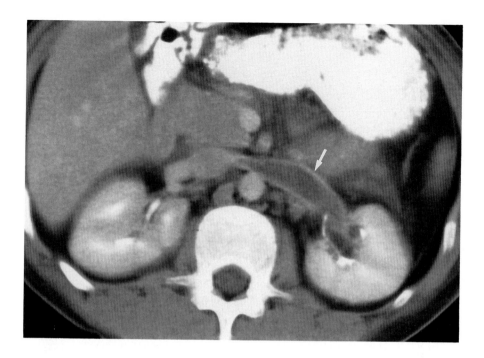

Figure 28-5. Acute renal vein thrombosis. Percutaneous CT shows a denser nephrogram on the left. Left renal vein thrombus is clearly demonstrated (arrow).

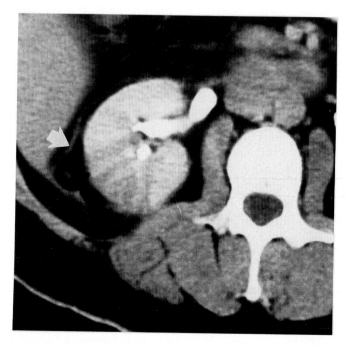

Figure 28-6. Acute pyelonephritis. Close-up CT view of the right kidney in a patient with clinical evidence of acute pyelonephritis. Narrow striate zones of diminished excretion of contrast material are present in the renal parenchyma. Minimal thickening of the renal fascia (arrow) is also demonstrated.

diminished excretion of contrast material, a persistent dense nephrogram, a diminished or absent pyelogram, and large wedge-shaped areas of decreased contrast enhancement on CT may be present.

Question 140

Concerning acute ureteral obstruction,

F (A) a significant irreversible loss of renal function occurs after as little as 48 hours of complete ureteral obstruction
T (B) backflow mechanisms (e.g., pyelolymphatic, pyelosinus, pyelotubular, and pyelovenous backflow) allow continued glomerular filtration in the early phase
F (C) increased enhancement of both the renal cortex and medulla is evident on CT
F (D) the "obstructive nephrogram" occurs principally because of leakage of contrast material into the renal interstitium
F (E) the most sensitive urographic sign is dilatation of the pyelocalyceal system

The degree to which renal function is permanently impaired by ureteral obstruction depends on the degree and length of the obstruction and whether other factors, such as infection, complicate the obstruction. In patients with acute obstruction there is an initial rise in renal blood flow, which is followed by a rise in ureteral pressure; as obstruction continues, both renal blood flow and ureteral pressure decline. There is a corresponding decrease in the glomerular filtration rate, because it is dependent on the difference between the glomerular capillary pressure and the sum of the colloid osmotic pressure of the plasma and the intratubular pressure.

The precise length of time that the kidney can tolerate acute ureteral obstruction without permanent loss of function is not known. Vaughn and Gillenwater demonstrated that in dogs, complete return of function was possible after periods of ureteral obstruction of up to 7 days; after 28 days of obstruction, renal function recovered to only 30% of its baseline value. The corresponding times in humans are not known; however, in patients suffering iatrogenic ureteral injury, return of renal function after periods of obstruction of up to several months has been described (Option (A) is false).

The development of hydronephrosis is strong evidence that there is continued urine formation even in the face of complete ureteral obstruction. The primary mechanism by which the kidney allows the continued formation of new urine is in the resorption of already formed urine. This resorption, termed "renal backflow," has four major components: pyelolymphatic backflow, pyelosinus backflow, pyelotubular backflow, and pyelovenous backflow **(Option (B) is true).**

Pyelovenous backflow is thought to represent the quantitatively most important route of backflow in acute ureteral obstruction. Experimentally, renal pelvic pressure in excess of 100 cm of H_2O is needed to establish this route of urine resorption; however, once it is established, much lower pressures are required to maintain it. Pyelovenous backflow occurs at the fornices of the calyces, where formed urine enters the venous plexus that surrounds the calyx. According to Hinman, after the second week of obstruction the fornices undergo histologic changes that diminish the role of pyelovenous backflow; at this time pyelotubular backflow becomes relatively more important as a protective mechanism for the kidney.

Pyelotubular backflow begins following the onset of hydronephrosis. High intrapelvic pressures allow opening of the normally closed papillary ducts and hence the flow of urine back into the renal tubules. Pyelotubular backflow may be demonstrated on retrograde pyelography and urography when high intrapelvic pressures are present.

Pyelolymphatic backflow is thought to augment pyelovenous backflow, though in smaller volumes, and represents the flow of formed urine into the renal lymphatic circulation. Pyelosinus backflow is occasionally observed on retrograde pyelography or on urography in the presence of acute ureteral obstruction. This phenomenon occurs when there is rupture of a fornix or fornices of the minor calyces, and it is demonstrated as a collection of contrast material that surrounds the renal hilus in the perinephric space (Figure 28-7). Pyelosinus extravasation serves to decompress the renal pelvis when urine escapes into the perinephric space, where resorption takes place. Occasionally, a uriniferous pseudocyst, termed a urinoma, forms as a result of this extravasation.

Elkin has investigated radiologic findings during urography in patients with acute ureteral obstruction. The affected kidney is usually enlarged. Initially, there is a diminished nephrogram, but on delayed radiographs there is a striking, progressively intensifying nephrogram, which is much more intense than normal. This phenomenon has been referred to as the "obstructive nephrogram." The appearance of contrast material in the collecting system (the renal medulla) is delayed, however, sometimes for as long as 24 hours after the injection of the contrast material. Thus on CT, increased enhancement of the renal cortex but decreased enhancement of the medulla will be present **(Option (C) is false)** (Figure 28-4). When the pyelogram is visualized, dilatation of the calyces and pelvis is usually present, even when the obstruction is of relatively short duration.

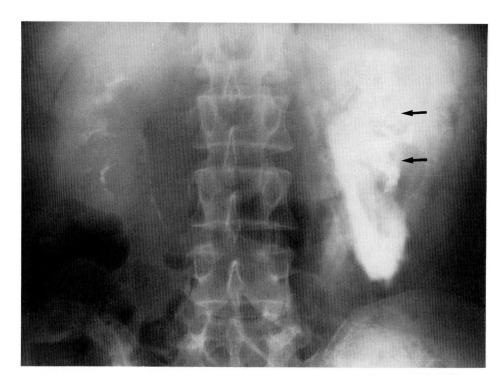

Figure 28-7. Pyelosinus extravasation. A 10-minute postinjection radiograph from an excretory urogram in a patient with acute ureteral obstruction secondary to a distal calculus demonstrates extensive contrast material extravasation into the perinephric space originating from ruptured fornices (arrows).

The aforementioned physiologic changes, however, represent a much more sensitive urographic sign of acute obstruction than the anatomic changes, which generally occur much more slowly **(Option (E) is false).**

The pathophysiology responsible for the obstructive nephrogram has not been completely explained. Some authorities believe that increasing tubular distension, which allows an increase in the volume of contrast material within each tubule, is primarily responsible for this phenomenon. Others believe that the increase in sodium and water resorption in the proximal tubule during ureteral obstruction leads to an increase in the concentration of contrast in the tubular lumen. Leakage of contrast material into the renal interstitium is not thought to play a significant role in this process **(Option (D) is false).**

Ultrasonography is not as reliable as urography for the detection of acute ureteral obstruction. In a study of 20 patients with proven acute ureteral obstruction secondary to ureteral calculi, Laing et al. found that sonography depicted the collecting system as normal in 35%. In a prospective study, Hill et al. found that urography led to a correct diagnosis in 85% of patients with acute flank pain; sonography was correct in 66%. The inaccuracy of sonography in this regard is related to the purely anatomic nature of the ultrasound study; in early obstruction, caliectasis may not have developed and thus the sonogram is falsely negative. Urography has the advantage of demonstrating both anatomic and functional information in patients with acute ureteral obstruction; further, the diuresis produced by the contrast material will enhance the amount of dilatation detected on the urographic study.

Recently, investigators have attempted to increase the sensitivity of sonography in patients with acute ureteral colic by color Doppler examination of the distal ureter. In normal individuals, a characteristic, bilaterally symmetric appearance of the jet of urine as it emanates from the distal ureter is seen on color Doppler studies. In patients with acute ureteral calculi, a significant decrease in the frequency or a change in the character of the jet is found on the affected side. In patients with nonobstructing stones or in those with a low level of obstruction, however, this asymmetry may not be present, and so the correct diagnosis of a ureteral calculus may be overlooked. Therefore, sonographic evaluation of suspected ureteral calculi is probably best limited to patients in whom urography poses increased risk.

Question 141

Concerning acute cortical necrosis,

(A) it generally occurs as a complication of pregnancy
(B) CT will demonstrate a thin zone of enhancement adjacent to the renal capsule
(C) radiographs demonstrate a characteristic pattern of tramlike cortical calcifications
(D) sonography in the early phase generally demonstrates a hyperechoic renal cortex
(E) bilateral involvement is invariable

Acute cortical necrosis (ACN) is an uncommon cause of acute renal failure that results from ischemic necrosis of the renal cortex, including the columns of Bertin, while sparing the medullary portion of the kidneys. It may occur diffusely throughout both kidneys, in a patchy distribution resulting in renal insufficiency rather than renal failure, or, rarely, as a unilateral condition **(Option (E) is false).** In virtually all of the reported unilateral cases, the unaffected kidney had coexisting ureteral obstruction or renal artery stenosis, which was thought to be protective of that kidney from the deleterious effects of the ischemia. Sparing of a thin rim of cortical tissue on the surface of the kidney is characteristic and is presumably related to preservation of the capsular blood supply. Although multiple etiologies for ACN have been described, the precise pathophysiology responsible for the condition remains obscure. Most authorities believe that the condition results from a transient episode of selective intrarenal vasospasm, possibly as a result of a circulating endotoxin. Other explanations include a selective form of intrarenal vascular thrombosis or damage to the glomerular capillary bed. On pathologic examination, extensive infiltration of the necrotic cortex by inflammatory cells is present within 3 to 4 days of the acute episode.

ACN has been found in association with a wide variety of conditions, including shock (particularly after trauma), renal transplantation, severe dehydration, venomous snake bite, transfusion reaction, hemolytic-uremic syndrome, pharyngitis, scarlet fever, pancreatitis, thrombotic thrombocytopenic purpura, and diabetic ketoacidosis. More than two-thirds of cases, however, are reported in association with pregnancy, especially those complicated by abruptio placentae, septic abortion, or placenta previa **(Option (A) is true).**

The radiographic findings depend on the stage of the disease. In the early stages, the kidneys are diffusely enlarged. On urography, there may be faint opacification of the collecting system, particularly if patchy involvement is present. Over the course of several months, there is smooth shrinkage of the renal parenchyma accompanied by a distinctive form of "tramlike" cortical calcification throughout the affected portions of the renal cortex. The calcification is characteristically dense and up to 2 mm thick, with extension into the columns of Bertin between the renal pyramids **(Option (C) is true).** These calcifications usually appear 1 to 2 months after the onset of the illness but can be seen as early as 18 days after the acute episode. Although generally considered to be characteristic of ACN, similar calcifications have also been found in patients with chronic glomerulonephritis.

On angiography, an abrupt termination of the vascularity of the interlobar and arcuate arteries may be found, with a prolongation of the transit time through the interlobar arteries. This results in a scalloped pattern of perfusion defects in the angiographic nephrogram. In addition, there may be hypertrophy of the capsular vessels. On sonography, the findings depend on the stage of the disease at the time of examination.

When imaged early in the course of the disease, the cortex is hypoechoic **(Option (D) is false);** however, at the later stage there is typically increased echogenicity of the septal cortex corresponding to the areas of radiographic calcification. The reported CT findings include (1) no enhancement of the renal cortex, (2) enhancement of the medulla, and (3) absence of excretion of contrast material into the collecting system. The necrotic cortex is characteristically represented by a radiolucent zone bordering the circumference of the kidneys adjacent to the renal capsule **(Option (B) is false).**

Question 142

Concerning acute pyelonephritis,

(A) CT or ultrasonography is generally required for diagnosis
(B) vesicoureteral reflux is commonly demonstrated in adult patients
(C) in adults, inadequately treated acute infection is the major cause of chronic pyelonephritis
(D) complicating abscesses most commonly occur in patients with altered host defense mechanisms

Inflammatory conditions involving the urinary tract are among the most common infectious disorders of humans. In most patients, the infection is confined to the lower urinary tract; the diagnosis is suspected on clinical grounds and confirmed by the finding of white blood cells and bacteria in the urine. There is usually a prompt response to appropriate antibiotic therapy.

Bacterial infections of the kidneys generally occur as a consequence of ascending infection from the lower urinary tract; the resulting condition is commonly known as acute pyelonephritis but is more properly referred to pathologically as acute infectious interstitial nephritis. Since women have a much higher incidence of lower urinary tract infection than men, bacterial infections of the kidneys are much more common in women. Beyond the age of 50, however, the incidence of urinary tract infection in men increases as a result of urinary stasis caused by prostatism, so that the incidence of urinary tract infection is equal for both sexes after this age. Despite evidence that the overwhelming majority of upper urinary tract infections involve spread of the infection from the lower urinary tract, it is distinctly uncommon for adults to have radiologically demonstrable vesicoureteral reflux **(Option (B) is false),** unless an abnormality of the bladder that causes the reflux (e.g., a neurogenic bladder) is also present. Other conditions that may predispose a patient with lower urinary tract infection to renal involvement include (1) urinary tract obstruction, (2) calculi, (3) altered bladder function, (4) altered host resistance, (5) pregnancy, and (6) the presence of congenital anomalies.

In most cases of acute pyelonephritis, the diagnosis is easily established by history, physical examination, and laboratory studies; there is usually a prompt response to antibiotic therapy, and imaging studies of the urinary tract either are not done or are performed after the fact **(Option (A) is false).** When response to therapy is slow, the precise diagnosis is in doubt, or the clinical picture is complicated by the presence of a systemic disease such as diabetes mellitus, more-immediate radiologic investigation is indicated (1) to look for an underlying abnormality that may have predisposed the patient to the infection; (2) to search for an abnormality, such as obstruction, calculus, or papillary necrosis, that may prevent a rapid response to therapy; or (3) to diagnose a complication of the parenchymal infection such as a renal or perinephric abscess.

The optimal approach to radiologic investigation in patients with bacterial infections involving the kidneys depends on several factors, including the acuity of the process; the presence or absence of complicating conditions such as altered host resistance, suspected urinary tract calculi, or known neurogenic bladder disease; and the degree, if any, to which renal function is compromised. Finally, the preference of the physician often determines the type and sequence of the evaluation. In patients with normal or near-normal renal function and in those with suspected calculi, urography is probably the best overall screening study. In patients in whom renal function is compromised, sonography is generally the initial study. CT, although more sensitive than either urography or sonography for the detection of parenchymal abnormalities associated with renal inflammatory disease, is probably best reserved for patients in whom a complicated form of renal inflammatory disease (i.e., renal or perinephric abscess) is suspected and for those not adequately evaluated by either urography or ultrasonography.

Before the availability of broad-spectrum antibiotics, most renal abscesses formed as a result of hematogenous dissemination of *Staphylococcus aureus* from a site usually in the skin or bone. With the widespread availability of antibiotics, most renal abscesses form as a result of the coalescence of small microabscesses that are present as a part of acute pyelonephritis or one of its variations. The predominant organisms responsible for abscesses today are gram-negative enteric species, and they are found in the setting of diabetes mellitus, drug abuse, alcoholism, or vesicoureteral reflux. However, an underlying renal calculus, usually of the staghorn variety, is probably the most common predisposing factor for the development of a renal abscess **(Option (D) is false).** These stones, usually formed of magnesium ammonium phosphate, generally occur in association with urea-splitting gram-negative organisms and commonly form the nidus for continuous urinary tract reinfection.

The term "chronic pyelonephritis" refers to a set of morphologic changes in the kidney that results from a previous episode of acute pyelonephritis. As such, this term may be a source of confusion in that it implies a state of indolent or ongoing infection when in fact none is present **(Option (C) is false).** To obviate such confusion, many authorities prefer the term "chronic atrophic pyelonephritis" or the etiologic appellation "reflux nephropathy" to refer to the set of morphologic changes known pathologically as chronic pyelonephritis.

The hallmark of chronic pyelonephritis is a cortical scar that overlies an associated blunted calyx. These changes are thought to occur as a result of reflux of infected urine back into the renal tubules, a process known as intrarenal reflux. The classic teaching is that such scarring generally occurs only in urinary tract infection during early childhood; the adult kidney had been thought to be relatively immune to permanent structural damage. Recent work, however, has demonstrated that in adults such scarring may occur as a result of renal calculi, severe episodes of pyelonephritis, or the healing of a renal abscess. The appreciation of subtle kidney damage following pyelonephritis has been facilitated by the increased use of CT to image patients with renal inflammatory disease; such studies are capable of detecting scarring that was easily overlooked by urography. In the past, urography was the only available method for the detection of such parenchymal abnormalities.

Question 143

Concerning acute renal infarction,

.[|] (A) the most common cause is embolism

T (B) the CT appearance is characteristic

T (C) when it is secondary to trauma, hematuria is frequently absent

F (D) hypertension is a common late complication

Acute renal infarction may occur as a result of renal artery thrombosis, embolism, aortic dissection, shock, vasculitis, or trauma. Clinically, there is the sudden onset of flank pain, hematuria, fever, nausea, and vomiting. There may be moderate leukocytosis, albuminuria, and microscopic hematuria on laboratory studies. These symptoms are relatively nonspecific, so the diagnosis was rarely established before death prior to the advent of CT imaging.

The most common cause of a sudden renal infarction is embolism (42% of the cases reported by Wong et al.), usually secondary to cardiac disease, particularly in patients with atrial fibrillation **(Option (A) is true).** Renal infarctions may be global (involving the main renal artery) or focal (involving a segmental or smaller branch renal vessel). Patients with focal infarction are generally asymptomatic.

The radiologic findings in patients with renal infarction depend on both the extent and the age of the process at the time of imaging. Classically, in patients with global infarction a nonfunctioning kidney is seen on urography. A cortical rim sign, as discussed above, may be present on high-dose nephrotomography. Retrograde pyelography, which was often performed in the past because of the nonspecific nature of the clinical symptoms, is normal. On ultrasonography, an acute global renal infarction appears as a normal kidney; however, on Doppler studies no flow in the renal artery or vein is found. In studies performed several weeks after the acute event, a shrunken, echogenic kidney is found.

In patients with segmental infarction, a wedge-shaped nephrographic defect may be detected on urography when the study is performed shortly after the acute event; after several weeks, a scar is present in the intercalyceal cortex. The sonographic appearance of a segmental infarct is variable; a focal echogenic mass, a hypoechoic mass, or normal renal architecture may be found depending on the age of the process.

On angiography, the vascular occlusion responsible for the infarction can be demonstrated directly. There will be a sharply defined cut-off vessel in the distribution of the infarction with segmental occlusions; in patients with global infarction, the main renal artery is occluded shortly after its origin.

In addition to the cortical rim sign described in the discussion to Question 139, the CT findings in renal infarction are characteristic **(Option (B) is true).** In patients with global infarction, more than 50% of the affected kidney demonstrates low attenuation and absence of contrast enhancement. Focal infarctions are demonstrated as wedge-shaped areas of absent contrast enhancement. Infarcted kidneys are generally normal in size and contour; extrarenal fluid collections and thickening of the renal fascia may be present as additional findings in a minority of cases. Retrograde opacification of the renal vein on the affected side has been reported as a secondary finding on CT, especially if an infusion technique of contrast enhancement has been used.

Traumatic renal artery thrombosis is reported to occur in approximately 3% of patients with renal injuries. The injury occurs as a result of tearing of the intima of the renal artery after acute deceleration. The resulting intimal flap causes thrombosis of the renal artery. The injury may involve the main renal artery and result in global renal infarction or, more commonly, may involve a segmental branch vessel and result in focal infarction. The injury generally occurs in patients who have fallen from a height or as a result of an auto-pedestrian accident. Either gross or microscopic hematuria is usually present; however, Cass and co-workers reported the absence of hematuria in as many as 40% of their patients **(Option (C) is true).**

With main renal artery occlusion, a nonfunctioning kidney (unilateral absence of excretion) is demonstrated on urography. Stables reported that a renal vascular injury was present in most patients demonstrating this finding following blunt trauma and suggested that immediate angiography be undertaken for confirmation. Cass and Luxenberg, however, reported that an injury of the renal pedicle was present in only 16 of their 53 patients with unilateral absence of excretion; the remainder were found to have a variety of other renal parenchymal injuries.

Most patients with main renal artery occlusion eventually develop irreversible loss of renal function and parenchymal atrophy. There are, however, a few isolated reports of spontaneous recovery of renal function. It is presumed that in such cases, renal function returns because the renal artery has recanalized or collateral renal circulation has developed.

Renovascular hypertension has been reported as a consequence of both segmental and global renal infarction following trauma. Bertini et al. studied 24 patients with segmental arterial occlusions demonstrated by angiography and found that although transient hypertension was common initially, none of the 10 patients monitored for up to 5 years suffered sustained elevation of blood pressure. Similarly, Cass et al. studied seven patients who survived renal pedicle injuries for up to 7 years after injury; no sustained hypertension was reported **(Option (D) is false).**

The management of patients suffering main renal artery occlusion following blunt trauma is controversial and is related to the variable reports of the kidney's tolerance for warm ischemia. Critical warm-ischemia times for human kidneys have been reported to be as short as 1 to 6 hours by some investigators, whereas others report successful revascularization after more than 20 hours. Even when revascularization is attempted, reports of successful return of renal function are sporadic; the precise frequency of success is not known because it is likely that most unsuccessful attempts are not reported. Because the majority of renal pedicle injuries occur in patients suffering multisystem trauma and because the nonrenal injuries are often more life-threatening, it is not uncommon for several hours of warm ischemia to have occurred before consideration of kidney-sparing surgery is even possible. In such circumstances, and in view of the low frequency of late complications associated with renal infarction, many authorities now believe that attempts at revascularization should be limited to the uncommon patient with bilateral renal artery thrombosis. For the same reasons, routine removal of infarcted kidneys is also deemed unnecessary. In addition, the chance for spontaneous recovery of some renal function, albeit small, would be obviated by such surgery.

Carl M. Sandler, M.D.

SUGGESTED READINGS

RENAL INFARCTION

1. Bankoff MS, Sarno RC, Mitcheson HD. Computed tomography differentiation of pyelonephritis and renal infarction. J Comput Tomogr 1984; 8:239–243
2. Bertini JE, Flechner SM, Miller P, et al. The natural history of traumatic branch renal artery injury. J Urol 1985; 135:228
3. Braedel HU, Schindler E, Cullen P, Hoene E. Demonstration of residual contrast medium in renal parenchyma using computerized tomography. J Urol 1987; 137:11–14
4. Cass AS, Luxenberg M. Unilateral nonvisualization on excretory urography after external trauma. J Urol 1984; 132:225–227

5. Cass AS, Susset J, Khan A, Godec CJ. Renal pedicle injury in the multiple injured patient. J Urol 1979; 122:728–730

6. Cates JD, Foley WD, Lawson TL. Retrograde opacification of the renal vein: a CT sign of renal artery avulsion. Urol Radiol 1986; 8:92–94

7. Demos TC, Gadwood K, Love L, Engel G. The rim nephrogram in renovascular compromise. Urol Radiol 1982; 4:227–230

8. Frank PH, Nuttall J, Brander WL, Prosser D. The cortical rim sign of renal infarction. Br J Radiol 1974; 47:875–878

9. Gatewood OM, Fishman EK, Burrow CR, Walker WG, Goldman SM, Siegelman SS. Renal vein thrombosis in patients with nephrotic syndrome: CT diagnosis. Radiology 1986; 159:117–122

10. Glazer GM, Francis IR, Brady TM, Teng SS. Computed tomography of renal infarction: clinical and experimental observations. AJR 1983; 140:721–727

11. Greweldinger J, Bufalini B, Adler J. Left renal pedicle injury diagnosed by computed axial tomography. Urol Radiol 1983; 5:55–56

12. Hann L. Renal subcapsular rim sign: new etiologies and pathogenesis. AJR 1982; 138:51–54

13. Lupetin AR, Mainwaring BL, Daffner RH. CT diagnosis of renal artery injury caused by blunt abdominal trauma. AJR 1989; 153:1065–1068

14. Martin KW, McAlister WH, Shackelford GD. Acute renal infarction: diagnosis by Doppler ultrasound. Pediatr Radiol 1988; 18:373–376

15. Mitchell W, Venable D. Segmental renal artery infarction: a case report with computerized tomography scan and angiographic correlation. J Urol 1987; 37:93–94

16. Paul GJ, Stephenson TF. The cortical rim sign in renal infarction. Radiology 1977; 122:338

17. Peterson NE. Traumatic bilateral renal infarction. J Trauma 1989; 29:158–167

18. Sant GR, Bankoff MS. Computed tomography in evaluation of blunt renal trauma. Potential for misdiagnosis of renal infarction. Urol Int 1988; 43:321–323

19. Stables DP. Unilateral absence of excretion at urography after abdominal trauma. Radiology 1976; 121:609–615

20. Steinberg DL, Jeffrey RB, Federle MP, McAninch JW. The computerized tomography appearance of renal pedicle injury. J Urol 1984; 132:1163–1164

21. Wong WS, Moss AA, Federle MP, Cochran ST, London SS. Renal infarction: CT diagnosis and correlation between CT findings and etiologies. Radiology 1984; 150:201–205

URETERAL OBSTRUCTION

22. Burge HJ, Middleton WD, McClennan BL, Hildebolt CF. Ureteral jets in healthy subjects and in patients with unilateral ureteral calculi: comparison with color Doppler US. Radiology 1991; 180:437–442

23. Elkin M. Radiological observations in acute ureteral obstruction. Radiology 1963; 81:484–491

24. Elkin M, Boyarsky S, Martinez J, et al. Physiology of ureteral obstruction as determined by roentgenologic studies. AJR 1964; 92:291–301

25. Hill MC, Rich JI, Mardiat JG, Finder CA. Sonography vs. excretory urography in acute flank pain. AJR 1985; 144:1235–1238

26. Hinman F Jr. The pathophysiology of urinary obstruction. In: Campbell MF, Harris JH (eds), Urology, vol 1, 3rd ed. Philadelphia: WB Saunders; 1970:313–348

27. Laing FC, Jeffrey BR Jr, Wing VW. Ultrasound versus excretory urography in evaluating acute flank pain. Radiology 1985; 154:613–616

28. Vaughan ED Jr, Gillenwater JY. Recovery following complete chronic unilateral ureteral occlusion: functional, radiographic and pathologic alterations. J Urol 1971; 106:27–35

ACUTE CORTICAL NECROSIS

29. Blumhardt R, Growcock G, Lasher JC. Cortical necrosis in a renal transplant. AJR 1983; 141:95–96

30. Goergen TG, Lindstrom RR, Tan H, Lilley JJ. CT appearance of acute renal cortical necrosis. AJR 1981; 137:176–177

31. Jordan J, Low R, Jeffrey RB Jr. CT findings in acute renal cortical necrosis. J Comput Assist Tomogr 1990; 14:155–156

32. Laupacis A, Ulan RA, Rankin RN, Stiller CR, Keown PA. CT findings in postpartum renal cortical necrosis. J Can Assoc Radiol 1983; 34:53–55

33. McAlister WH, Nedelman SH. The roentgen manifestations of bilateral renal cortical necrosis. AJR 1961; 86:129–135

34. Sefczek RJ, Beckman I, Lupetin AR, Dash N. Sonography of acute renal cortical necrosis. AJR 1984; 142:553–554

35. Sty JR, Starshak RJ, Hubbard AM. Acute renal cortical necrosis in hemolytic uremic syndrome. J Clin Ultrasound 1983; 11:175–178

36. Tuttle RJ, Minielly JA. The angiographic diagnosis of acute hemorrhagic renal cortical necrosis. Radiology 1978; 126:637–638

37. Whelan JG Jr, Ling JT, Davis LA. Antemortem roentgen manifestations of bilateral renal cortical necrosis. Radiology 1967; 89:682–689

RENAL INFLAMMATORY DISEASE

38. Corriere JN Jr, Sandler CM. The diagnosis and immediate therapy of acute renal and perirenal infections. Urol Clin North Am 1982; 9:219–228

39. Gold RP, McClennan BL, Rottenberg RR. CT appearance of acute inflammatory disease of the renal interstitium. AJR 1983; 141:343–349

40. Goldman SM. Acute and chronic urinary infection: present concepts and controversies. Urol Radiol 1988; 10:17–24

41. Goldman SM, Fishman EK. Upper urinary tract infection: the current role of CT, ultrasound, and MRI. Semin US CT MR 1991; 12:335–360

42. Morehouse HT, Weiner SN, Hoffman JC. Imaging in inflammatory disease of the kidney. AJR 1984; 143:135–141

43. Newhouse JH, Amis ES Jr. The relationship between renal scarring and stone disease. AJR 1988; 151:1153–1156

44. Piccirillo M, Rigsby CM, Rosenfield AT. Sonography of renal inflammatory disease. Urol Radiol 1987; 19:66–78

45. Rauschkolb EN, Sandler CM, Patel S, Childs TL. Computed tomography of renal inflammatory disease. J Comput Assist Tomogr 1982; 6:502–506
46. Soulen MC, Fishman EK, Goldman SM. Sequelae of acute renal infections: CT evaluation. Radiology 1989; 173:423–426
47. Soulen MC, Fishman EK, Goldman SM, Gatewood OM. Bacterial renal infection: role of CT. Radiology 1989; 171:703–707
48. Thornbury JR. Acute renal infections. Urol Radiol 1991; 12:209–213

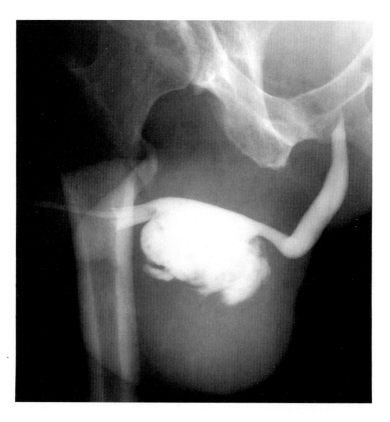

Figure 29-1. This 33-year-old man presented with pain and marked scrotal swelling. You are shown a retrograde urethrogram.

Case 29: Periurethral Abscess

Question 144

Which *one* of the following is the MOST likely diagnosis?

(A) Periurethral abscess
(B) Carcinoma of the anterior urethra
(C) Megalourethra
(D) Congenital saccular urethral diverticulum
(E) Cowper's duct cyst

Figure 29-1 is a retrograde urethrogram of a 33-year-old man who presented with a markedly swollen painful scrotum. An irregular collection of contrast material is present on the inferior aspect of the penile urethra, which communicates broadly with the urethral lumen. The bulbous urethra appears normal, and the posterior urethra is not filled. The scrotum and penis are markedly swollen. Periurethral abscess is the most likely dignosis **(Option (A) is correct).**

Carcinoma of the urethra (Option (B)) is unlikely because when this lesion involves the anterior urethra, it typically appears as a long, irregular urethral stricture (Figure 29-2) and scrotal swelling is not a feature. Megalourethra (Option (C)) is a rare congenital anomaly that results in dilatation of the penile urethra and the phallus itself (Figure 29-3). The disorder is usually relatively easily identified shortly after birth and may be associated with a variety of other congenital anomalies (see Question 146).

Congenital diverticula of the floor of the urethra are generally classified as either diffuse or saccular. The diffuse variety is the same as megalourethra. A congenital saccular urethral diverticulum (Option (D)) is an outpocketing of the ventral aspect of the anterior urethra; it usually occurs in the penile urethra (Figure 29-4) or, less commonly, in the bulbous urethra. The diverticulum communicates with the urethral lumen via a broad-based neck, but it generally has a smooth outline and is not associated with the diffuse swelling of the scrotum that is present

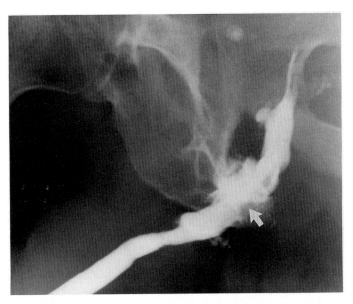

Figure 29-2. Squamous cell carcinoma of the urethra. There is a moderate stricture in the distal bulbous urethra. A long, irregular area of narrowing associated with perineal extravasation secondary to a urethral perineal fistula that partially obscures the stricture (arrow) is present in the mid-bulbous urethra. On biopsy, the irregular midbulbar stricture was demonstrated to represent a squamous cell carcinoma.

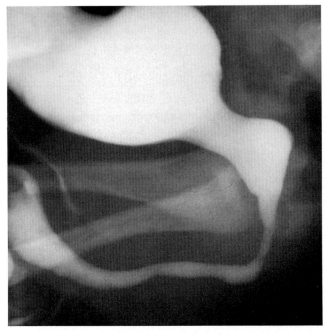

Figure 29-3. Scaphoid megalourethra. Retrograde urethrogram in a child with prune-belly syndrome showing mild dilatation of the distal penile urethra.

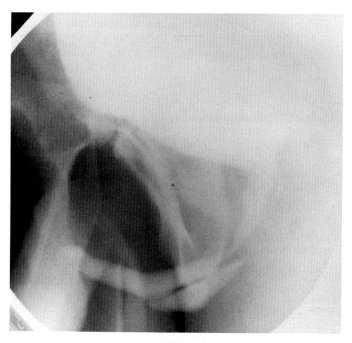

Figure 29-4. Congenital saccular anterior urethral diverticulum in a young boy who presented with post-voiding dribbling.

in the test case. A dilated posterior urethra, because of concomitant urethral obstruction caused by the diverticulum, is present in 75% of cases. As such, the condition has frequently been confused with an anterior urethral valve (Figure 29-5). In fact, the obstruction associated with a congenital diverticulum occurs because of a valvelike mechanism caused by the anterior lip of the diverticulum. As the patient voids, the diverticulum fills; this in turn produces compression of the urethra because the lip of the diverticulum forms an acute angle with the ventral floor of the urethra.

A Cowper's duct cyst (Option (E)) is caused by obstruction of Cowper's duct at its orifice, leading to proximal dilatation; on urethrography, the abnormality is usually demonstrated as an extrinsic mass that compresses the lumen of the bulbous urethra on its ventral surface. In cases in which the orifice of the duct remains patent or the cyst has ruptured into the urethra, contrast material will reflux into the duct, which can be recognized as a tubular structure that extends toward the urogenital diaphragm. As with congenital urethral diverticula, these lesions generally present in children, but they have occasionally been reported as presenting in adulthood.

Normal Male Anterior Urethra

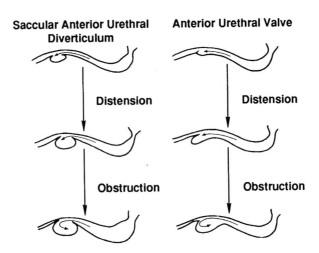

Saccular Anterior Urethral Diverticulum	Anterior Urethral Valve
Distension	Distension
Obstruction	Obstruction

Figure 29-5. Diagrammatic representation of the differences between a congenital saccular anterior urethral diverticulum and an anterior urethral valve. See text. (Adapted with permission from Kirks and Grossman [18].)

Periurethral abscesses are often life-threatening infections; they originate in the periurethral glands of Littré. If the ostium of one of the glands becomes sealed by inspissated pus or by fibrosis, a periurethral abscess is formed. The tunica albuginea tends to resist the spread of infection dorsally, and so the abscess tends to spread ventrally into the corpus spongiosum, where it may be confined by Buck's fascia. If, however, Buck's fascia is perforated, the resulting infection can spread into the buttocks, the thighs, or the anterior abdominal wall. If the abscess drains into the urethra, it can be demonstrated radiologically, as in the test case, by retrograde urethrography. When such abscesses heal, the lining of the abscess cavity may epithelialize, resulting in an acquired anterior urethral diverticulum (Figure 29-6).

The presenting signs of a periurethral abscess include scrotal swelling, which is present in 90% of cases; fever; and acute urinary retention. In one series, approximately 10% of abscesses had drained spontaneously at the time of presentation. A history of either venereal disease or

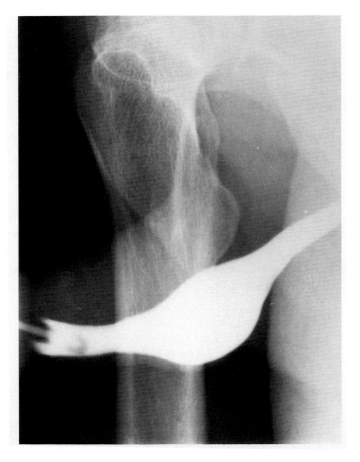

Figure 29-6. Acquired urethral diverticulum. Retrograde urethrogram demonstrating a smooth focal area of dilatation in the penile urethra after prolonged Foley catheterization.

previous urethral stricture disease is present in about 80% of the cases. A significant number of cases are associated with recent urethral instrumentation or prolonged Foley catheterization; in such cases, the abscess is presumed to result from a combination of infection and pressure necrosis of the urethra. The most common organisms found are gram-negative rods, enterococci, and anaerobes. A periurethral abscess has been the presenting complaint in some patients with squamous cell carcinoma of the urethra.

Question 145

Concerning carcinoma of the urethra,

(A) the bulbous urethra is the most common site in men
(B) the most common cell type is adenocarcinoma
(C) when it involves the anterior urethra in men, it generally is associated with underlying stricture disease
(D) it is more common in women than in men
(E) the most common presenting complaint is voiding difficulty

Malignant tumors of the urethra are relatively uncommon, making up less than 1% of all malignant urinary tract tumors. Carcinoma of the urethra is twice as common in women as in men **(Option (D) is true)**, and, according to McCallum, 80% of the reported cases occur in Caucasians. The tumor generally presents in patients between 55 and 60 years of age.

The histologic characteristics of the lesion depend on its anatomic locations. Squamous cell carcinoma is the most common cell type in the male anterior urethra and in women; it accounts for between 70 and 80% of the cases altogether **(Option (B) is false).** Transitional cell carcinoma accounts for approximately 15% of cases overall and is the most common cell type in the prostatic urethra; adenocarcinoma, undifferentiated tumors, metastatic disease, and benign tumors are less common. More than 60% of tumors in men occur in the bulbomembranous region **(Option (A) is true)** and are thought to be related to squamous metaplasia that occurs as a result of chronic irritation, usually in association with long-standing urethral stricture disease **(Option (C) is true).**

The disease in men progresses insidiously, and because so many of the patients have underlying urethral stricture disease, their symptoms are often attributed to that diagnosis. The most common presenting complaint is obstructive voiding dysfunction **(Option (E) is true),** but a palpable mass, a urethroperineal fistula, or a periurethral abscess may be the initial finding. Most patients with transitional cell carcinoma have a history of a urothelial tumor, generally involving the bladder. Hematuria or a urethral discharge is reported, surprisingly, in only 25% of cases. A combination of surgery, radiation therapy, and chemotherapy is used in most centers for management; neoplasms involving the distal urethra generally have a better prognosis than do the more proximal tumors.

On urethrography, squamous cell tumors cause an irregular stricture with or without a fistula (Figure 29-2). It is often difficult to differentiate a malignant urethral stricture from a benign lesion based on the radiographic appearance alone. A history of recurrent stricture disease or a stricture that requires frequent dilatation, however, should raise the suspicion of cancer. In patients with transitional cell carcinoma, a filling defect in the prostatic urethra is the typical finding.

Carcinoma of the female urethra, although more common than carcinoma of the male urethra, is nonetheless considered rare. Almost 70% of the reported cases are squamous cell carcinoma, with transitional cell carcinoma and adenocarcinoma representing most of the remaining cases. There are no rigidly defined anatomic divisions of the female urethra, so most authors divide the tumors into those confined to the distal one-third (anterior) and those involving the proximal two-thirds (posterior). Anterior lesions have a better prognosis, but approximately 33% of the patients have clinically palpable inguinal lymph nodes at the time of presentation. Radiology plays a limited role in the initial diagnosis since most patients present with bleeding or a palpable mass, but CT or MRI is often used to evaluate the extent of pelvic lymph node involvement.

Question 146

Which *one* of the following is MOST closely associated with megalourethra?

(A) Seminal vesicle cyst
(B) Congenital megacalyces
(C) Prune-belly syndrome
(D) Megacystis-microcolon syndrome
(E) Hirschsprung's disease

A megalourethra (sometimes also referred to as a congenital diffuse urethral diverticulum) is a congenital anomaly of the male urethra associated with a deficiency in the formation of the penile corpora. Two types of megalourethra have been described: scaphoid megalourethra, associated with a deficiency of the corpus spongiosum, and fusiform megalourethra, generally attributed to a deficiency of both the corpus spongiosum and the corpus cavernosum. Fusiform megalourethra is associated with diffuse mesenchymal abnormalities and multiple urinary tract anomalies including renal dysplasia/hypoplasia, extrophy of the bladder, congenital rectovesical fistula, and other sometimes lethal fetal anomalies. Scaphoid megalourethra, which is less severe, is also associated with a wide variety of congenital anomalies (Table 29-1). Of the

Table 29-1. Anomalies associated with scaphoid megalourethra

Prune-belly syndrome	Supernumerary digits
Renal aplasia/dysplasia/	Ventricular septal defects
hypoplasia	Microcephalus
Megaureter	Cleft palate
Megacystis	Imperforate anus
Posterior urethral valves	Esophageal atresia

options listed, however, only prune-belly syndrome (Eagle-Barrett syndrome), in which the incidence of scaphoid megalourethra approaches 50%, has been consistently associated with this anomaly **(Option (C) is correct).** Fusiform megalourethra has also been described in patients with prune-belly syndrome; indeed, the more recent literature has viewed scaphoid and fusiform megalourethra as forming a continuum with a variable degree of expression and severity. Thus, rather than two distinct entities, it is probably best to view the condition as a single disorder with a spectrum of presentations.

The penile urethra forms during embryologic development as a result of closure of the urogenital groove. The urethra is then invested by vascular elements and connective tissue, which will form the corpus spongiosum. Failure of these elements to invert produces a scaphoid megalourethra. Failure of the mesoderm to form erectile tissue (corpus cavernosum) causes the urethral epithelial layer to develop directly on the tunica albuginea. Thus, both the dorsal and ventral supports for the urethra are absent, resulting in a fusiform megalourethra.

Prune-belly syndrome is a congenital anomaly characterized by the triad of absent abdominal musculature, urinary tract anomalies, and undescended testes. Variants of the syndrome have been described in female infants, but the full-blown syndrome develops only in male infants. The syndrome is typically recognized at birth because of the characteristic appearance of the abdomen produced by the absence of the abdominal musculature. The skin overlying the abdomen has a wrinkled appearance reminiscent of a prune; in older children the wrinkling tends to disappear and is replaced by a more "pot-bellied" appearance. The cause of prune-belly syndrome is unknown; some authorities believe it to be related to a mesodermal deficiency, whereas others believe that the primary defect is in the urinary system and that this defect causes the abnormal development of the abdominal wall.

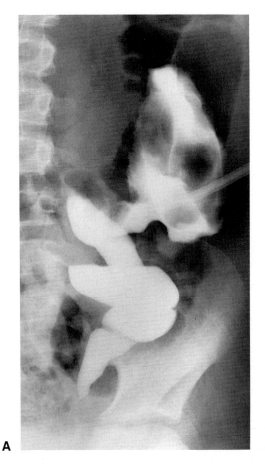

A

Figure 29-7. Prune-belly syndrome. (A) Nephrostogram in a 10-year-old boy showing marked ureteral tortuosity and dilatation. The distal portion of the ureter appears tapered. (B) CT scan of the pelvis in a different patient. The bladder (B) is displaced by the markedly tortuous and dilated ureter (U). The abdominal musculature is essentially absent.

The urinary tract abnormalities affect the kidneys, the ureters, and the bladder, as well as the urethra. The kidneys may be normal or dysplastic. The ureteral abnormalities (Figure 29-7) tend to be the most constant feature and include ureteral tortuosity and dilatation, frequently in a segmental distribution. Vesicoureteral reflux is common, but the ureteral abnormalities may be present in the absence of this finding. The bladder tends to be large and may be associated with a patent urachus. In addition to the abnormality of the penile urethra,

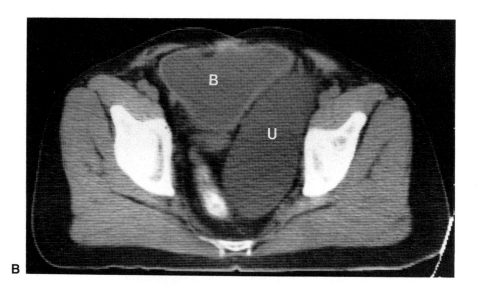

B

dilatation of the prostatic urethra, associated with prostatic hypoplasia, is characteristically present. The cryptorchid testes are usually located within the abdomen.

Besides the urinary tract abnormalities, anomalies of the heart, limbs, and gastrointestinal tract have been found in patients with this syndrome.

Seminal vesicle cysts (Option (A)) are commonly associated with ipsilateral absence of the kidney, ureter, and trigone. Rarely, a seminal vesicle cyst may be associated with an ipsilateral blind-ending ureter.

Congenital megacalyces (Option (B)) is an uncommon condition in which the number of calyces is increased and each has a dilated, cauliflowerlike configuration, but no obstruction is present and the renal parenchyma and renal functions are normal. Other urinary tract anomalies associated with megacalyces include medullary sponge kidney, duplication of the collecting system, and primary megaureter.

Megacystis-microcolon syndrome (Option (D)) presents with abdominal distension and decreased bowel movements in the neonatal period. There may be deficient (but nonetheless present) abdominal musculature. In contrast to the Eagle-Barrett syndrome, a female predominance has been reported in megacystis-microcolon syndrome. The most important manifestations are a dilated urinary bladder and a small, contracted colon associated with decreased intestinal peristalsis. Hydronephrosis and vesicoureteral reflux may also be present.

Hirschsprung's disease (Option (E)) results in aganglionosis of the colon, but there are no associated genitourinary manifestations.

Question 147

Concerning Cowper's duct cyst,

T (A) it most commonly presents in childhood
T (B) post-voiding dribbling is the most common presenting complaint
F (C) it appears as a filling defect in the bulbous urethra
T (D) urethral obstruction is uncommon

Cowper's glands are small, paired glands located in the urogenital diaphragm; they communicate with the mid-bulbous urethra via paired ducts. They provide mucinous secretions that lubricate spermatozoa during ejaculation. If there is obstruction of the proximal duct as a result of either fibrosis or inflammation, a Cowper's duct cyst (also known as Cowper's syringocele or retention cyst) may be formed. Maizels et al. have classified these lesions into four types (Figure 29-8), each with a different radiographic appearance: (1) simple syringocele (a minimally dilated duct); (2) imperforate syringocele (a dilated duct that presents as an extrinsic mass that compresses the bulbous urethra); (3) perforate syringocele (a bulbous duct that drains into the urethra via a patulous ostium); and (4) ruptured syringocele (the fragile membrane that remains after a dilated duct ruptures). These authors reported eight cases in boys ranging in age from 2 to 17 years. Similarly, Moskowitz et al. reported five cases in boys aged from 3 to 9 years. Thus, although the condition has been reported to present initially in adulthood, these studies show that it most commonly presents in the pediatric age group **(Option (A) is true)**. A variety of presenting complaints, including hematuria, dysuria, frequency, enuresis, urinary tract infection, and the presence of a perineal mass, have been described. The most common symptom, however, is post-voiding dribbling **(Option (B) is true)**, apparently related to reflux of urine into the duct during voiding. Frank urethral obstruction is uncommon **(Option (D) is true)**.

The abnormality may be demonstrated on voiding cystourethrography or retrograde urethrography. The imperforate variety appears as an extrinsic mass that compresses the bulbous urethra. The other varieties demonstrate reflux of contrast material into a tubular structure, which can be identified as Cowper's duct. In none of the reported cases has the lesion been demonstrated as a filling defect in the bulbous urethra **(Option (C) is false)**.

The exact etiology of Cowper's duct cyst has not been precisely identified. Because it may occur in very young infants, many investigators have presumed it to be congenital. Others have postulated that it is

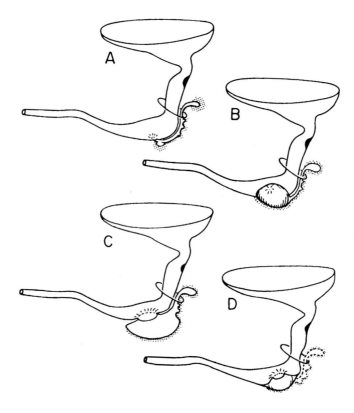

Figure 29-8. Diagrammatic representation of Cowper's duct cyst. Cowper's glands (stippled area) are located in the urogenital diaphragm (black circle). (A) Simple syringocele. (B) Imperforate syringocele with dilated distal duct impinging on the midbulbar urethra. (C) Perforate syringocele with a patulous orifice, allowing free reflux of contrast material in a dilated duct. (D) Ruptured syringocele with membranes as remnants in its wall. (Reprinted with permission from Maizels et al. [21].)

caused by an inflammatory process either in the urethra or in Cowper's gland itself, leading to stenosis at the orifice of the duct.

Carl M. Sandler, M.D.

SUGGESTED READINGS

PERIURETHRAL ABSCESS

1. Bhandari M, Palaniswamy R. Management of complicated strictures of the urethra in men. Br J Urol 1984; 56:410–412
2. Davidson KC, Garlow WB, Brewer J. Computerized tomography of prostatic and periurethral abscesses: 2 case reports. J Urol 1986; 135:1257–1258
3. Dickinson AJ, Hastie KJ, Charlton CA. Primary squamous carcinoma of the male urethra presenting as a periurethral abscess. Br J Urol 1990; 65:217
4. Malatinsky E. Sepsis caused by periurethral abscess. Int Urol Nephrol 1991; 23:485–488
5. McCallum RW, Rogers JM, Alexander MW. The radiologic assessment of iatrogenic urethral injury. J Can Assoc Radiol 1985; 36:122–126
6. Walther MM, Mann BB, Finnerty DP. Periurethral abscess. J Urol 1987; 138:1167–1170

CARCINOMA OF THE URETHRA

7. Anderson KA, McAninch JW. Primary squamous cell carcinoma of anterior male urethra. Urology 1984; 23:134–140
8. Baskin LS, Turzan C. Carcinoma of male urethra: management of locally advanced disease with combined chemotherapy, radiotherapy, and penile-preserving surgery. Urology 1992; 39:21–25
9. Hahn P, Krepart G, Malaker K. Carcinoma of female urethra. Manitoba experience: 1958–1987. Urology 1991; 37:106–109
10. Hopkins SC, Nag SK, Soloway MS. Primary carcinoma of male urethra. Urology 1984; 23:128–133
11. Kaplan GW, Bulkley GJ, Grayhack JT. Carcinoma of the male urethra. J Urol 1967; 98:365–371
12. McCallum RW. Urethral neoplasms. In: Pollack HM (ed), Clinical urography. Philadelphia: WB Saunders; 1990:1404–1413
13. Sailer SL, Shipley WU, Wang CC. Carcinoma of the female urethra; a review of results with radiation therapy. J Urol 1988; 140:1–5

MEGALOURETHRA AND PRUNE-BELLY SYNDROME

14. Appel RA, Kaplan GW, Brock WA, Streit D. Megalourethra. J Urol 1986; 135:747–751
15. Berdon WE, Baker DH, Wigger HJ, Blanc WA. The radiologic and pathologic spectrum of the prune belly syndrome. The importance of urethral obstruction in prognosis. Radiol Clin North Am 1977; 15:83–92
16. Greskovich FJ III, Nyberg LM Jr. The prune belly syndrome: a review of its etiology, defects, treatment and prognosis. J Urol 1988; 140:707–712
17. Shrom SH, Cromie WJ, Duckett JW Jr. Megalourethra. Urology 1981; 17:152–156

CONGENITAL URETHRAL DIVERTICULA

18. Kirks DR, Grossman H. Congenital saccular anterior urethral diverticulum. Radiology 1981; 140:367–372
19. Netto NR Jr, Lemos GC, Claro JF, Hering FL. Congenital diverticulum of male urethra. Urology 1984; 24:239–242
20. Tank ES. Anterior urethral valves resulting from congenital urethral diverticula. Urology 1987; 30:467–469

COWPER'S DUCT CYST

21. Maizels M, Stephens FD, King LR, Firlit CF. Cowper's syringocele: a classification of dilatations of Cowper's gland duct based upon clinical characteristics of 8 boys. J Urol 1983; 129:111–114
22. Moskowitz PS, Newton NA, Lebowitz RL. Retention cysts of Cowper's duct. Radiology 1976; 120:377–380
23. Redman JF, Rountree GA. Pronounced dilatation of Cowper's gland duct manifest as a perineal mass: a recommendation for management. J Urol 1988; 139:87–88
24. Sant GR, Kaleli A. Cowper's syringocele causing incontinence in an adult. J Urol 1985; 133:279–280

Notes

Index

Where there are multiple page references, **boldface** indicates the main discussion of a topic.

Bladder *(cont'd)*
combined intraperitoneal bladder and urethral rupture, 261–62
exstrophy of, 70
extraperitoneal bladder rupture, 187, 189, 261–64, **266–69**
intraperitoneal bladder rupture, 261, **264–65**
lymphomas and, 37
neurofibroma of, 40
"pie-in-the-sky," 192
salvage rates, 39
schistosomiasis of, 66–68
squamous cell carcinoma of, 65–66
transitional cell carcinoma of, 63, 65
Bladder dome
intraperitoneal bladder rupture and, 264
lesions, 63
Bladder flap, 313
Blind-ending ureteral bud, **234–35**
imaging of, 223
Blood dyscrasias, renal sinus hemorrhage and, 126
Blood tests, renovascular hypertension screening, 472–74
Boari flap, 313
Bone spicules
extraperitoneal bladder rupture and, 266
intraperitoneal bladder rupture and, 269
urethral injury and, 192
Bowel herniation into the scrotum, 13
Bowel loop structure, 207
BPH. *See* Benign prostatic hyperplasia
Brunn's cell nests, 227
Brush biopsy, 229
Buck's fascia, 198, 199, 506
Bull's eye pattern of testicular torsion, 15
Burkitt's lymphoma
description, 323, 326
differential diagnosis
candidiasis, 323–24
leukemia, 325
medullary cystic disease, 324–25
renal metastases, 325
Wilms' tumor, 426

C

Café-au-lait spots, 176
Caisson disease, 3–4
Calcification, and
acquired cystic kidney disease, 91
autosomal dominant polycystic kidney disease, 95
genitourinary tuberculosis, 52
phleboliths, 52

Calcification, and *(cont'd)*
squamous cell carcinoma, 65–66
urachal carcinoma, 74
Calculi. *See* Stones
Candida albicans, 323–24
Candida pyelonephritis, 335
Candidiasis, **334–36**
differential diagnosis
Burkitt's lymphoma, 323–24
immunocompromised patients and, 324, 334–35
leukemia and, 324
Captopril, 459–69, 471, **474–77**
Captopril test, 473
Carcinoma. *See also* Adenocarcinomas; Squamous cell carcinoma; Transitional cell carcinoma
adrenal cortical, 374
bladder, 37, 63, 65–66
breast, 128, 325, 330, 374, 382
cervical, 127
embryonal cell, 444
gastrointestinal tract, 325
lung, 325, 330, 374, 382
ovarian, 53
prostatic, 289–303
renal, 174
renal cell, 88–89, 155–56, 241, **248–50**
urachal, 65–68, **72, 74**
urethral, 503, 507, **508–9**
Cardiovascular disease
acute renal infarction secondary to, 496
renovascular hypertension and, 469
Catheterization
bladder tumors and, 230
for embolization, 250
retrograde urethrography, 192
Cavernosography
of corpora, **398–400**
penile arterial blood flow, 390
Cavernosometry, penile arterial blood flow and, 390
Cellular atypism, 233–34
Cerebellar hemangioblastomas, 88, 178
Cervical ectropion, 45
Chlamydia trachomatis, 57, 444
Chronic pyelonephritis, 495
Cigarette smoking, transitional cell carcinoma and, 70, 351
Clear cell adenocarcinoma, DES exposure and, 45
Clear cell sarcoma
differential diagnosis
mesoblastic nephroma, 432
Clitoral hypertrophy, neurofibromatosis and, 40

Goblet sign, 225, 229
Gonorrhea, pelvic inflammatory disease and, 47
Gray-scale ultrasonography
  acute testicular torsion, 15
  endometriosis, 52–53
  intrascrotal pathology and, 8

H

Hamartomas, 178
Hematogenous spread
  renal metastases, 330
  tuberculosis, 375
  ureteral metastatic disease, 343–44
Hematomas. *See* Butterfly hematomas; Pelvic hematomas; Subcapsular hematomas
Hematuria, and
  extracorporeal shock wave lithotripsy, 146
  lymphomas, 37
  nutcracker phenomenon, 242, 253
  renal cell carcinoma, 241
  urachal carcinoma, 74
Hemihypertrophy, 177–78
Hemodialysis, and
  acquired cystic kidney disease, 91
  autosomal dominant polycystic kidney disease, 173
  ureteral obstruction, 129
Hemorrhage. *See* Adrenal hemorrhage; Renal sinus hemorrhage; Suburothelial hemorrhage
Heparin
  renal sinus hemorrhage and, 131
  renal vein thrombosis treatment, 286
  venous thrombosis treatment, 408
Hepatic fibrosis, 176
Herald sign for Crohn's disease, 68
Hereditary factors. *See* Genetic factors
Hermaphrodites, 218
Heroin, 255–56
High scrotal testis, 207, 214
Hirschsprung's disease, 512
Histoplasmosis
  differential diagnosis
    Addison's disease, 374
HM3 Dornier lithotriptor, 142, 145–46
Hodgkin's disease
  adrenal involvement, 383
  Burkitt's lymphoma and, 323, 326
  incidence, 37
HSG. *See* Hysterosalpingograms

Hydroceles
  differential diagnosis
    scrotal hernia, 8, 10
  imaging, 450, 453
Hydronephrosis, **362–66**
  differential diagnosis
    renal vein thrombosis, 359
  prune belly syndrome and, 114
  ureteral obstruction and, 488
Hypertension. *See also* Hypotension; Renovascular hypertension
  autosomal dominant polycystic kidney disease, 79, 173
  extracorporeal shock wave lithotripsy, 146–47
  medullary cystic disease, 90
  multilocular cystic nephroma, 182
  neurofibromatosis, 40
  tuberous sclerosis, 179
Hypertrophied periureteral collaterals, 344–45
Hypospadias, 218
Hypotension, 476
Hysterosalpingograms
  DES exposure patterns, 45
  endometriosis, 50
  pelvic inflammatory disease, 45, 47
  salpingitis isthmica nodosa, 45, 57

I

Ileal conduits, ureteral stents and, 319
Ileal interposition, 313
Iliac artery structure, 203
Iliac vein compression
  differential diagnosis
    pelvic lymphocele, 407
Iliac vein structure, 203
Iliac vein thrombosis
  differential diagnosis
    pelvic lymphocele, 407
Immediate, dense, persistent nephrograms, 134
Immunocompromised patients, candidiasis and, 324, 334–35
Impotence, **387–403**
Incidence. *See also* Prevalence
  adenocarcinomas, 228
  anomalies additional to multicystic dysplastic kidney, 118
  bladder cancer, 70
  endometriosis, 54
  genitourinary tuberculosis, 51
  posterior urethral injury, 193
  post-ESWL hypertension, 146–47
  post-ESWL subcapsular hematoma, 142

O

Obstructed testis, 207, 214
Obstructive nephrogram, 489
Obstructive uropathy, renography for, 363
Optic nerve atrophy, 325, 329
Ovaries
   carcinoma of, 53
   cysts, 53
   tubo-ovarian abscesses, 53

P

Papaverine
   impotence treatment, 401
   penile arteriography and, 396
   response of cavernosal arteries, 390
Papillary necrosis, 335
Parasitic diseases, 66–68
Pathognomonic retinal phakomas, tuberous
      sclerosis and, 178
PBS. *See* Prune belly syndrome
Pelvic fractures, and
   anterior urethral injuries, 198
   combined intraperitoneal and extraperi-
         toneal bladder rupture, 267
   extraperitoneal bladder rupture, 187,
         189, 266
   intraperitoneal bladder rupture, 264
   posterior urethral injury, 191–97
Pelvic hematomas, **417–19**
   differential diagnosis
      pelvic lymphocele, 409
Pelvic inflammatory disease, **57–58**
   differential diagnosis
      salpingitis isthmica nodosa, 45, 47
Pelvic lipomatosis, **414–17**
   differential diagnosis
      pelvic lymphocele, 408
Pelvic lymphoceles, **413–14**
   differential diagnosis
      iliac vein compression, 407
      iliac vein thrombosis, 407
      pelvic hematoma, 409
      pelvic lipomatosis, 408
   percutaneous aspiration, 413, 414
   urinomas and, 413–14
Penile arteriography, **394–97**
Penile artery disease
   differential diagnosis
      veno-occlusive disease, 387
Penile enlargement, neurofibromatosis and,
      40
Peripheral plasma renin assay, 473
Perirenal cobwebs, 486

Periurethral abscesses, **506–7**
   differential diagnosis
      carcinoma of the urethra, 503
      congenital saccular urethral diverticu-
            lum, 503, 505
      Cowper's duct cyst, 505
      megalourethra, 503
Peyronie's disease, **401–3**
   differential diagnosis
      veno-occlusive disease, 387
Phantom calyx, 229
Pharmacologic maintenance erectile flow,
      398
Phenacetin abuse
   squamous cell carcinoma and, 353
   transitional cell carcinoma and, 228, 351–
         52
Pheochromocytomas, 177
Phleboliths, calcification and, 52
PID. *See* Pelvic inflammatory disease
Pie-in-the-sky bladder, 192
Polycystic ovaries, 53
Polyglandular autoimmune syndrome
   type I, 380
   type II, 380, 382
Posterior urethral valves, **111–13**
   differential diagnosis
      urine ascites, 104–5
   prune belly syndrome and, 116
Post-traumatic erectile failure, 396–97
Potter type IV cystic disease, 105
Pregnancy. *See also* Ectopic pregnancies
   acute cortical necrosis and, 492
Prevalence. *See also* Incidence
   renovascular hypertension, 470
Primary ureteral neoplasms, **351–53**
Primary urothelial tumor
   differential diagnosis
      ureteral metastatic disease, 341
Prostaglandin E1, 401
Prostate dislocation, 191, 192
Prostate gland description, 295
Prostate-specific antigen, 303
Prostatic acid phosphatase, 303
Prostatic carcinoma, **302–3**
   iliac vein compression and, 407
   imaging of, 291–93, 296, **298–302**
   nodal metastasis sequence, 299–300
   screening program, 297
   staging, 289–97
   treatment, 295
   tumor involvement of the seminal vesi-
         cles, 292
Proteus mirabilis, and
   renal abscess, 162
   struvite calculi, 149

Renal sinus hemorrhage *(cont'd)*
  differential diagnosis
    shock, 125
    uric acid nephropathy, 125
Renal tubular ectasia, medullary sponge kidneys and, 86
Renal vascular malformation
  differential diagnosis
    nutcracker phenomenon, 242
    renal cell carcinoma, 241
    substance abuse, 243
    transitional cell carcinoma, 242–43
  substance abuse and, **255–56**
Renal vein renin sampling, 473–74
Renal vein thrombosis, **283–86**
  dense nephrogram and, 134
  differential diagnosis
    hydronephrosis, 359
    mesoblastic nephroma, 360
    multicystic dysplastic kidney, 361
    renal infarction, 274, 360–61, 486
  imaging, **366–70**
  subcapsular hematoma and, 140
  ureteral notching and, 347
Renin-angiotensin-aldosterone system, 475
Renography, for obstructive uropathy, 363
Renovascular hypertension, **469–74**. *See also* Hypertension
  renal infarction and, 497–98
Retention cyst. *See* Cowper's duct cyst
Retinal angiomas, von Hippel-Lindau disease and, 176
Retinal angiomatosis, 88
Retinitis pigmentosa, 325, 329
Retrograde pyelography
  candidiasis, 335
  cortical rim sign, 496
  medullary cystic disease, 329
  pelvic lymphocele, 410
  renal infarction, 279
  transitional cell carcinoma, 353
Retrograde urethrography
  catheter placement and, 192
  Cowper's duct cyst, 513
  extraperitoneal bladder rupture, 187, 189
  periurethral abscess, 503
  posterior urethral valves, 111–12
  pre-surgical, 197
  straddle injury, 189
  urethral injury, 189, 191
Retroperitoneal disease, renal lymphoma and, 328
Retroperitoneal fibrosis, bilateral ureteral obstruction and, 127
Revascularization, 468, 498

Rhabdomyosarcomas, **29–30, 38–39**
  differential diagnosis
    lymphomas, 26
    neurofibromatosis, 26–27
    sacrococcygeal teratomas, 25
Rim sign. *See* Cortical rim sign
RVH. *See* Renovascular hypertension
RVT. *See* Renal vein thrombosis

S

Sacrococcygeal dermoids. *See* Sacrococcygeal teratomas
Sacrococcygeal teratomas
  differential diagnosis
    rhabdomyosarcomas, 25
Salpingitis isthmica nodosa, **56–57**
  differential diagnosis
    DES exposure, 45
    endometriosis, 50
    genitourinary tuberculosis, 47, 49–50
    pelvic inflammatory disease, 45, 47
Scaphoid megalourethra, 509, 510
SCC. *See* Squamous cell carcinoma
Schistosoma haematobium, 66
Schistosomiasis
  differential diagnosis
    urachal carcinoma, 66–68
    squamous cell carcinoma relationship, 65–66, 67–68
Schmidt's syndrome, 380, 382
Scout radiograph, for ureteral metastatic disease, 341
Scrotal air causes, 4
Scrotal gangrene. *See* Fournier's gas gangrene
Scrotal hernia
  differential diagnosis
    adenomatoid tumor of the epididymis, 13
    Fournier's gas gangrene, 3
    gas-containing scrotal abscess secondary to Crohn's disease, 4
    hydrocele, 8, 10
    spermatocele, 10–11, 13
    sperm granuloma, 13
    varicocele, 8
Scrotum, imaging of, **450–56**
Seat belts, intraperitoneal bladder rupture and, 264
Segmental infarction
  differential diagnosis
    renal abscess, 158–59
Seminal vesicle cysts, 512

Transitional cell carcinoma (cont'd)
  differential diagnosis
    renal vascular malformation, 242–43
    urachal carcinoma, 63, 65
  epithelial ureteral tumors and, 351–53
  goblet sign, 225, 229
  histologic types, 352
  imaging of, 223, 224
  multiple papillary
    differential diagnosis
      ureteritis cystica, 227
  predisposing factors, 70–71
  renal sinus hemorrhage and, 132
  risk factors, 351–52
  ureteritis cystica and, 227
  of the urethra, 508, 509
Transplantation. See also Autotransplantation
  acquired cystic kidney disease and, 91
Transrectal ultrasonography, for prostatic carcinoma, 300–302
Transureteroureterostomy, 309–10, 313
Transurethral resection of the prostate, 289
Transuterine fallopian tube recanalization, 58
TRUS. See Transrectal ultrasonography
T-shaped uterus, DES exposure and, 45, 49
Tubal occlusion, salpingitis isthmica nodosa and, 57
Tuberculosis. See also Adrenal tuberculosis
  differential diagnosis
    Addison's disease, 373–74
  genitourinary
    differential diagnosis
      salpingitis isthmica nodosa, 47, 49–50
      ureteritis cystica, 228
    female genital tract, **51–52**
Tuberous sclerosis, **178–80**
  differential diagnosis
    von Hippel-Lindau disease, 171, 172
Tubo-ovarian abscesses, endometriosis and, 53
Tubular necrosis. See Acute tubular necrosis
Tubular nephrograms, 134

U

Ultrasonography. See also Color-flow Doppler ultrasonography; Duplex Doppler ultrasonography; Gray-scale ultrasonography; Transrectal ultrasonography
  acquired cystic kidney disease, 172
  acute cortical necrosis, 492–93

Ultrasonography (cont'd)
  acute pyelonephritis, 158, 281
  acute tubular necrosis and ureteral obstruction differentiation, 276
  angiomyolipomas, 179
  autosomal dominant polycystic kidney disease, 95, 173
  autosomal recessive polycystic kidney disease, 81, 83
  cortical rim sign, 496
  endometriosis, 50
  epididymal cysts, 448
  intratesticular tumors, 444–45
  leukemia, 333
  lymphomas, 125
  medullary cystic disease, 90, 330
  neuroblastomas, 28
  pelvic hematoma, 418
  pelvic inflammatory disease, 58
  pelvic lymphocele, 410, 413
  posterior urethral valves, 111
  renal abscess, 159
  renal cell carcinoma staging, 249
  renal infarction, 279
  renal lymphoma, 326–27
  renal vein thrombosis, 283, 284–85, 366–67
  rhabdomyosarcomas, 38
  scrotum, 451–52, 453–545
  spermatoceles, 446
  undescended testes, 211, 216
  ureteral endometriosis, 351
  ureteral obstruction, 490–91
  varicoceles, 455
  Wilms' tumor, 423–24, 425
  xanthogranulomatous pyelonephritis, 166
Undescended testes, **207–9**
  fetal weight and, 208
  histologic differences from normal testes, 217
  hypospadias and, 218
  imaging of, **211–16**
  infertility and, 217–18
  prune belly syndrome and, 114, 218
  structure of, 203, 205
  testis development, 208–9
Unguinal hernias, 217
UPJ obstruction. See Ureteropelvic junction obstruction
Urachal carcinoma, **72, 74**
  differential diagnosis
    Crohn's disease, 68
    schistosomiasis of the bladder, 66–68
    squamous cell carcinoma of the bladder, 65–66